Nanomedicine in the Treatment and Management of Alzheimer's Disease

This book aims to discuss the various drug delivery approaches of neuroprotective medicines via nanoparticles, such as enzymes, monoclonal antibodies, neurotrophic factors, pharmaceutical drugs, and nucleic acid-based medication, to manage Alzheimer's disease.

Nanomedicine in the Treatment and Management of Alzheimer's Disease investigates drug administration approaches, either separately or in combination, to improve neuroprotection in Alzheimer's disease. The book examines various novel therapeutic applications of nanomaterials in drug delivery for the central nervous system in Alzheimer's disease treatment. The book explores the role of nanoparticles in crossing the blood–brain barrier and blood-CSF barrier in the treatment and management of Alzheimer's disease. The authors also explain the nanoparticle-based delivery of therapeutic molecules including phytochemicals, peptides, siRNA, enzymes, and monoclonal antibodies in the treatment of Alzheimer's disease. Finally, the book also discusses the various challenges and future perspectives of nanomedicine in the management of Alzheimer's disease.

The book will help in bridging the gap of knowledge in neurosciences, neurotherapeutics, nanotechnology, and nanomedicine domains. The book chapter may be useful to educators, researchers, legislators, and medical professionals including pharmacologists, biochemists, corporate pharma R&D researchers, neurologists, and scientists involved in neurodegenerative diseases and nanomedicine.

Dr Nidhi Puranik is a Research Assistant Professor in the Department of Life Science at Yeungnam University in Gyeongsan, South Korea. She did her PhD work at the Defence Research & Development Establishment-DRDO (Research Center), and her degree was awarded from Bharathair University, Coimbatore, Tamil Nadu, India. She has more than 10 years of research and teaching experience in the field of disease therapeutics and diagnostics. Her current research is focused on the screening and development of plant-based drugs for various diseases.

Professor Shiv Kumar Yadav is currently working as an Assistant Professor in the Department of Zoology at Government Lal Bahadur Shastri PG College, Sironj, Vidisha, Madhya Pradesh, India. He has more than 8 years of R&D experience. He is currently working on computational biology and phytochemical-based drug development.

Nanomedicine in the Treatment and Management of Alzheimer's Disease

Edited by
Nidhi Puranik and Shiv Kumar Yadav

CRC Press
Taylor & Francis Group
Boca Raton London New York

CRC Press is an imprint of the
Taylor & Francis Group, an **informa** business

First edition published 2026
by CRC Press
2385 NW Executive Center Drive, Suite 320, Boca Raton, FL 33431

and by CRC Press
4 Park Square, Milton Park, Abingdon, Oxon, OX14 4RN

CRC Press is an imprint of Taylor & Francis Group, LLC

ISBN: 978-1-032-89551-2 (hbk)
ISBN: 978-1-032-89554-3 (pbk)
ISBN: 978-1-003-54338-1 (ebk)

DOI: 10.1201/9781003543381

Typeset in Times
by KnowledgeWorks Global Ltd.

Dedicated to Almighty, who gave us the strength to complete this work.

Contents

About the Editors

Nidhi Puranik is a Research Assistant Professor in the Department of Life Science at Yeungnam University in Gyeongsan, South Korea. She did her PhD at Defence Research & Development Establishment-DRDO (Research Center), and her degree was awarded from Bharathiar University, Coimbatore, Tamil Nadu, India. She has more than 10 years of research and teaching experience in the field of disease therapeutics and diagnostics. Her current research is focused on the screening and development of plant-based drugs for various diseases. She has been awarded the prestigious GATE, CSIR-NET, ICAR-NET, DRDO Junior research fellowship, MPCST Young Scientist award, MPCST Young Scientist training fellowship (National), and Young Investigator award (International). She has worked in various prestigious institutes of India- ICMR-NIREH, Bhopal, ICAR-IISR, Indore, Jiwaji University, Gwalior, and Barkatullah University, Bhopal. She has published over 40 high-impact research articles and has edited five books with international publishers, including Springer (02) and IOP Publishing (03). Her work holds significant relevance in clinical medicine, particularly in the diagnosis and treatment of human diseases.

Shiv Kumar Yadav is currently working as an Assistant Professor at Government Lal Bahadur Shastri PG College, Sironj, Vidisha, Madhya Pradesh, India. He has more than seven years of R&D experience. He has published more than ten articles in SCI journals. He received his MSc degree in Biotechnology from Jiwaji University, Madhya Pradesh, India, in 2010 and has submitted a PhD in Biological Sciences at Bharathiar University, Coimbatore, Tamil Nadu. He received an ICMR-JRF fellowship for his PhD. He has qualified for various national exams in the life sciences, such as CSIR-NET-JRF, ICMR-JRF, UGC-NET, GATE, ASRB NET, and South Asian University PhD entrance exam. He has worked in reputed research and academic institutes such as DRDO-DRDE (Gwalior), Jiwaji University (Gwalior), and Barkatullah University (Bhopal). He is currently working on Disease diagnosis and treatment.

Contributors

Ekansh Agrawal
Amity Institute of Biotechnology, Amity University, Gwalior, India

Binu Bhat
Shriram Institute for Industrial Research, Delhi, India

Divya Bisht
Biochemistry Discipline, School of Sciences, Indira Gandhi National Open University, New Delhi, India

Suruchi Chaudhary
Amity Institute of Biotechnology, Amity University, Gwalior, India

Mukul Das
Shriram Institute for Industrial Research, Delhi, India

Mohan Muttanahally Eraiah
Department of Medicine, BGS Global Institute of Medical Sciences, Bengaluru, India

Prakash Goudanavar
Department of Pharmaceutics, Sri Adichunchanagiri College of Pharmacy, Adichunchanagiri University, B. G. Nagara, India

Sagarkumar Joshi
Department of Microbiology and Biotechnology, Gujarat University, Ahmedabad, India
Department of Microbiology, Darshan Institute of Science, Darshan University, Rajkot, India

Puja Panwar Hazari
Department of Cyclotron and Radiopharmaceuticals Research, Advanced Radioisotope Production Center, Institute of Nuclear Medicine and Allied Sciences, Timarpur, Delhi, India.

Raju Koneri
Research Institute, BGS Global Institute of Medical Sciences, Bengaluru, India

Anamika Kulshrestha
Arya College of Pharmacy, Kukus, Jaipur, India

Meenakshi Kumari
Department of Botany, Career Point University, Kota, India

Ankita Lakra
Govt. Physiotherapy College, Raipur, India

Dibyananda Majhi
Department of Chemistry, IIT Hyderabad, Kandi, Telangana, India

Vijay Bahadur Maurya
Institute of Pharmacy, V.B.S. Purvanchal University, Jaunpur, India

Pawan Ganesh Nayak
Department of Pharmacology, Manipal College of Pharmaceutical Sciences, Manipal Academy of Higher Education, Manipal, India

Ethirajulu Nirmala
Departtment of Pharmaceutics, Shri Venktaswara College of Pharmacy, Ariyur, Puducherry, India

Saish Pawar
Department of Pharmaceutical Sciences, School of Health Sciences and Technology, MIT World Peace University, Pune, India

Deena Prakash
Biochemistry Discipline, School of Sciences, Indira Gandhi National Open University, New Delhi, India

Moqbel Ali Moqbel Redhwan
Department of Pharmacology, KLE College of Pharmacy, Bengaluru, India
KLE Academy of Higher Education and Research, Belgavi, India

Bharti Sahu
Department of Pharmacy, Ram Krishna Dharmarth Foundation University, Bhopal, India

Pravat Kumar Sahu
Department of Chemistry, IIT Hyderabad, Kandi, Telangana, India

Suman Samaddar
Research Institute, BGS Global Institute of Medical Sciences, Bengaluru, India

Nidhi Saxena
Department of Microbiology, Atmiya University, Rajkot, India

Anushri Sharma
Department of Biochemistry, Barkatullah University, Bhopal, India

Arun Sharma
Department of Chemistry, School of Basic and Applied Sciences, Career Point University, Kota, India

Neha Sharma
Amity Institute of Biotechnology, Amity University, Gwalior, India

Sarika Sharma
Sri Aurobindo Institute of Pharmacy, Indore, India

Manish Shrivastava
Amity Institute of Biotechnology, Amity University, Gwalior, India

Vikas Shrivastava
Amity Institute of Biotechnology, Amity University, Gwalior, India

Ch. Subrahmanyam
Department of Chemistry, IIT Hyderabad, Kandi, Telangana, India

Niharika Singh
Amity Institute of Biotechnology, Amity University, Gwalior, India

Ragini Singh
Amity Institute of Biotechnology, Amity University, Gwalior, India

Pooja Singh
Department of Biochemical Engineering, HBTU, Kanpur, India

Rohit Kumar Singh
Agricultural Research Organization, Volcani Institute, Israel

Surabhi Singh
EARS Pvt. Ltd., Bhopal, India

Nagaraja Sreeharsha
Department of Pharmaceutical Sciences, College of Clinical Pharmacy, King Faisal University, Al Hofuf, Saudi Arabia

Rajesh Singh Tomar
Amity Institute of Biotechnology, Amity University, Gwalior, India

Jayachandran Venkatesan
Department of Biomaterials and Transplant Sciences, School of Dental Sciences and Technology, Malla Reddy Vishwavidyapeeth (Deemed to be University), Hyderabad, Telangana, India

Oshin Verma
Department of Biotechnology, Bundelkhand University, Jhansi, India

Priyanka Yadav
Department of Biotechnology, IIT Hyderabad, Kandi, Telangana, India

Acknowledgment

The editors extend their heartfelt gratitude to all contributors for their valuable efforts in the respective chapters of this book. Their dedication, hard work, and analytical insights are deeply appreciated and recognized.

Dr Nidhi Puranik expresses sincere thanks to Yeungnam University, Gyeongsan, South Korea, for its infrastructure support and assistance. Professor Shiv Kumar Yadav extends his gratitude to Government Lal Bahadur Shastri PG College, Sironj, Vidisha, Madhya Pradesh, India, for providing the necessary facilities and support.

Preface

Alzheimer's disease (AD) is a debilitating condition that primarily affects the elderly. It is marked by a gradual and progressive deterioration of the brain brought on by extracellular plaques that form in the hippocampus. AD cells are composed of plaque-encased tangles of twisted strands of accumulated microtubule-binding proteins. When administering matching medications to treat various clinical diseases, we must overcome the blood–brain barrier (BBB), a robust, naturally occurring barrier that separates blood from brain cells and keeps them safe. Innovative alternatives to traditional methods for resolving problems with drug transport across the BBB are offered by nanomedicines. The current study highlights the developments in nanomedicines' applications to AD diagnosis and treatment.

AD is a brain disorder that deteriorates cognitive function and is fatal, progressive, and irreversible. It currently affects 32.6 million people worldwide; if effective treatments are not found by 2050, that number might increase to 139 million. The current treatment plan does not stop or delay the disease's progression; instead, it improves cognitive function and momentarily alleviates symptoms. A possible approach based on nanotechnology may enhance the drug's specificity and bioavailability when it comes to brain targeting. Moreover, a thorough synopsis of the uses of nanomedicines for the efficient delivery of medications for the treatment of AD is provided in this paper.

The proposed book gives the idea of how nanotechnology has transformed AD management techniques, as well as points out the main roadblocks that are now being faced and future directions for this area. Additionally, the development of nanomedicines for the treatment of AD may encourage the rapid expansion of both clinical trials and research into these treatments.

The book compiles detailed literature on various novel therapeutic applications of nanomaterial in drug delivery for CNS in AD treatment. It gives enormous room for researchers to explore therapeutic targets and different approaches for the management of AD more deeply. There are many books available on the application of nanomaterials in drug delivery for CNS however no specific available that compiles the literature on therapeutic targets, therapeutic approaches, and the use of nanoparticles in the treatment and management of AD together therefore, the book has become one of its kind. The book will help in bridging the gap of knowledge in neurosciences, neurotherapeutics, nanotechnology, and nanomedicine domains. The book chapter may also be useful to educators, researchers, legislators, and medical professionals in the form of a better selection of nanomaterial and drug design.

1 Overview of Neuropathology of Alzheimer's Disease

Ethirajulu Nirmala, Vijay Bahadur Maurya, Anamika Kulshrestha, Surabhi Singh, Nidhi Puranik, and Arun Sharma

1.1 INTRODUCTION

Alzheimer's disease (AD) is a neurological disease that worsens with time and primarily affects elderly people. It causes significant memory loss and cognitive deterioration. With millions of people afflicted with AD and the number predicted to increase significantly with aging populations, there is an urgent need for effective therapeutic strategies [1–3]. AD, the most prevalent type of dementia, has emerged as a serious global public health concern in today's scenario. It is essential to comprehend the fundamental mechanisms of AD to develop effective therapies and treatments.

The hallmark of AD is a progressive loss of cognitive function that starts with mild memory loss and gradually advances to severe impairments in language, reasoning, and day-to-day functioning [4–6]. The development of amyloid-beta (Aβ) plaques, neurofibrillary tangles (NFTs) made of hyperphosphorylated tau protein, and extensive neuronal loss are among the neuropathological characteristics of AD (Figure 1.1) [7–9]. These pathological features are primarily observed in the hippocampus and cerebral cortex, regions critical for memory and cognitive function [1]. These pathogenic alterations are linked to detrimental cognitive dysfunctions, neuronal loss, and synaptic abnormalities. Although lipid receptors, dysregulated neurotransmitters and their receptors, oxidative stress, mitochondrial stress, and dysregulated calcium homeostasis are also major pathological characteristics of AD [10].

The exact aetiology of AD remains elusive, though it is widely accepted that a combination of genetic, environmental, and lifestyle factors eventually contribute to its development. Mutations in genes such as APP, PSEN1, and PSEN2 are known to cause familial forms of AD, while the APOE ε4 allele is a significant risk factor for sporadic AD [11–14]. Despite extensive research, the precise mechanisms by which these factors lead to the neuropathological changes observed in AD are still under investigation [15]. There is growing evidence that noncoding RNAs including long noncoding RNAs (lncRNA) and microRNAs (miRNAs) play a critical role in the molecular pathophysiology of AD [16–18]. It has been shown lncRNAs, which range in size from 200 nucleotides to more than 100 kilobytes, are essential

DOI: 10.1201/9781003543381-1

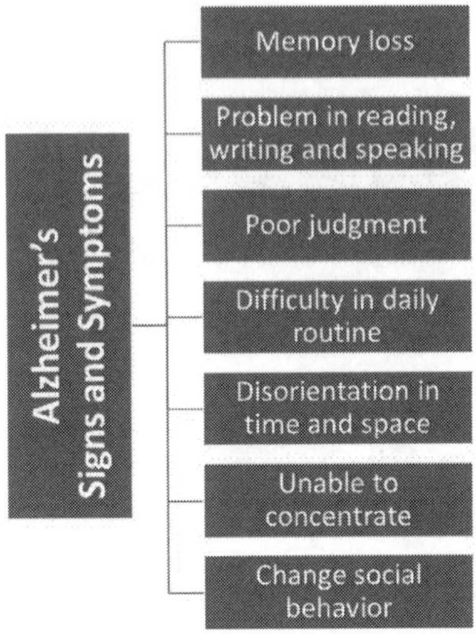

FIGURE 1.1 Signs and symptoms of Alzheimer's disease.

for several fundamental biological processes that are crucial for the development of AD. LncRNAs influence both transcriptional and posttranscriptional aspects of gene expression and are involved in the control of tau, Aβ peptide, inflammation, cell death, and other elements that are key to the pathophysiology of AD [18,19]. MiRNAs attach to target genes' 3′ and 5′ untranslated regions to silence them post-transcriptionally. More than 70% of all experimentally identified miRNAs are expressed in the brain, and these miRNAs are essential for certain signals during memory formation as well as synaptic function [20,21].

To identify potential therapeutic targets, such as reducing Aβ deposition or tau hyperphosphorylation, it is essential to get the neuropathology of AD. Additionally, understanding the progression of neuropathological changes can aid in predicting disease course and outcomes, which is crucial for patient care and planning [22]. Finally, research on neuropathology has led to the development of biomarkers for early diagnosis, which is essential for implementing interventions before significant brain damage occurs.

Understanding the underlying mechanisms and developing diagnostic and therapeutic tools are made possible by the study of neuropathology. By analysing the molecular and cellular changes that occur in the brain, researchers can devise ways to slow or even stop the disease's progression. Biomarkers that can identify the disease in its preclinical stages and enable earlier intervention are also made possible by this knowledge [23].

1.2 HISTORICAL CONTEXT

Over a century, several turning points in the study of AD have moulded our current knowledge of the neuropathology of the disease. Over the years, innovative observations and continuous research have contributed to our growing knowledge of AD, from its initial clinical description to the molecular discoveries of the late 20th and early 21st centuries. The term "Alzheimer's disease" has been used for over 100 years [24] and has a wide history as "Alzheimer's disease" has several distinctive meanings [25]. Dr. Alois Alzheimer reported the first example of what would become known as Alzheimer's Disease in 1906. The case of Auguste Deter, a 51-year-old lady who showed gradual memory loss, disorientation, and behavioural problems, was described by Alzheimer, a German physician, and neuropathologist. Alzheimer performed a detailed analysis of her brain following her passing and found specific neuropathological characteristics, such as NFTs and amyloid plaques [26]. These results, which were initially published in 1906 after being presented at a symposium, provided the disease's first clinical and pathological description. Significant developments in biochemistry, genetics, and neuroimaging provided information on the molecular and cellular mechanisms underlying the disease at the end of the 20th century [27,28].

1.2.1 Key Historical Milestones in AD Neuropathology

1.2.1.1 Discovery of Amyloid-Beta and Its Role in Plaque Formation (1984)

The discovery in the 1980s that Aβ is the main component of the plaques seen in Alzheimer's patients was one of the biggest advances in the field of AD research. The amyloid hypothesis was developed as a result of the isolation and characterization of Aβ [29–32]. According to this theory, the build-up of Aβ peptides in the brain sets off a series of actions that eventually result in neurodegeneration. Research on Aβsynthesis, aggregation, and clearance was redirected after its discovery and is still a major area of study for AD [7,33].

1.2.1.2 Identification of Tau Protein and Neurofibrillary Tangles (1986)

Not long after Aβ was discovered, scientists discovered that NFTs, another characteristic of AD, are primarily composed of tau protein [34]. Researchers discovered in 1986 that AD causes hyperphosphorylation of tau, a microtubule-associated protein, which results in the creation of tangles that impair brain function. The tau hypothesis was developed, which states that tau pathology is a major factor contributing to AD neurodegeneration [35–38]. This finding led to a dual focus in AD research on NFTs and amyloid plaques.

1.2.1.3 Genetic Discoveries and the Role of APOE (1993)

Another significant turning point in the study of AD is the discovery of genetic risk factors. The ε4 allele of the apolipoprotein E (APOE) gene was found to be a significant genetic risk factor for late-onset AD in 1993 [39–41]. This finding improved our knowledge of the heritability and population risk of AD by shedding light on the genetic predispositions that contribute to the disease.

1.2.1.4 Advancements in Neuroimaging Techniques (1990s–Present)

The research of AD neuropathology has changed dramatically with the introduction of sophisticated neuroimaging methods like magnetic resonance imaging (MRI) and positron emission tomography (PET). With the use of these technologies, scientists can now see NFTs and amyloid plaques in live patients, which helps with early diagnosis and disease progression monitoring. Particularly significant has been the creation of PET tracers that are specific for tau and amyloid, which have made it possible to investigate these diseases in vivo and how they relate to cognitive decline [42–45].

1.2.1.5 Emergence of the Amyloid Cascade Hypothesis (1992)

The amyloid cascade hypothesis, first put forth, rose to prominence as a key idea in the study of AD [46]. According to this theory, the first step in a series of events that eventually results in tau pathology, neuronal death, and clinical symptoms is the deposition of Aβ. The majority of studies and treatment initiatives that try to alter the course of the disease by focusing on Aβaggregation and production have been directed by this theory [47–49].

1.2.1.6 Discovery of Presenilin Mutations (1995)

In the mid-1990s, mutations in the presenilin 1 (PSEN1) and presenilin 2 (PSEN2) genes were identified as the cause of familial AD, a rare type of the disease with an early onset. The gamma-secretase complex, which is involved in the cleavage of amyloid precursor protein (APP) to create Aβ, is encoded by these genes [50–52]. The identification of presenilin mutations confirmed the important role of Aβ in AD pathogenesis by offering vital insights into the molecular mechanisms underlying Aβsynthesis and accumulation [31].

The historical background of AD reflects the combined efforts of innumerable researchers along with an overview of how our knowledge of AD has changed over time and its implications for ongoing and future studies [53].

1.3 BASIC NEUROPATHOLOGICAL FEATURES

A variety of neuropathological characteristics that are specific to AD all work together to cause the disease's progressive neurodegeneration in affected people. NFTs and senile plaques, commonly referred to as amyloid plaques, are two of the most common [54–56]. These lesions are essential to the pathophysiology of the disease and have a major impact on neuronal malfunction and cognitive decline, along with other pathological indicators such as granulovacuolar degeneration (GVD) [57–59] and neuritic plaques [60].

1.3.1 Neurofibrillary Tangles

Intracellular clumps known as NFTs are mostly made of hyperphosphorylated tau protein. Tau is a protein that is connected with microtubules and helps to stabilize them, which is necessary for preserving the form and functionality of neurons. Tau experiences aberrant hyperphosphorylation in AD, which impairs tau's capacity to attach to microtubules. PHFs, or paired helical filaments, are formed as a result, and they eventually combine to produce NFTs [61].

The hyperphosphorylation of tau at particular serine and threonine sites is the first step in the development of NFT. These changes cause tau to self-assemble into insoluble fibrils by changing its shape to build up into thick, twisted bundles called NFTs [62]. The entorhinal cortex, hippocampal regions, and other brain areas related to memory and cognition are the most frequently affected by these tangles, which are associated with AD symptoms [63].

In AD, NFTs are closely linked to cell death and neuronal dysfunction. NFTs interfere with neurons' ability to operate normally in several ways. First, the destabilization of microtubules brought on by tau sequestration into NFTs affects axonal transport, which is essential for the passage of nutrients, organelles, and signalling chemicals through neurons. The result of this disturbance is synapse malfunction and ultimately neuronal death [64,65].

Moreover, the build-up of NFTs is linked to the degeneration of neural networks and synapses, both of which are necessary for cognitive processes like memory and learning. Similar to the clinical course of AD, tau pathology spreads recognizably, starting in the entorhinal cortex and moving on to the hippocampus and neocortex [2]. The extent of NFT pathology plays a critical role in the pathogenesis of dementia, as evidenced by its stronger correlation with dementia severity than amyloid plaque load.

1.3.2 Senile Plaques (Amyloid Plaques)

Amyloid plaques, sometimes referred to as senile plaques, are extracellular deposits mainly made up of Aβ peptides from the amyloid protein. The cerebral cortex and hippocampal regions are the primary locations of these plaques, which are characteristic features of AD [66]. The cleavage of the transmembrane protein known as APP by the enzyme's beta-secretase and gamma-secretase initiates the production of amyloid plaques. Aβ peptides, whose lengths might vary, are released by this successive cleavage; Aβ42 is especially prone to aggregation [66,67].

The oligomers formed by the aggregation of Aβ peptides eventually form fibrils and dense, intractable plaques. Dystrophic neurites, activated microglia, and reactive astrocytes frequently encircle these plaques, suggesting a localized inflammatory response [68,69]. The amyloid cascade theory, which suggests that the build-up of Aβ is the initial event in the pathogenesis of AD, is cantered on the process of amyloid plaque development.

In AD, amyloid plaques are linked to several neurodegenerative processes. Particularly harmful to neurons are Aβ oligomers, which are byproducts of the intermediate stages of plaque development. By interfering with synaptic signalling and plasticity, these oligomers can impair synaptic function and cause cognitive impairments. Moreover, it has been demonstrated that they cause calcium dysregulation, oxidative stress, and mitochondrial dysfunction—all of which are factors in the death of neurones [60,70].

Apart from their immediate neurodegenerative consequences, amyloid plaques are thought to initiate a series of actions culminating in persistent neuroinflammation. Neuronal injury is aggravated by pro-inflammatory cytokines released by activated microglia and astrocytes surrounding plaques. Prolonged inflammation and oxidative stress accelerate AD development and increase tau pathology dissemination [71,72].

1.3.2.1 Neuritic Plaques

Dystrophic neurites, or abnormally enlarged and injured nerve cell processes, are a specific subtype of amyloid plaques that are seen inside and surrounding the amyloid

TABLE 1.1
Neuritic Plaques and Neurofibrillary Tangles of Alzheimer's Disease

S. No.	Neuritic Plaques	Neurofibrillary Tangles
1	Commonly found in the brains of elderly people but appears in excessive numbers in the cortex of AD patients.	Twisted remains of a protein which is essential for maintaining proper cell structure.
2	Surrounded by deteriorating neurons that produce acetylcholine (neurotransmitter essential for processing memory and learning)	It is still not confirmed that plaques and tangles are the cause of Ad or part of the results of the disorder.

core. Compared to diffuse plaques, which mostly consist of loosely distributed Aβ fibrils without accompanying neuritic disease, these plaques are usually larger and more complicated. Neuritic plaques are frequently observed in the temporal and parietal lobes, two regions of the brain linked to higher cognitive abilities [73–75].

These plaques show significant disruption of synaptic connections and neuronal architecture due to the presence of dystrophic neurites. Hyperphosphorylated tau is also commonly linked to these plaques, establishing a connection between the tau and amyloid diseases [8]. A major comparison of neuritic plaques and neurofibrillary tangles is presented in Table 1.1.

1.3.2.2 Granulovacuolar Degeneration

Granulovacuolar degeneration, a condition characterized by the accumulation of large membrane-bound vacuoles containing a central granule, is hippocampal pyramidal neurons of AD and other dementias individuals. The cytoplasm of neurons with GVD is marked by the presence of tiny, membrane-bound vacuoles containing dense granules [76–78]. The CA1 area of the hippocampal pyramidal neurons, which is essential for memory formation, is where these vacuoles are most frequently detected. They are also found beyond the hippocampal formation and can be detected in various brain regions, including the entorhinal cortex, temporal neocortex, hypothalamus, amygdala, and frontal and parietal cortical areas [77].

Though its precise aetiology and relevance in AD are yet unknown, GVD is thought to be a cellular reaction to long-term stress or trauma [57].

The investigation of these neuropathological aspects by the study of the complex link between these pathological indicators and the clinical symptoms of the disorder provides vital insights into the mechanisms underlying AD [79].

1.4 MOLECULAR AND CELLULAR MECHANISMS

Neurons gradually deteriorate as a result of intricate molecular and cellular processes that underlie AD. The amyloid cascade and tau theories, which explain the functions of aberrant tau and Aβproteins, respectively, are fundamental to these pathways. The immune system and inflammation, especially when it comes to glial cells, also significantly contribute to the disease's aggravation. Comprehending these pathways is essential for formulating treatment approaches intended to prevent or reverse the advancement of AD [80].

1.4.1 Amyloid Cascade Hypothesis

One of the most well-known theories describing the molecular pathophysiology of AD is the amyloid cascade theory. According to this theory, the build-up of Aβ peptides in the brain is what sets off a series of degenerative events that eventually result in neurodegeneration.

The transmembrane protein known as APP, which is extensively produced in neurones, is the source of Aβpeptides. The processing of APP can occur via two primary routes: the non-amyloidogenic pathway, which is cleaved by alpha-secretase, and the amyloidogenic pathway, which is cleaved sequentially by gamma-secretase and beta-secretase (BACE1). Aβ peptides are produced by the latter process; Aβ40 and Aβ42 are the most prevalent types. Because it is hydrophobic, aggregation is especially likely to occur in Aβ42 [81].

According to the amyloid cascade theory, the build-up of Aβ42 is a crucial occurrence. These peptides combine to generate highly neurotoxic oligomers, which are soluble, tiny versions of Aβ. These oligomers build up into fibrils, which then further aggregate into the insoluble amyloid plaques that are indicative of AD. It is observed that Aβ aggregation causes damage to cell membranes, obstructs synaptic function, and starts a chain of harmful events that eventually result in neuronal death [70].

The effects of Aβon the health of neurons are extensive and diverse. The most hazardous form of the peptide is thought to be in the form of Aβ oligomers, which interfere with neurotransmitter receptors, change calcium homeostasis, and reduce synaptic plasticity. These disturbances correlate with the early cognitive signs of AD and are especially harmful to the hippocampal and other memory and learning regions [82].

Moreover, the formation of Aβ causes oxidative stress by producing reactive oxygen species (ROS), which harm DNA, lipids, and proteins within the cell. Moreover, Aβ ruins mitochondrial processes, making neuronal energy deficiencies worse. The progressive loss of synapses, neuronal death, and cognitive decline seen in AD patients are caused by these combined consequences [83].

1.4.2 Tau Hypothesis

The tau hypothesis, which emphasizes the part anomalies of tau protein in AD, is a complement to the amyloid cascade concept. Tau is a protein that is connected with microtubules and is vital for the stability and proper operation of neuronal microtubules, which are necessary for intracellular transport [84].

The tau protein experiences aberrant hyperphosphorylation at several different locations in AD. Due to this hyperphosphorylation, tau is less able to connect to microtubules, which causes it to detach and then aggregate into NFTs and PHFs. These tangles are a defining feature of AD and are directly linked to the illness's severity [34,84].

Normal biological activities are disrupted when hyperphosphorylated tau accumulates abnormally. It reduces the cell's capacity to maintain microtubule stability, which is essential for the movement of vesicles, organelles, and other payloads inside neurons. Particularly in areas of the brain important for memory and cognition, the existence of NFTs is highly correlated with neuronal loss and dysfunction [85].

Tau's function in microtubule stabilization is essential for preserving the form and functionality of neurons. The cytoskeletal "highways" that motor proteins use to move vital components between the cell body and synaptic terminals, like mitochondria and synaptic vesicles, are made up of microtubules. These transport systems break down as a result of microtubule destabilization brought on by hyperphosphorylated tau in AD [86].

Because of the ensuing disruption in the delivery of essential components to synapses, axonal transport impairment results in synaptic dysfunction. As one of the main characteristics of AD and a factor in the clinical symptoms of memory loss and cognitive decline, this leads to the breakdown of synaptic connections. Furthermore, a prion-like process appears to underpin the transmission of tau disease from one area of the brain to another, with misfolded tau causing normal tau in linked neurones to misfold, which in turn facilitates the spread of NFTs.

1.4.3 Inflammation and Immune Response

The immune system and chronic inflammation are important factors in the development of AD. The immune system of the brain reacts to the build-up of tau and Aβ pathology, mainly through the action of glial cells like microglia and astrocytes. However, this response frequently makes the damage to neurons worse rather than better.

The immune cells known as microglia, which dwell in the central nervous system, are in charge of identifying and eliminating infections, dead cells, and other detritus. In the context of AD, tau tangles and amyloid plaques cause microglia to become activated. But instead of efficiently removing these pathogenic deposits, persistent microglia activation results in an ongoing inflammatory state. Neuroinflammation is facilitated by the release of pro-inflammatory cytokines, chemokines, and other mediators by activated microglia. This inflammatory reaction can worsen the course of AD by causing further neuronal damage.

AD pathogenesis now includes chronic neuroinflammation as a major component. Acute inflammation serves as a defence mechanism, but prolonged inflammation—as in AD—causes more immune activation and brain damage in a vicious cycle. Activated microglia and astrocytes continuously emit pro-inflammatory cytokines, which lead to oxidative stress, disruption of the blood-brain barrier, and increased immune cell recruitment to the brain [87].

In addition to harming neurons, this persistent inflammation impairs the brain's capacity to eliminate Aβ and restore tissue. Amyloid plaque and neurofibrillary tangle build-up are accelerated over time by neuroinflammation, which adds to the unstoppable development of AD.

1.5 REGIONAL BRAIN CHANGES

Particular and progressive alterations occur in the brain's cortical and subcortical regions in AD. The clinical symptoms of memory loss, cognitive decline, and behavioural abnormalities that patients experience are closely associated with these alterations. The regional brain changes involve cortical regions (temporal, parietal, and frontal lobes) and subcortical structures (hippocampus, amygdala, and basal forebrain) [8].

1.5.1 Cortical Areas Affected

AD has a major influence on the cortical parts of the brain, most notably the temporal, parietal, and frontal lobes, which are crucial for memory, language, attention, and executive functioning.

1.5.1.1 Temporal Lobe

One of the first brain areas to be impacted by AD is the temporal lobe, more specifically the medial temporal lobe. The typical memory loss observed in the early stages of AD is caused by the degradation of neurons in the temporal lobe [88].

Language and auditory processing are similarly impacted by atrophy in the temporal lobe. As the illness worsens, patients may have problems naming objects (anomia) and understanding language (Wernicke's aphasia), which are indicative of lateral temporal cortex involvement.

1.5.1.2 Parietal Lobe

AD also affects the parietal lobe, a region critical to attention, sensory integration, and spatial orientation. In the later stages of AD, visuospatial impairments are frequently caused by damage to this region. Patients suffering from prosopagnosia (the inability to recognize faces) may find it challenging to perform tasks requiring spatial awareness, such as navigating familiar areas.

Additionally, the integration of sensory data from many modalities is facilitated by the parietal lobe. Patients may find it difficult to perform tasks requiring the synchronization of motor, auditory, and visual information as their AD worsens. This can show up as apraxia, a condition in which people with the physical capacity to complete learnt motor tasks struggle. Parietal lobe atrophy is linked to deficits in complex attention and executive function and contributes to the overall cognitive deterioration in AD [89].

1.5.1.3 Frontal Lobe

Higher-order cognitive processes including decision-making, problem-solving, personality expression, and executive functions are controlled by the frontal lobe. The frontal lobe of Alzheimer's dementia is impacted later in the disease course than the temporal and parietal lobes.

Planning, organizing, and controlling improper behaviour are examples of executive function deficiencies brought on by frontal lobe damage. Apathy, disinhibition, and alterations in social behaviour are possible in patients, which may indicate prefrontal brain involvement. The capacity to carry out difficult tasks and make decisions is progressively compromised as the disease advances. Frontal release indicators, including the grab reflex, which is suggestive of advanced AD, are also a result of frontal lobe atrophy [90].

TABLE 1.2
Effects of Alzheimer's Disease on Cortical and Sub-Cortical Areas

S. No.	Cortical	Sub-Cortical
1	Disorder affecting the cortex, the outer portion or layers of the brain	Dysfunction in parts of the brain that are beneath the cortex
2	Alzheimer's and Creutzfeldt-Jacob are its two forms	Huntington's disease and AIDS dementia complex are its two forms
3	Memory and language difficulties (Aphasia) most pronounced symptoms	Memory loss and language difficulties not present or less severe
4	Aphasia is the inability to recall words and understand common language	Thinking slows down with changes in their personality and attention span

1.5.2 Subcortical Structures

AD affects not only cortical areas but also several important subcortical structures, such as the basal forebrain, amygdala, and hippocampal regions. Major effects of AD on cortical and sub-cortical areas are listed in Table 1.2. These structures play a major role in the clinical signs of AD, and their degradation is crucial for memory, emotional processing, and neurotransmitter control.

1.5.2.1 Hippocampal

One of the most important brain areas for memory and learning is the hippocampus, which is badly damaged by AD. One of the first indications of AD is hippocampal shrinkage, which is closely linked to the memory impairments that define the illness. The formation of long-term memories is mostly dependent on the hippocampus, and its degeneration results in anterograde amnesia, which is the inability to form new memories [91].

The memory problems are made worse by the expansion of hippocampal injury in AD, which affects nearby areas like the entorhinal cortex and parahippocampal gyrus. Additionally, when involved in spatial navigation, the hippocampal atrophy can cause confusion and make it harder to navigate familiar situations. In neuroimaging investigations, the extent of hippocampal atrophy is frequently utilized as a diagnostic marker and is correlated with the severity of cognitive impairment.

1.5.2.2 Amygdala

An important component of emotional processing, the amygdala is implicated in fear, anger, and the creation of emotional memories. The amygdala experiences considerable shrinkage in AD, which adds to the patients' emotional and behavioural symptoms.

Changes in emotional responses, including elevated anxiety, anger, and depression, are frequent in AD and can result from damage to the amygdala. The intricate emotional and behavioural abnormalities associated with AD may be caused by interactions between the amygdala and other damaged brain areas, like the prefrontal cortex [92].

1.5.2.3 Basal Forebrain

Acetylcholine is produced in the basal forebrain, which contains the nucleus basalis of Meynert. Acetylcholine is a neurotransmitter that is necessary for memory, attention, and learning. One of the first areas of neuronal death in AD is the basal forebrain, which results in a marked decrease in cholinergic transmission throughout the brain.

Apart from the main cause of the extensive cognitive deficits associated with AD is the loss of cholinergic neurons in the basal forebrain. These deficits include problems with memory, attention, and executive function. The impairment of acetylcholine exacerbates the disease's cognitive and behavioural symptoms by altering the modulation of other neurotransmitter systems. One of the main treatments for AD is cholinesterase inhibitors, which raise acetylcholine levels; this emphasizes the significance of basal forebrain atrophy in the pathophysiology of the illness [93].

1.6 GENETIC AND ENVIRONMENTAL FACTORS

AD is impacted by both environmental and hereditary factors. These elements influence the disease's beginning, course, and severity. Environmental and lifestyle variables also play a major influence, especially in late-onset AD, even if certain genetic variants are highly connected with AD, especially in cases with an early onset [94].

1.6.1 Genetic Factors

AD is mostly hereditary, with different genetic profiles linked to early- and late-onset variants of the illness. It has been determined that some genetic variants and mutations greatly raise the likelihood of getting AD.

1.6.1.1 Early-Onset and Late-Onset AD

Less than 5% of cases of AD are early-onset Alzheimer's disease (EOAD), which usually results before the age of 65. One mutant copy of the gene is enough to induce EOAD, which is frequently inherited in an autosomal dominant fashion. Three genes APP, PSEN1, and PSEN2 are the main sites of alterations linked to EOAD [95]. The most prevalent type of AD, known as late-onset Alzheimer's disease (LOAD), develops beyond the age of 65 and is impacted by both environmental and hereditary factors. In contrast to EOAD, LOAD is usually brought on by a confluence of environmental variables and genetic risk factors rather than a single gene mutation.

1.6.1.2 Amyloid Precursor Protein

Aβ peptides are produced in greater amounts or with altered cleavage when mutations occur in the APP gene, which is found on chromosome 21. A characteristic feature of AD neuropathology, amyloid plaque development, is closely associated with these mutations [70].

1.6.1.3 Presenilin 1 (PSEN1) and Presenilin 2 (PSEN2)

PSEN1 and PSEN2 are genes encoding elements of the gamma-secretase complex, implicated in the conversion of Aβ from APP. Alterations in gamma-secretase activity caused by mutations in PSEN1 (located on chromosome 14) and PSEN2 (located on chromosome 1) result in an increase in the generation of the hazardous Aβ42 peptide, which is more prone to aggregation [70,96].

APOE: The main genetic risk factor for LOAD is the APOE gene, which is found on chromosome 19. APOE is composed of three common alleles: ε2, ε3, and ε4. The APOE ε4 allele has been linked to an elevated risk of AD; two to three times higher risk for people with one copy of the allele, and eight to twelve times higher risk for those with two copies. The ε4 version of APOE is less effective in promoting the clearance of Aβ from the brain, which can contribute to its accumulation and plaque development. APOE is involved in lipid metabolism and the clearance of Aβ [97].

1.6.1.4 Key Genetic Mutations (APP, PSEN1, PSEN2, APOE)

To understand the pathophysiology of AD requires knowledge of the particular genetic abnormalities linked to the disease. Each of these mutations has a role in the pathogenic mechanisms underlying AD, specifically in the generation, accumulation, and removal of Aβ.

1.6.1.5 APP Mutations

Changes in the APP gene might result in an excess of Aβ or longer, more prone to aggregation versions of Aβ, like Aβ42. This excess Aβbuilds up in the brain to create amyloid plaques, a major component of the pathophysiology of AD and harmful to neurons [98].

1.6.1.6 Mutations in PSEN1 and PSEN2

These changes cause the gamma-secretase complex to function improperly, which increases the synthesis of the Aβ42 peptide. Aβ42 build-up plays a role in the development of amyloid plaques, which set off a series of pathogenic occurrences such as tau hyperphosphorylation, the creation of NFTs, and neuronal death [52].

APOE ε4: Increased brain Aβ deposition, compromised synaptic function, and neuroinflammation are linked to the APOE ε4 genotype. While APOE ε4's precise mechanisms of action in AD are still being investigated, its function in Aβmetabolism and clearance is well-known [99]. AD risk is markedly increased among carriers of the ε4 allele, especially in later life.

1.6.2 Environmental and Lifestyle Factors

Environmental and lifestyle factors are important in the development and progression of AD, in addition to hereditary risk. These variables may have an impact on the severity and progression of AD in addition to influencing the likelihood of getting the illness [100].

Diet and Nutrition: It has been demonstrated that dietary factors affect the likelihood of getting AD. Heavy intake of sugar and saturated fats has been linked to a higher risk of AD and cognitive decline, whereas those abundant in antioxidants, omega-3 fatty acids, and other neuroprotective nutrients like those in the Mediterranean diet have been linked to a lower risk [101]. Nutritional variables may impact inflammation, oxidative stress, and Aβmetabolism, which can all have an impact on brain health.

Physical Activity: There is a clear and constant correlation between regular physical activity and a decreased risk of AD. Exercise lowers inflammation, strengthens the heart, and may even increase neural plasticity and neurogenesis [102]. The danger of Aβformation and neurodegeneration are believed to be decreased by these preventive effects.

Social Engagement: A higher risk of cognitive decline and AD has been linked to social isolation and low involvement. On the other hand, by lowering stress, fostering mental stimulation, improving emotional well-being, preserving close social links, and taking part in fulfilling social activities may prevent cognitive decline [103].

Sleep Quality: An elevated risk of AD has been associated with poor sleep quality, especially in cases of sleep disorders such as insomnia and sleep apnea. Sleep is essential for the removal of Aβ from the brain, and irregular sleep patterns can cause amyloid plaques to build up and trigger more neuroinflammation [104,105].

Cardiovascular Diseases (CVD) and Health: Recent studies support the hypothesis that CVD may contribute to AD progression, as the diseases often coexist. AD risk has been linked to cardiovascular risk factors, including obesity, diabetes, hypertension, and hypercholesterolemia. These illnesses worsen vascular injury, which can worsen tau pathology and amyloid deposition, which increases neurodegeneration [106].

1.7 DIAGNOSTIC APPROACHES

A multidisciplinary approach involving clinical evaluation, neuroimaging techniques, and biomarker analysis is necessary for the diagnosis of AD [107]. With early intervention and better care planning, the main methods of diagnosing AD-like biomarker analysis, neuroimaging methods, and clinical diagnosis are given below:

1.7.1 Clinical Diagnosis

Clinical diagnosis, which entails extensive cognitive evaluations and neurological exams, is frequently the initial stage in the identification of AD. These techniques aid in distinguishing AD from other forms of dementia and mental illnesses.

1.7.1.1 Cognitive Assessments

The primary step in diagnosing AD is often clinical diagnosis, which involves comprehensive cognitive tests and neurological exams. These methods help to differentiate AD from other types of dementia and mental diseases [108].

Mini-Mental State Examination (MMSE): The MMSE is a cognitive tool used for the assessment of a variety of cognitive disorders that provides an overview of cognitive function [109,110]. An extensively used screening instrument, the MMSE evaluates language, orientation, recollection, attention, math, and visuospatial abilities. With scores ranging from 0 to 30, it offers a summary of cognitive function; scores less than 24 may indicate cognitive impairment [111].

1.7.1.2 Montreal Cognitive Assessment (MoCA)

MoCA is a cognitive screening tool for AD in both research and clinical settings [112,113]. A more sensitive measure than the MMSE is the MoCA, especially when it comes to identifying moderate cognitive impairment (MCI), which frequently occurs before AD [114,115]. Although it includes more difficult activities, the MoCA covers similar topics and is beneficial for identifying early cognitive changes.

1.7.1.3 Neuropsychological Testing

Neuropsychological testing is done when a more thorough evaluation is needed. A wide range of cognitive abilities, including memory, language, attention, executive function, and visuospatial skills, are assessed by this extensive assessment. The findings may aid in distinguishing AD from other neurodegenerative diseases [116].

1.7.1.4 Neuroimaging Techniques: MRI, PET, and CT Scans

Neuroimaging is crucial in diagnosing dementia, particularly AD, to rule out structural causes like strokes, brain tumours, infectious diseases, and rare vascular issues. MRI and PET are commonly used imaging techniques; however, CT scan can also be recommended, especially when MRI cannot be accomplished [117]. These techniques shed light on the anatomical and functional alterations in the brain linked to AD.

1.7.1.5 Magnetic Resonance Imaging

MRI can produce high-resolution images of brain regions; it is the recommended imaging modality for AD. Particular brain regions that are frequently impacted by AD, such as the entorhinal cortex and hippocampal regions, can be detected for atrophy using MRI. Additionally, it aids in ruling out other dementia causes such as vascular lesions or tumours [118].

1.7.1.6 Positron Emission Tomography

PET scans are used to evaluate the brain's functioning characteristics. When it comes to AD, there are two primary kinds of PET scans:

- **FDG-PET**: This scan gauges the brain's glucose metabolism. FDG-PET visualizes neural injury or synaptic dysfunction distribution, identifying distinct dementia phenotypes from AD, Lewy bodies, and frontotemporal lobar degeneration [119]. AD is distinguished from other dementias by the distinctive finding of hypometabolism in the temporal and parietal lobes [120].
- **Amyloid-PET**: This scan shows the presence of amyloid deposition in the brain by binding radiotracers to amyloid plaques. Amyloid-PET imaging is expected to aid in early or preclinical diagnosis of AD by monitoring disease progression and measuring Aβ accumulation in the brain. Amyloid-PET is especially helpful in the early detection of AD, even before the onset of clinical symptoms [121,122].
- **Computed Tomography (CT)**: Although MRI is the preferred method, in certain cases, CT scans are utilized in place of MRIs. Brain atrophy can be

detected by CT, which can also rule out other potential causes of cognitive impairment such as brain haemorrhages or strokes. The presence of ventricular enlargement can be detected by a CT scan [123].

1.7.2 Biomarkers

Because they offer objective measurements of the underlying pathophysiology of the disease, biomarkers are becoming more and more significant in the diagnosis of AD. Blood samples and, more recently, cerebrospinal fluid (CSF) can be used for biomarker analysis [124].

1.7.3 Cerebrospinal Fluid Analysis

Examining particular proteins and other components that represent the biochemical alterations in the brain that occur during AD is part of the CSF analysis process.

Amyloid-beta: Amyloid plaques in the brain are formed by the peptide Aβ42. As the peptide accumulates in plaques, the amount of Aβ42 in the CSF falls in AD. Hence, decreased CSF Aβ42 levels suggest the presence of amyloid disease [125].

Total Tau (t-tau) and Phosphorylated Tau (p-tau): A further characteristic of AD is NFTs, which are linked to tau proteins. Increased t-tau levels signify overall neuronal injury, but p-tau is more closely associated with tau pathology. AD is characterized by high levels of these proteins in the CSF [126].

Aβ42/t-tau ratio: To improve diagnostic precision, the CSF's Aβ42 to t-tau ratio is frequently utilized. Ratios of p-tau/Aβ42 and t-tau/Aβ42 ratios are excellent [127]. Clinical practice uses a low ratio to support the diagnosis of AD since it is highly indicative of the illness.

1.7.4 Blood-based Biomarkers

Research on blood-based biomarkers is just getting started, but it offers a less intrusive option to CSF analysis. These biomarkers hold potential for early AD diagnosis and surveillance, even though they are still being studied [128,129].

Plasma Aβ: The amount of this protein in the blood can indicate the existence of amyloid plaques in the brain. Though they are still being developed, blood-based Aβ tests are less precise than CSF biomarkers [130].

Plasma Tau: Raised blood levels of tau, especially phosphorylated tau, are linked to AD, just like CSF indicators. Tau biomarkers derived from blood are being developed as a readily available diagnostic modality [128].

Neurofilament Light Chain (NfL): NfL is a neurodegenerative marker that can be found in blood and CSF. Increased NfL levels may be a general indicator of neuronal damage and are linked to several neurodegenerative illnesses, including AD [131,132].

The main methods for diagnosing AD are described in this part, with a focus on the significance of a multidisciplinary strategy that integrates biomarker analysis, neuroimaging, and clinical assessment to produce a precise and timely diagnosis.

1.8 CONCLUSION AND FUTURE PROSPECTS

The exploration of AD neuropathology concluded in a complex interplay of factors that contribute to its progression, from the accumulation of Aβ plaques and NFTs to disruptions in synaptic function, neuroinflammation, and vascular health. The neuropathological explanation of AD extends beyond traditional Aβ and tau pathology with the importance of synaptic dysfunction, vascular contributions, neuroinflammation, and disruptions in proteostasis as critical elements in disease progression. Recent advances have identified several novel therapeutic targets, including strategies aimed at preserving synaptic function, modulating neuroinflammation, improving vascular health, and enhancing proteostasis. Gene and RNA-based therapies also offer reliable approaches to treatment.

Ongoing research and clinical trials are at the forefront of converting scientific discoveries into practical treatments. From Aβ and tau-targeting therapies to multidomain lifestyle interventions and novel biomarker development, these efforts are critical in advancing our knowledge of AD and improving patient outcomes.

The continued evolution of AD research demands a sustained focus on cohesive and effective treatment strategies. Future research should emphasize embracing a more holistic view of AD that includes the interplay between genetic, environmental, and pathological factors. Early intervention remains a key strategy for minimizing the impact of AD with an advanced personalized medicine approach to individual patient profiles, including genetic, biochemical, and clinical characteristics.

In a nutshell, while significant progress has been made in understanding and addressing AD, much work remains to be done. By continuing to build on recent advances and exploring new research directions, the scientific community can hope to make meaningful strides towards effective treatments and ultimately, a cure for this devastating disease.

REFERENCES

1. Deture MA, Dickson DW. The neuropathological diagnosis of Alzheimer's disease. Molecular Neurodegeneration 2019 14:1 2019;14:1–18. https://doi.org/10.1186/S13024-019-0333-5.
2. Kamatham PT, Shukla R, Khatri DK, Vora LK. Pathogenesis, diagnostics, and therapeutics for Alzheimer's disease: Breaking the memory barrier. Ageing Res Rev 2024;101:102481. https://doi.org/10.1016/J.ARR.2024.102481.
3. Puranik N, Yadav D, Song M. Advancements in the application of nanomedicine in Alzheimer's disease: A therapeutic perspective. International Journal of Molecular Sciences 2023, Vol 24, Page 14044 2023;24:14044. https://doi.org/10.3390/IJMS241814044.
4. Alzheimer's Association. Alzheimer's disease facts and figures. Alzheimer's and Dementia 2015;11:332–84. https://doi.org/10.1016/J.JALZ.2015.02.003
5. Castro M, Smith GE. Mild cognitive impairment and Alzheimer's disease. APA Handbook of Clinical Geropsychology, Vol 2: Assessment, Treatment, and Issues of Later Life 2015:173–207. https://doi.org/10.1037/14459-007.
6. Tarawneh R, Holtzman DM. The clinical problem of symptomatic Alzheimer disease and mild cognitive impairment. Cold Spring Harb Perspect Med 2012;2:a006148. https://doi.org/10.1101/CSHPERSPECT.A006148.

7. Sadigh-Eteghad S, Sabermarouf B, Majdi A, Talebi M, Farhoudi M, Mahmoudi J. Amyloid-Beta: A crucial factor in Alzheimer's disease. Medical Principles and Practice 2014;24:1. https://doi.org/10.1159/000369101.
8. Serrano-Pozo A, Frosch MP, Masliah E, Hyman BT. Neuropathological alterations in Alzheimer disease. Cold Spring Harb Perspect Med 2011;1:a006189. https://doi.org/10.1101/CSHPERSPECT.A006189.
9. Rajmohan R, Reddy PH. Amyloid Beta and phosphorylated tau accumulations cause abnormalities at synapses of Alzheimer's disease neurons. J Alzheimers Dis 2017; 57:975. https://doi.org/10.3233/JAD-160612.
10. Puranik N, Song M. Glutamate: Molecular mechanisms and signaling pathway in Alzheimer's disease, a potential therapeutic target. Molecules 2024, Vol 29, Page 5744 2024;29:5744. https://doi.org/10.3390/MOLECULES29235744.
11. Raulin AC, Doss SV, Trottier ZA, Ikezu TC, Bu G, Liu CC. ApoE in Alzheimer's disease: Pathophysiology and therapeutic strategies. Molecular Neurodegeneration 2022 17:1 2022;17:1–26. https://doi.org/10.1186/S13024-022-00574-4.
12. Bekris LM, Yu CE, Bird TD, Tsuang DW. Genetics of Alzheimer disease. J Geriatr Psychiatry Neurol 2010;23:213. https://doi.org/10.1177/0891988710383571.
13. Neuner SM, Goate AM. Genetic architecture of Alzheimer's disease. Neurobiol Dis 2020;143:104976. https://doi.org/10.1016/J.NBD.2020.104976.
14. Tanzi RE, Bertram L. New frontiers in Alzheimer's disease genetics. Neuron 2001;32: 181–4. https://doi.org/10.1016/S0896-6273(01)00476-7.
15. Selkoe DJ. Alzheimer's disease: Genes, proteins, and therapy. Physiol Rev 2001;81:741–66. https://doi.org/10.1152/PHYSREV.2001.81.2.741.
16. Zhang Y, Zhao Y, Ao X, Yu W, Zhang L, Wang Y et al. The role of non-coding RNAs in Alzheimer's disease: From regulated mechanism to therapeutic targets and diagnostic biomarkers. Front Aging Neurosci 2021;13:654978. https://doi.org/10.3389/FNAGI.2021.654978/BIBTEX
17. Canoy RJ, Sy JC, Deguit CD, Castro CB, Dimaapi LJ, Panlaqui BG et al. Non-coding RNAs involved in the molecular pathology of Alzheimer's disease: A systematic review. Front Neurosci 2024;18:1421675. https://doi.org/10.3389/FNINS.2024.1421675/BIBTEX
18. Wu X, Xia P, Yang L, Lu C, Lu Z The roles of long non-coding RNAs in Alzheimer's disease diagnosis, treatment, and their involvement in Alzheimer's disease immune responses. Noncoding RNA Res 2024;9:659–66. https://doi.org/10.1016/J.NCRNA.2024.03.008.
19. Li D, Zhang J, Li X, Chen Y, Yu F, Liu Q Insights into lncRNAs in Alzheimer's disease mechanisms. RNA Biol 2021;18:1–11. https://doi.org/10.1080/15476286.2020.1788848.
20. Puranik N, Song M Insights into the role of microRNAs as clinical tools for diagnosis, prognosis, and as therapeutic targets in Alzheimer's disease. International Journal of Molecular Sciences 2024, Vol 25, Page 9936 2024;25:9936. https://doi.org/10.3390/IJMS25189936.
21. Samadian M, Gholipour M, Hajiesmaeili M, Taheri M, Ghafouri-Fard S. The eminent role of microRNAs in the pathogenesis of Alzheimer's disease. Front Aging Neurosci 2021;13:641080. https://doi.org/10.3389/FNAGI.2021.641080.
22. Golde TE disease-modifying therapies for Alzheimer's disease: More questions than answers. Neurotherapeutics 2022;19:209. https://doi.org/10.1007/S13311-022-01201-2.
23. Fiandaca MS, Mapstone ME, Cheema AK, Federoff HJ The critical need for defining preclinical biomarkers in Alzheimer's disease. Alzheimer's & Dementia 2014;10:S196–212. https://doi.org/10.1016/J.JALZ.2014.04.015
24. Yang HD, Kim DH, Lee SB, Young LD History of Alzheimer's disease. Dement Neurocogn Disord 2016;15:115. https://doi.org/10.12779/DND.2016.15.4.115.

25. Knopman DS, Petersen RC, Jack CR A brief history of "Alzheimer disease": Multiple meanings separated by a common name. Neurology 2019;92:1053. https://doi.org/10.1212/WNL.0000000000007583.
26. Hippius H, Neundörfer G The discovery of Alzheimer's disease. Dialogues Clin Neurosci 2003;5:101–8. https://doi.org/10.31887/DCNS.2003.5.1/HHIPPIUS.
27. Holtzman DM, Morris JC, Goate AM. Alzheimer's disease: The challenge of the second century. Sci Transl Med 2011;3:77sr1. https://doi.org/10.1126/SCITRANSLMED.3002369
28. Nehls M Unified theory of Alzheimer's disease (UTAD): Implications for prevention and curative therapy. Journal of Molecular Psychiatry 2016 4:1 2016;4:1–52. https://doi.org/10.1186/S40303-016-0018-8.
29. Glenner GG, Wong CW Alzheimer's disease: Initial report of the purification and characterization of a novel cerebrovascular amyloid protein. Biochem Biophys Res Commun 1984;120:885–90. https://doi.org/10.1016/S0006-291X(84)80190-4.
30. Cline EN, Bicca MA, Viola KL, Klein WL The amyloid-β oligomer hypothesis: Beginning of the third decade. Journal of Alzheimer's Disease 2018;64:S567–610. https://doi.org/10.3233/JAD-179941.
31. Tanzi RE, Bertram L Twenty years of the Alzheimer's disease amyloid hypothesis: A genetic perspective. Cell 2005;120:545–55. https://doi.org/10.1016/J.CELL.2005.02.008.
32. Zhang Y, Chen H, Li R, Sterling K, Song W Amyloid β-based therapy for Alzheimer's disease: Challenges, successes and future. Signal Transduction and Targeted Therapy 2023 8:1 2023;8:1–26. https://doi.org/10.1038/s41392-023-01484-7.
33. Murphy MP, Levine H Alzheimer's disease and the β-amyloid peptide. J Alzheimers Dis 2010;19:311. https://doi.org/10.3233/JAD-2010-1221.
34. Boutajangout A, Sigurdsson EM, Krishnamurthy PK Tau as a therapeutic target for Alzheimer's disease. Curr Alzheimer Res 2011;8:666. https://doi.org/10.2174/156720511796717195.
35. Grundke-Iqbal I, Iqbal K, Tung YC, Quinlan M, Wisniewski HM, Binder LI Abnormal phosphorylation of the microtubule-associated protein tau (tau) in Alzheimer cytoskeletal pathology. Proc Natl Acad Sci U S A 1986;83:4913–7. https://doi.org/10.1073/PNAS.83.13.4913.
36. Kosik KS, Joachim CL, Selkoe DJ Microtubule-associated protein tau (tau) is a major antigenic component of paired helical filaments in Alzheimer disease. Proceedings of the National Academy of Sciences 1986;83:4044–8. https://doi.org/10.1073/PNAS.83.11.4044.
37. Iqbal K, Zaidi T, Wen GY, Grundke-Iqbal I, Merz PA, Shaikh SS et al. Defective brain microtubule assembly in Alzheimer's disease. Lancet 1986;2:421–6. https://doi.org/10.1016/S0140-6736(86)92134-3.
38. Grundke-Iqbal I, Iqbal K, Quinlan M, Tung YC, Zaidi MS, Wisniewski HM Microtubule-associated protein tau. A component of Alzheimer paired helical filaments. Journal of Biological Chemistry 1986;261:6084–9. https://doi.org/10.1016/S0021-9258(17)38495-8.
39. Chartier-hariln MC, Parfitt M, Legrain S, Pérez-tur J, Brousseau T, Evans A et al. Apolipoprotein e, ε4 allele as a major risk factor for sporadic early and late-onset forms of Alzheimer's disease: Analysis of the 19q13.2 chromosomal region. Hum Mol Genet 1994;3:569–74. https://doi.org/10.1093/HMG/3.4.569.
40. Corder EH, Saunders AM, Gaskell PC, Pericak-Vance MA, Strittmatter WJ, Roses AD et al. Gene Dose of apolipoprotein e type 4 allele and the risk of Alzheimer's disease in late onset families. Science (1979) 1993;261:921–3. https://doi.org/10.1126/SCIENCE.8346443.
41. Saunders AM, Strittmatter WJ, Schmechel D, St. George-Hyslop PH, Pericak-Vance MA, Joo SH et al. Association of apolipoprotein e allele ϵ4 with late-onset familial and sporadic Alzheimer's disease. Neurology 1993;43:1467–72. https://doi.org/10.1212/WNL.43.8.1467.

42. McKay NS, Gordon BA, Hornbeck RC, Dincer A, Flores S, Keefe SJ et al. Positron emission tomography and magnetic resonance imaging methods and datasets within the dominantly inherited Alzheimer network (DIAN). Nature Neuroscience 2023 26:8 2023;26:1449–60. https://doi.org/10.1038/s41593-023-01359-8.
43. Márquez F, Yassa MA Neuroimaging biomarkers for Alzheimer's disease. Molecular Neurodegeneration 2019 14:1 2019;14:1–14. https://doi.org/10.1186/S13024-019-0325-5.
44. Dustin D, Hall BM, Annapragada A, Pautler RG Neuroimaging in Alzheimer's disease: Preclinical challenges toward clinical efficacy. Translational Research 2016;175:37–53. https://doi.org/10.1016/J.TRSL.2016.03.005.
45. Del Sole A, Malaspina S, Magenta BA. Magnetic resonance imaging and positron emission tomography in the diagnosis of neurodegenerative dementias. Funct Neurol 2017;31:205. https://doi.org/10.11138/FNEUR/2016.31.4.205.
46. Hardy JA, Higgins GA Alzheimer's disease: The amyloid Cascade hypothesis. Science 1992;256:184–5. https://doi.org/10.1126/SCIENCE.1566067.
47. Sehar U, Rawat P, Reddy AP, Kopel J, Reddy PH Amyloid Beta in aging and Alzheimer's disease. International Journal of Molecular Sciences 2022, Vol 23, Page 12924 2022;23: 12924. https://doi.org/10.3390/IJMS232112924.
48. Zhang X, Fu Z, Meng L, He M, Zhang Z The early events that initiate β-amyloid aggregation in Alzheimer's disease. Front Aging Neurosci 2018;10:359. https://doi.org/10.3389/FNAGI.2018.00359
49. Gulisano W, Maugeri D, Baltrons MA, Fà M, Amato A, Palmeri A et al. Role of amyloid-β and tau proteins in Alzheimer's disease: Confuting the amyloid Cascade. J Alzheimers Dis 2018;64:S611. https://doi.org/10.3233/JAD-179935.
50. Dai M-H, Zheng H, Zeng L-D, Zhang Y, Dai M-H, Zheng H et al. The genes associated with early-onset Alzheimer's disease. Oncotarget 2018;9:15132–43. https://doi.org/10.18632/ONCOTARGET.23738.
51. Cacace R, Sleegers K, Van Broeckhoven C Molecular genetics of early-onset Alzheimer's disease revisited. Alzheimer's & Dementia 2016;12:733–48. https://doi.org/10.1016/J.JALZ.2016.01.012.
52. Lanoiselée HM, Nicolas G, Wallon D, Rovelet-Lecrux A, Lacour M, Rousseau S et al. APP, PSEN1, and PSEN2 mutations in early-onset Alzheimer disease: A genetic screening study of familial and sporadic cases. PLoS Med 2017;14:e1002270. https://doi.org/10.1371/JOURNAL.PMED.1002270.
53. Bertram L, Tanzi RE Thirty years of Alzheimer's disease genetics: The implications of systematic meta-analyses. Nat Rev Neurosci 2008;9:768–78. https://doi.org/10.1038/NRN2494.
54. Nelson PT, Braak H, Markesbery WR Neuropathology and cognitive impairment in Alzheimer disease: A complex but coherent relationship. J Neuropathol Exp Neurol 2009;68:1. https://doi.org/10.1097/NEN.0B013E3181919A48.
55. Silva MVF, Loures CDMG, Alves LCV, De Souza LC, Borges KBG, Carvalho MDG Alzheimer's disease: Risk factors and potentially protective measures. Journal of Biomedical Science2019 26:1 2019;26:1–11. https://doi.org/10.1186/S12929-019-0524-Y.
56. Zheng Q, Wang X Alzheimer's disease: Insights into pathology, molecular mechanisms, and therapy. Protein Cell 2025;16:83–120. https://doi.org/10.1093/PROCEL/PWAE026.
57. Köhler C, Dinekov M, Götz J Granulovacuolar degeneration and unfolded protein response in mouse models of tauopathy and aβ amyloidosis. Neurobiol Dis 2014;71:169–79. https://doi.org/10.1016/J.NBD.2014.07.006.
58. Hondius DC, Koopmans F, Leistner C, Pita-Illobre D, Peferoen-Baert RM, Marbus F et al. The proteome of granulovacuolar degeneration and neurofibrillary tangles in Alzheimer's disease. Acta Neuropathol 2021;141:341–58. https://doi.org/10.1007/S00401-020-02261-4/FIGURES/7.

59. Puladi B, Dinekov M, Arzberger T, Taubert M, Köhler C The relation between tau pathology and granulovacuolar degeneration of neurons. Neurobiol Dis 2021;147:105138. https://doi.org/10.1016/J.NBD.2020.105138.
60. Villemagne VL, Burnham S, Bourgeat P, Brown B, Ellis KA, Salvado O et al. Amyloid β deposition, neurodegeneration, and cognitive decline in sporadic Alzheimer's disease: A prospective cohort study. Lancet Neurol 2013;12:357–67. https://doi.org/10.1016/S1474-4422(13)70044-9.
61. Brion JP, Anderton BH, Authelet M, Dayanandan R, Leroy K, Lovestone S et al. Neurofibrillary tangles and tau phosphorylation. Biochem Soc Symp 2001;67:81–8. https://doi.org/10.1042/BSS0670081/77612
62. Alonso ADC, Zaidi T, Novak M, Grundke-Iqbal I, Iqbal K Hyperphosphorylation induces self-assembly of tau into tangles of paired helical filaments/straight filaments. Proc Natl Acad Sci U S A 2001;98:6923–8. https://doi.org/10.1073/PNAS.121119298.
63. Igarashi KM Entorhinal cortex dysfunction in Alzheimer's disease. Trends Neurosci 2022;46:124. https://doi.org/10.1016/J.TINS.2022.11.006.
64. Pritchard SM, Dolan PJ, Vitkus A, Johnson GVW The toxicity of tau in Alzheimer disease: Turnover, targets and potential therapeutics. J Cell Mol Med 2011;15:1621–35. https://doi.org/10.1111/J.1582-4934.2011.01273.X.
65. Kopeikina KJ, Hyman BJ, Spires-Jones TL Soluble forms of tau are toxic in Alzheimer's disease. Transl Neurosci 2012;3:223. https://doi.org/10.2478/S13380-012-0032-Y.
66. Chen GF, Xu TH, Yan Y, Zhou YR, Jiang Y, Melcher K et al. Amyloid beta: Structure, biology and Structure-based therapeutic development. Acta Pharmacologica Sinica 2017 38:9 2017;38:1205–35. d.
67. Cole SL, Vassar R The Alzheimer's disease β-secretase enzyme, BACE1. Mol Neurodegener 2007;2:22. https://doi.org/10.1186/1750-1326-2-22.
68. Sondag CM, Dhawan G, Combs CK Beta amyloid oligomers and fibrils stimulate differential activation of primary microglia. J Neuroinflammation 2009;6:1–13. https://doi.org/10.1186/1742-2094-6-1/FIGURES/4
69. Mitsubori M, Takeda K, Nagashima S, Ishido S, Matsuoka M, Inatome R et al. Identification of highest neurotoxic amyloid-β plaque type showing reduced contact with astrocytes. Biochem Biophys Res Commun 2021;549:67–74. https://doi.org/10.1016/J.BBRC.2021.02.081.
70. Hampel H, Hardy J, Blennow K, Chen C, Perry G, Kim SH et al. The amyloid-β pathway in Alzheimer's disease. Molecular Psychiatry 2021 26:10 2021;26:5481–503. https://doi.org/10.1038/s41380-021-01249-0.
71. Miao J, Ma H, Yang Y, Liao Y, Lin C, Zheng J et al. Microglia in Alzheimer's disease: Pathogenesis, mechanisms, and therapeutic potentials. Front Aging Neurosci 2023;15:1201982. https://doi.org/10.3389/FNAGI.2023.1201982/BIBTEX
72. Andronie-Cioara FL, Ardelean AI, Nistor-Cseppento CD, Jurcau A, Jurcau MC, Pascalau N et al. Molecular mechanisms of neuroinflammation in aging and Alzheimer's disease progression. International Journal of Molecular Sciences 2023, Vol 24, Page 1869 2023;24:1869. https://doi.org/10.3390/IJMS24031869.
73. Tsering W, Prokop S Neuritic plaques — Gateways to understanding Alzheimer's disease. Mol Neurobiol 2023;61:2808. https://doi.org/10.1007/S12035-023-03736-7.
74. Hansra GK, Popov G, Banaczek PO, Vogiatzis M, Jegathees T, Goldbury CS et al. The neuritic plaque in Alzheimer's disease: Perivascular degeneration of neuronal processes. Neurobiol Aging 2019;82:88–101. https://doi.org/10.1016/J.NEUROBIOLAGING.2019.06.009.
75. Jang J, Yeo S, Baek S, Jung HJ, Lee MS, Choi SH et al. Abnormal accumulation of extracellular vesicles in hippocampal dystrophic axons and regulation by the primary cilia in Alzheimer's disease. Acta Neuropathol Commun 2023;11:1–30. https://doi.org/10.1186/S40478-023-01637-3/FIGURES/6

76. Funk KE, Mrak RE, Kuret J Granulovacuolar degeneration bodies of Alzheimer's disease resemble late-stage autophagic organelles. Neuropathol Appl Neurobiol 2011;37:295. https://doi.org/10.1111/J.1365-2990.2010.01135.X.
77. Wiersma VI, Hoozemans JJM, Scheper W Untangling the origin and function of granulovacuolar degeneration bodies in neurodegenerative proteinopathies. Acta Neuropathologica Communications2020 8:1 2020;8:1–21. https://doi.org/10.1186/S40478-020-00996-5.
78. Funk KE, Mrak RE, Kuret J Granulovacuolar degeneration (GVD) bodies of Alzheimer's disease (AD) resemble late-stage autophagic organelles. Neuropathol Appl Neurobiol 2011;37:295–306. https://doi.org/10.1111/J.1365-2990.2010.01135.X.
79. Sperling RA, Aisen PS, Beckett LA, Bennett DA, Craft S, Fagan AM et al. Toward defining the preclinical stages of Alzheimer's disease: Recommendations from the national institute on aging-Alzheimer's association workgroups on diagnostic guidelines for Alzheimer's disease. Alzheimers Dement 2011;7:280–92. https://doi.org/10.1016/J.JALZ.2011.03.003.
80. De Strooper B, Karran E The cellular phase of Alzheimer's disease. Cell 2016;164:603–15. https://doi.org/10.1016/J.CELL.2015.12.056.
81. O'Brien RJ, Wong PC Amyloid precursor protein processing and Alzheimer's disease. Annu Rev Neurosci 2011;34:185. https://doi.org/10.1146/ANNUREV-NEURO-061010-113613.
82. Selkoe DJ, Hardy J The amyloid hypothesis of Alzheimer's disease at 25 years. EMBO Mol Med 2016;8:595–608. https://doi.org/10.15252/EMMM.201606210.
83. Olufunmilayo EO, Gerke-Duncan MB, Holsinger RMD Oxidative stress and antioxidants in neurodegenerative disorders. Antioxidants2023, Vol 12, Page 517 2023;12:517. https://doi.org/10.3390/ANTIOX12020517.
84. Medeiros R, Baglietto-Vargas D, Laferla FM The role of tau in Alzheimer's disease and related disorders. CNS Neurosci Ther 2010;17:514. https://doi.org/10.1111/J.1755-5949.2010.00177.X.
85. Li B, Chohan MO, Grundke-Iqbal I, Iqbal K Disruption of microtubule network by Alzheimer abnormally hyperphosphorylated tau. Acta Neuropathol 2007;113:501–11. https://doi.org/10.1007/S00401-007-0207-8.
86. Davidson R, Krider RI, Borsellino P, Noorda K, Alhwayek G, Vida TA Untangling tau: Molecular insights into neuroinflammation, pathophysiology, and emerging immunotherapies. Curr Issues Mol Biol 2023;45:8816. https://doi.org/10.3390/CIMB45110553.
87. Heneka MT, Carson MJ, Khoury JE, Landreth GE, Brosseron F, Feinstein DL et al. Neuroinflammation in Alzheimer's disease. Lancet Neurol 2015;14:388–405. https://doi.org/10.1016/S1474-4422(15)70016-5.
88. Schwab S, Afyouni S, Chen Y, Han Z, Guo Q, Dierks T et al. Functional connectivity alterations of the temporal lobe and hippocampus in semantic dementia and Alzheimer's disease. Journal of Alzheimer's Disease 2020;76:1461. https://doi.org/10.3233/JAD-191113.
89. Jobson DD, Hase Y, Clarkson AN, Kalaria RN The role of the medial prefrontal cortex in cognition, ageing and dementia. Brain Commun 2021;3:fcab125. https://doi.org/10.1093/BRAINCOMMS/FCAB125
90. Shukla A, Tiwari R, Tiwari S Analyzing subcortical structures in Alzheimer's disease using ensemble learning. Biomed Signal Process Control 2024;87:105407. https://doi.org/10.1016/J.BSPC.2023.105407.
91. Rao YL, Ganaraja B, Murlimanju BV, Joy T, Krishnamurthy A, Agrawal A Hippocampus and its involvement in Alzheimer's disease: A review. 3 Biotech 2022;12:1–10. https://doi.org/10.1007/S13205-022-03123-4/FIGURES/2
92. Stouffer KM, Grande X, Düzel E, Johansson M, Creese B, Witter MP et al. Amidst an amygdala renaissance in Alzheimer's disease. Brain 2023;147:816. https://doi.org/10.1093/BRAIN/AWAD411.

93. Hampel H, Mesulam MM, Cuello AC, Farlow MR, Giacobini E, Grossberg GT et al. The cholinergic system in the pathophysiology and treatment of Alzheimer's disease. Brain 2018;141:1917. https://doi.org/10.1093/BRAIN/AWY132.
94. Reitz C, Mayeux R Alzheimer disease: Epidemiology, diagnostic criteria, risk factors and biomarkers. Biochem Pharmacol 2014;88:640–51. https://doi.org/10.1016/J.BCP.2013.12.024.
95. Valdez-Gaxiola CA, Rosales-Leycegui F, Gaxiola-Rubio A, Moreno-Ortiz JM, Figuera LE Early- and late-onset Alzheimer's disease: Two sides of the Same coin? Diseases 2024;12:110. https://doi.org/10.3390/DISEASES12060110.
96. Xiao X, Liu H, Liu X, Zhang W, Zhang S, Jiao B APP, PSEN1, and PSEN2 variants in Alzheimer's disease: Systematic re-evaluation according to ACMG guidelines. Front Aging Neurosci 2021;13:695808. https://doi.org/10.3389/FNAGI.2021.695808/FULL
97. Yamazaki Y, Painter MM, Bu G, Kanekiyo T Apolipoprotein e as a therapeutic target in Alzheimer's disease: A review of basic research and clinical evidence. CNS Drugs 2016;30:773. https://doi.org/10.1007/S40263-016-0361-4.
98. Tcw J, Goate AM Genetics of β-amyloid precursor protein in Alzheimer's disease. Cold Spring Harb Perspect Med 2017;7:a024539. https://doi.org/10.1101/CSHPERSPECT.A024539.
99. Li W, Li R, Yan S, Zhao Z, Shan Y, Qi Z et al. Effect of APOE ε4 genotype on amyloid-β, glucose metabolism, and gray matter volume in cognitively normal individuals and amnestic mild cognitive impairment. Eur J Neurol 2023;30:587–96. https://doi.org/10.1111/ENE.15656.
100. Kivipelto M, Mangialasche F, Ngandu T Lifestyle interventions to prevent cognitive impairment, dementia and Alzheimer disease. Nat Rev Neurol 2018;14:653–66. https://doi.org/10.1038/S41582-018-0070-3.
101. Hu N, Yu JT, Tan L, Wang YL, Sun L, Tan L Nutrition and the risk of Alzheimer's disease. Biomed Res Int 2013;2013:524820. https://doi.org/10.1155/2013/524820.
102. Lin T-W, Tsai S-F, Kuo Y-M Physical exercise enhances neuroplasticity and delays Alzheimer's disease. Brain Plasticity 2018;4:95. https://doi.org/10.3233/BPL-180073.
103. Ren Y, Savadlou A, Park S, Siska P, Epp JR, Sargin D The impact of loneliness and social isolation on the development of cognitive decline and Alzheimer's disease. Front Neuroendocrinol 2023;69:101061. https://doi.org/10.1016/J.YFRNE.2023.101061.
104. Brzecka A, Leszek J, Ashraf GM, Ejma M, Ávila-Rodriguez MF, Yarla NS et al. Sleep disorders associated with Alzheimer's disease: A perspective. Front Neurosci 2018;12:330. https://doi.org/10.3389/FNINS.2018.00330
105. Gonzales PNG, Villaraza SG, Rosa JACD The association between sleep and Alzheimer's disease: A systematic review. Dement Neuropsychol 2024;18:e20230049. https://doi.org/10.1590/1980-5764-DN-2023-0049.
106. Leszek J, Mikhaylenko EV, Belousov DM, Koutsouraki E, Szczechowiak K, Kobusiak-Prokopowicz M et al. The links between cardiovascular diseases and Alzheimer's disease. Curr Neuropharmacol 2021;19:152. https://doi.org/10.2174/1570159X18666200729093724.
107. Dubois B, Feldman HH, Jacova C, DeKosky ST, Barberger-Gateau P, Cummings J et al. Research criteria for the diagnosis of Alzheimer's disease: Revising the NINCDS-ADRDA criteria. Lancet Neurol 2007;6:734–46. https://doi.org/10.1016/S1474-4422(07)70178-3.
108. Chapman RM, Mapstone M, Porsteinsson AP, Gardner MN, McCrary JW, Degrush E et al. Diagnosis of Alzheimer's disease using neuropsychological testing improved by multivariate analyses. J Clin Exp Neuropsychol 2010;32:793. https://doi.org/10.1080/13803390903540315.

109. Mitchell AJ. The mini-mental state examination (MMSE): Update on its diagnostic accuracy and clinical utility for cognitive disorders. Cognitive Screening Instruments: A Practical Approach 2016;37–48. https://doi.org/10.1007/978-3-319-44775-9_3.
110. Arevalo-Rodriguez I, Smailagic N, Roquéi Figuls M, Ciapponi A, Sanchez-Perez E, Giannakou A et al. Mini-mental state examination (MMSE) for the detection of Alzheimer's disease and other dementias in people with mild cognitive impairment (MCI). Cochrane Database of Systematic Reviews 2015;2015. https://doi.org/10.1002/14651858.CD010783.PUB2/MEDIA/CDSR/CD010783/REL0002/CD010783/IMAGE_N/NCD010783-TST-003.PNG
111. Su Y, Dong J, Sun J, Zhang Y, Ma S, Li M et al. Cognitive function assessed by mini-mental state examination and risk of all-cause mortality: A community-based prospective cohort study. BMC Geriatr 2021;21:524. https://doi.org/10.1186/S12877-021-02471-9.
112. Costa AS, Reich A, Fimm B, Ketteler ST, Schulz JB, Reetz K Evidence of the sensitivity of the MoCA alternate forms in monitoring cognitive change in early Alzheimer's disease. Dement Geriatr Cogn Disord 2014;37:95–103. https://doi.org/10.1159/000351864.
113. Tsai CF, Lee WJ, Wang SJ, Shia BC, Nasreddine Z, Fuh JL Psychometrics of the Montreal cognitive assessment (MoCA) and its subscales: Validation of the Taiwanese version of the Moca and an item response theory analysis. Int Psychogeriatr 2012;24:651–8. https://doi.org/10.1017/S1041610211002298.
114. Hoops S, Nazem S, Siderowf AD, Duda JE, Xie SX, Stern MB et al. Validity of the MoCA and MMSE in the detection of MCI and dementia in Parkinson disease. Neurology 2009;73:1738. https://doi.org/10.1212/WNL.0B013E3181C34B47.
115. Pinto TCC, Machado L, Bulgacov TM, Rodrigues-Júnior AL, Costa MLG, Ximenes RCC et al. Is the Montreal cognitive assessment (MoCA) screening superior to the mini-mental state examination (MMSE) in the detection of mild cognitive impairment (MCI) and Alzheimer's disease (AD) in the elderly? Int Psychogeriatr 2019;31:491–504. https://doi.org/10.1017/S1041610218001370.
116. Nelson PT, Alafuzoff I, Bigio EH, Bouras C, Braak H, Cairns NJ et al. Correlation of Alzheimer disease neuropathologic changes with cognitive status: A review of the literature. J Neuropathol Exp Neurol 2012;71:362–81. https://doi.org/10.1097/NEN.0B013E31825018F7.
117. Morris JC, Raji CA, Benzinger TLS The value of neuroimaging in dementia diagnosis. Continuum (Minneap Minn) 2022;28:800. https://doi.org/10.1212/CON.0000000000001133.
118. Aramadaka S, Mannam R, Narayanan RS, Bansal A, Yanamaladoddi VR, Sarvepalli SS et al. Neuroimaging in Alzheimer's disease for early diagnosis: A comprehensive review. Cureus 2023;15:e38544. https://doi.org/10.7759/CUREUS.38544.
119. Kato T, Inui Y, Nakamura A, Ito K Brain fluorodeoxyglucose (FDG) PET in dementia. Ageing Res Rev 2016;30:73–84. https://doi.org/10.1016/J.ARR.2016.02.003.
120. Ishii K PET approaches for diagnosis of dementia. AJNR Am J Neuroradiol 2014;35:2030. https://doi.org/10.3174/AJNR.A3695.
121. Chun KA Beta-amyloid imaging in dementia. Journal of Yeungnam Medical Science 2018;35:1–6. https://doi.org/10.12701/YUJM.2018.35.1.1.
122. Mosconi L, McHugh PF. FDG- and amyloid-PET in Alzheimer's disease: Is the whole greater than the sum of the parts? The Quarterly Journal of Nuclear Medicine and Molecular Imaging 2011;55:250.
123. Mendez MF, Mastri AR, Zander BA, Frey WH A clinicopathological study of CT scans in Alzheimer's disease. J Am Geriatr Soc 1992;40:476–8. https://doi.org/10.1111/J.1532-5415.1992.TB02014.X.

124. Jack CR, Knopman DS, Jagust WJ, Shaw LM, Aisen PS, Weiner MW et al. Hypothetical model of dynamic biomarkers of the Alzheimer's pathological cascade. Lancet Neurol 2010;9:119–28. https://doi.org/10.1016/S1474-4422(09)70299-6.
125. Bloom GS Amyloid-β and tau: The trigger and bullet in Alzheimer disease pathogenesis. JAMA Neurol 2014;71:505–8. https://doi.org/10.1001/JAMANEUROL.2013.5847.
126. Hampel H, Blennow K, Shaw LM, Hoessler YC, Zetterberg H, Trojanowski JQ Total and phosphorylated tau protein as biological markers of Alzheimer's disease. Exp Gerontol 2009;45:30. https://doi.org/10.1016/J.EXGER.2009.10.010.
127. van Harten AC, Wiste HJ, Weigand SD, Mielke MM, Kremers WK, Eichenlaub U et al. Detection of Alzheimer's disease amyloid beta 1-42, p-tau, and t-tau assays. Alzheimer's & Dementia 2021;18:635. https://doi.org/10.1002/ALZ.12406.
128. Delaby C, Hirtz C, Lehmann S Overview of the blood biomarkers in Alzheimer's disease: Promises and challenges. Rev Neurol (Paris) 2023;179:161–72. https://doi.org/10.1016/J.NEUROL.2022.09.003.
129. Leuzy A, Mattsson-Carlgren N, Palmqvist S, Janelidze S, Dage JL, Hansson O Blood-based biomarkers for Alzheimer's disease. EMBO Mol Med 2021;14:e14408. https://doi.org/10.15252/EMMM.202114408.
130. Shin HS, Lee S-K, Kim S, Kim H-J, Chae WS, Park SA The correlation study between plasma aβ proteins and cerebrospinal fluid Alzheimer's disease biomarkers. Dement Neurocogn Disord 2016;15:122–8. https://doi.org/10.12779/DND.2016.15.4.122.
131. Nabizadeh F, Balabandian M, Rostami MR, Kankam SB, Ranjbaran F, Pourhamzeh M Plasma neurofilament light levels correlate with white matter damage prior to Alzheimer's disease: Results from ADNI. Aging Clin Exp Res 2022;34:2363–72. https://doi.org/10.1007/S40520-022-02095-Y/METRICS
132. Alcolea D, Delaby C, Muñoz L, Torres S, Estellés T, Zhu N et al. Use of plasma biomarkers for AT(n) classification of neurodegenerative dementias. J Neurol Neurosurg Psychiatry 2021;92:1206–14. https://doi.org/10.1136/JNNP-2021-326603.

2 Current Therapeutic Targets and Approaches in the Treatment of Alzheimer's Disease

Shiv Kumar Yadav, Puja Panwar Hazari, Binu Bhat, and Mukul Das

2.1 INTRODUCTION

Alzheimer's disease (AD) is considered one of the most common neurodegenerative diseases and remains a clinical concern among the elderly population (Choonara et al., 2009). It is a progressive neurodegenerative disorder characterized by distinctive pathological changes including the abnormal buildup of extracellular amyloid-beta (Aβ) peptide and the aggregation of an abnormal tau protein within neurons. Amyloid-beta and tau proteins are essential diagnostic biomarkers that can be measured in cerebrospinal fluid (CSF) (Scheltens et al., 2016; Lane et al., 2018). An important objective of AD research is to discover precise and reliable biomarkers that enable early detection and timely intervention. In the past decade, substantial progress has been made in developing biomarkers that enable the *in vivo* assessment of AD (Wattmo et al., 2020). Imaging techniques like magnetic resonance imaging (MRI), positron emission tomography (PET), and single-photon emission computed tomography (SPECT) can play a role in diagnosing AD and aid in developing more effective treatments (Coimbra et al., 2006; Mittal et al., 2021). Neuroimaging shows changes in the brain of AD patients, but early computed tomography (CT) scan detection can be difficult. However, advanced techniques such as PET and MRI can detect significant changes in the structure and function of the brain. PET scans often show decreased brain metabolism in specific regions, while MRI can identify chemical changes and early signs of brain atrophy. Functional MRI is useful in understanding brain activity and connections (Zeng et al., 2021). AD is marked by diverse neurodegenerative changes and pathological features in the brain. The important characteristics of AD include memory loss, degeneration of cholinergic neurons, and a progressive decline in cognitive functions leading to dementia. In AD patients, the treatment strategies have primarily focused on alleviating cognitive and behavioral symptoms (Qaseem et al., 2008). According to a recent study, there are 6.9 million older adults in the USA with AD, and around 200,000 people under 65 years of age have symptoms of onset AD (Alzheimer's Association 2024). The

DOI: 10.1201/9781003543381-2

estimated overall cost of healthcare in 2024 was $360 billion, which was $15 billion increase over 2023. Therefore, the Alzheimer's Association projects that healthcare expenses for AD alone in the US will approach $1 trillion by 2050 if progress in prevention, management, and treatment does not occur (Alzheimer's Association 2024).

The primary approaches for the management of AD have focused on improving the symptoms associated with cognitive and behavioral changes (Qaseem et al., 2008). The current therapeutic strategies encompass pharmacological and non-pharmacological interventions designed to slow cognitive decline, enhance memory, improve daily functioning, and minimize behavioral disturbances including anxiety, depression, and aggression. However, these treatments do not stop or reverse the disease progression. Despite extensive research, an effective treatment for AD has yet to be found due to complex neurodegenerative processes, which are not completely understood by current therapies (Parums, 2024).

2.2 DISEASE-MODIFYING TREATMENTS IN AD

Cholinesterase inhibitors are among the most widely used disease-modifying drugs, frequently used as a first line of treatment for people with mild to moderate AD patients. These drugs work by blocking cholinesterase at the synaptic level, which increases cholinergic transmission (Birks, 2006). However, there is no evidence that cholinesterase inhibitors have a neuroprotective effect or delay the progression of AD (Birks, 2006; Parums, 2024). In individuals with mild, moderate, or severe AD-related dementia, treatment with donepezil, galantamine, or rivastigmine at the recommended doses over six months to a year led to modest improvements in cognitive function, daily living activities, and behavioral symptoms (Birks, 2006). The main excitatory neurotransmitter in the brain is glutamate. It activates several postsynaptic receptors, including the N-methyl-D-aspartate (NMDA) receptor, which is particularly associated with memory functions, dementia, and the development of AD (Reisberg et al., 2003). Memantine, an NMDA receptor antagonist, has shown potential benefits in reducing clinical deterioration in patients with moderate-to-severe AD, providing a therapeutic option in a field with limited alternatives (Reisberg et al., 2003). Cholinesterase inhibitors and glutamate regulators approved by the US Food and Drug Administration (FDA) for AD treatment are listed in Table 2.1.

Over the recent years, the drug development for AD has focused on disease-modifying immunotherapies and oral small-molecule drugs. The main targets of these therapies are to eliminate Aβ, prevent the formation of neurofibrillary tangles caused by tau protein, reduce cellular oxidation, and regulate neuronal metabolism in AD patients. Amyloid-beta and tau have emerged as the most promising targets for disease-modifying treatments (Parums, 2021; Cummings et al., 2023). Aducanumab, a human monoclonal antibody for targeting Aβ, was the first disease-modifying therapy for AD to receive accelerated approval from the FDA in June 2021 for the treatment of AD. However, its approval sparked significant debate, as many scientists doubted its effectiveness in slowing cognitive decline (Heidebrink and Paulson, 2024; Kiani and Hodson, 2024). Aducanumab was developed from the lymphocytes of elderly blood donors who exhibited little to no cognitive decline with age (Arndt et al., 2018). Preclinical research showed

TABLE 2.1
FDA-Approved Drugs for Alzheimer's Disease

Drug class	Drugs	Mechanism	Indication	References
Cholinesterase inhibitors	Tacrine	AChE-I, BuChE-I	First drug to receive FDA approval for the treatment of mild-to-moderate AD. It showed limited cognitive benefits without halting disease progression. Its use was discontinued due to significant side effects, mainly hepatotoxicity.	Grutzendler and Morris, 2001; Bautista-Aguilera et al., 2021
	Donepezil	AChE-I	Mild-to-moderate AD/ Moderate-to-severe AD	Birks, 2006; Marucci et al., 2021
	Rivastigmine	AChE-I, BuChE-I	Mild-to-moderate AD oral and transdermal/Moderate-to-severe transdermal	Birks, 2006; Marucci et al., 2021
	Galantamine	AChE-I, BuChE-I	Mild-to-moderate AD	Birks, 2006; Marucci et al., 2021
Glutamate regulator	Memantine	NMDA receptor antagonist	Moderate-to-severe AD	Johnson and Kotermanski, 2006; Lamptey et al., 2022

Note: Acetylcholinesterase inhibitor (AChE-I), Butyrylcholinesterase inhibitor (BuChE-I); *N-methyl-d-aspartate (NMDA) receptor.*

that it selectively binds to aggregated Aβ while exhibiting low affinity for soluble monomers (Sevigny et al., 2016; Arndt et al., 2018). Moreover, aducanumab has also been shown to cross the blood–brain barrier (BBB) in a mouse model of AD, binding to parenchymal Aβ and reducing both soluble and insoluble Aβ levels in a dose-dependent manner (Sevigny et al., 2016). The phase Ib PRIME trial studied aducanumab in 165 AD participants, who received a placebo or aducanumab (1, 3, 6, or 10 mg/kg) for a year. A significant dose- and time-dependent reduction in brain amyloid was reported using PET scans after 1 year. However, this trial reported a dose-dependent side effect such as amyloid-related imaging abnormalities (ARIA). Biogen conducted two phase III trials of aducanumab, EMERGE and ENGAGE, focusing on early symptomatic AD. These trials were initially scheduled to last 18 months. However, in March 2019, Biogen terminated both trials early based on an interim futility analysis that showed aducanumab would be ineffective. After six months, Biogen in Cambridge, Massachusetts announced that their prediction was incorrect and EMERGE high-dose group had achieved its primary endpoint. In both trials, ARIA was the most prevalent adverse event (Heidebrink and Paulson, 2024).

By 2024, aducanumab was discontinued making way for newer anti-amyloid therapies such as lecanemab and donanemab, which have demonstrated greater promise (Eisenstein, 2024; Kiani and Hodson, 2024). Lecanemab has been shown to slow cognitive decline and received full approval from US FDA in July 2023. In a 2022 phase III study, lecanemab reduced cognitive decline by 27% in individuals with early-stage AD. However, ARIA was reported in 21.5% of individuals, and the overall clinical benefit was limited (Van Dyck et al., 2023; Eisenstein, 2024). Another anti-amyloid antibody, donanemab revealed that 36% of participants with early-stage AD showed no disease progression after one year compared to 23% in the placebo group. Despite its promise, ARIA emerged as a significant adverse effect, contributing to three deaths during the trial (Sims et al., 2023; Eisenstein, 2024). The FDA approved donanemab in July 2023, following a delayed decision to allow an independent advisory committee to review the drug, likely reflecting lessons learned from prior controversies (Eisenstein, 2024). A timeline of AD research is shown in Figure 2.1.

2.3 NANOMEDICINE APPROACHES IN THE TREATMENT OF AD

Currently, standard therapeutic approaches have shown limited success in mitigating cognitive decline, both in Phase III clinical trials and in real-world clinical practice (Avgerinos et al., 2021; Roghani et al., 2024). The challenges posed by the BBB, along with the drawbacks of existing therapeutic approaches, have created a significant unmet need for innovative treatment strategies in addressing neurodegenerative disorders (NDs) (Teleanu et al., 2019). Among the many strategies explored, nanotechnology has emerged as a promising and secure means of delivering medications directly to the central nervous system (CNS). Nanotechnology can overcome traditional therapy limitations and improve therapeutic outcomes for NDs by allowing for more targeted and efficient administration (Lamptey et al., 2022).

2.3.1 Nanoparticle-based Drug Delivery

Nanoparticle-based drug delivery offers a promising approach to improving treatments for neurological disorders involving cognitive impairment. These nanoparticles (NPs) effectively overcome difficulties associated with the physicochemical properties of drugs that limit their ability to reach the CNS (Wilar et al., 2024). Nanoparticle-based drug delivery systems (NDDSs) can encapsulate a diverse range of therapeutic agents including natural compounds, biological molecules (proteins, peptides, and nucleic acids), and FDA-approved medicines. These systems are designed to efficiently deliver their payloads to specific target sites and significantly improve the precision of treatment. Furthermore, NDDSs can influence the pharmacokinetic profiles of encapsulated medicines, increasing their stability, bioavailability, and therapeutic efficacy while decreasing systemic toxicity and associated side effects (Ashok et al., 2022; Duan et al., 2023). The progression and development of AD are influenced by numerous critical pathological mechanisms including the accumulation of Aβ plaques, which disrupt neuronal communication and trigger neurotoxicity, and hyperphosphorylation of tau proteins leading to the formation of neurofibrillary tangles that compromise neuronal stability (Fang et al., 2019). Moreover,

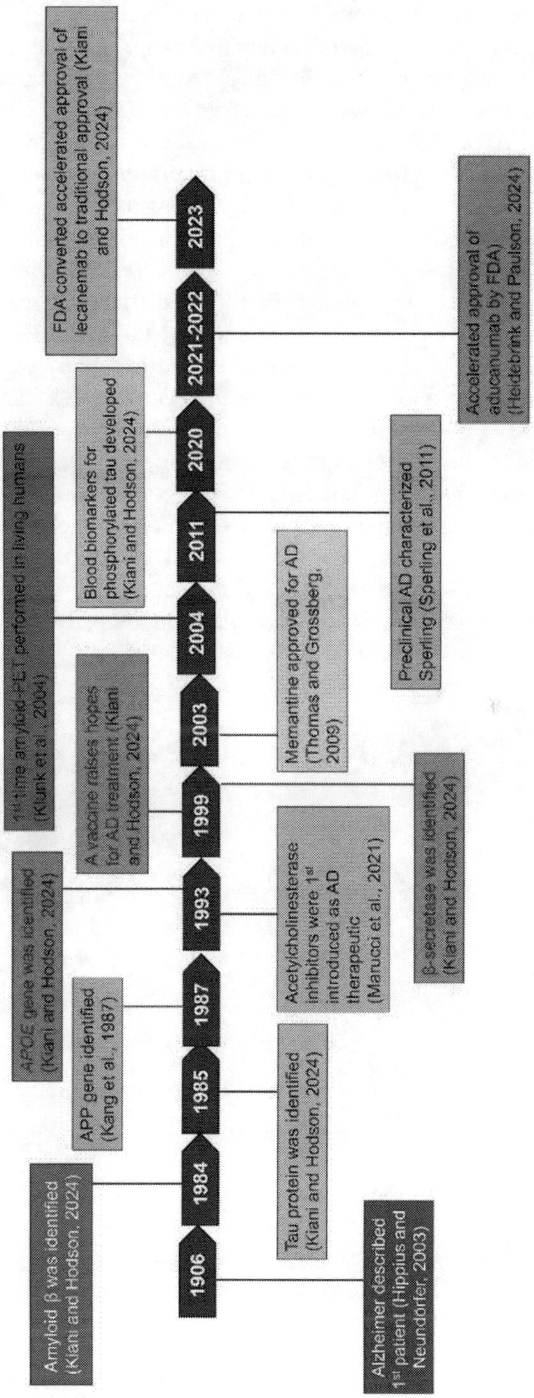

FIGURE 2.1 Timeline of advancements in Alzheimer's disease research.

neuroinflammation, and metabolic dysfunction characterized by impaired glucose metabolism, and energy production in the brain also contribute to AD progression. The important pathological events associated with AD are shown in Figure 2.2. The effective targeting of interconnected pathological pathways is essential for developing therapeutic strategies in treating AD (Butterfield and Halliwell, 2019; Duan et al., 2023). In a sporadic AD model in rats induced by intracerebroventricular injection of streptozotocin, gold NPs were found to prevent impairments in mitochondrial ATP production, reduce neuroinflammation, and alleviate oxidative stress (Muller et al., 2017). Maize tetrapeptide-anchored gold NPs (nanopeptides) exhibit neuroprotective effects in cellular and murine AD models. Nanopeptides inhibited intracellular reactive oxygen species (ROS), promoted PC12 cell differentiation, and improved cognitive and motor functions in an AD mouse model. Moreover, these nanopeptides enhanced acetylcholine levels, cholineacetyltransferase activity, and antioxidant defenses while reducing acetylcholinesterase (Zhang et al., 2021). Yang et al. (2021) demonstrated that PLGA-PEG-encapsulated fucoxanthin NPs effectively crossed the BBB and provided sustained release of fucoxanthin, showing superior efficacy in preventing cognitive deficits in Aβ-induced AD mice compared to free fucoxanthin. In the recent past, a study developed self-fluorescent solo tryptophan nanoparticles (TNPs) as nanotheranostic agents to target the amyloidogenic core. TNPs effectively inhibited and disrupted Aβ42 and another amyloid model dipeptide, phenylalanine-phenylalanine, protected neurons from cytotoxicity, and rescued spatial and learning

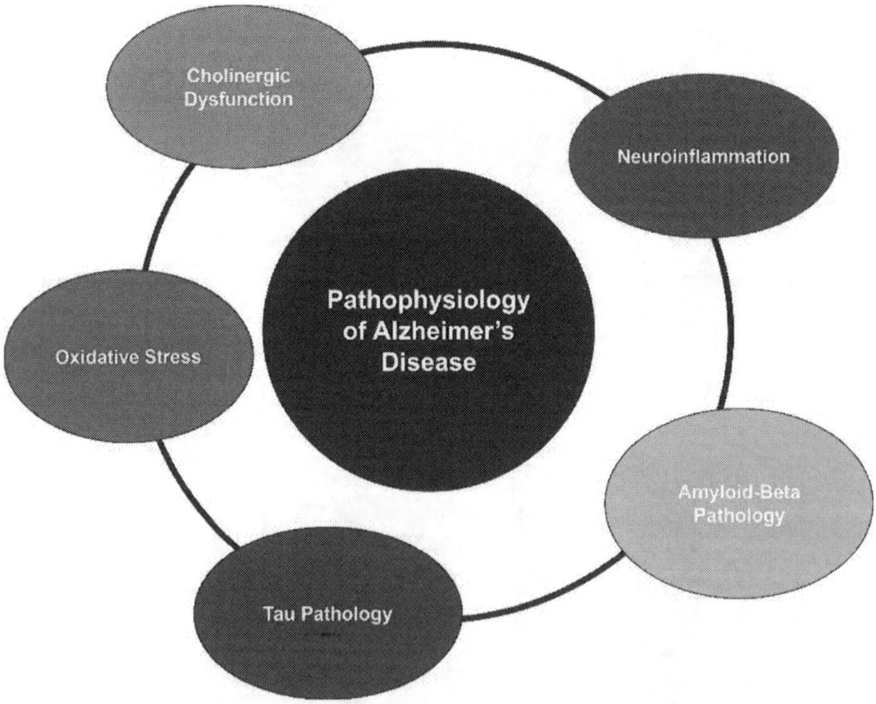

FIGURE 2.2 The important pathological events associated with Alzheimer's disease.

memory in an AD rat model. TNPs, with their BBB permeability and imaging capabilities, represent an appropriate therapeutic and diagnostic method for AD (Sharma et al., 2022).

2.3.2 Targeted Therapies

Targeted immunotherapy using NPs represents an innovative and promising strategy for addressing AD by targeting its two primary pathological features such as Aβ plaques and tau protein tangles. These NPs can be engineered to deliver therapeutic molecules directly to the brain, overcoming the challenges posed by the BBB. NPs can modulate immune responses by encapsulating antibodies, peptides, or small molecules in order to clear Aβ aggregates and inhibit tau protein hyperphosphorylation (Mashal et al., 2022). This approach also allows for specific targeting of affected regions in the brain and reduces unintended interactions with healthy tissues. Recent advances in nanotechnology have empowered the development of multifunctional NPs that combine diagnostic and therapeutic capabilities, facilitating early detection and monitoring of treatment efficacy (La Barbera et al., 2022; Mashal et al., 2022). Liu et al. (2016) reported a multifunctional nanocarrier based on PEGylated dendrigraft poly-L-lysines (DGLs) for AD treatment. The system co-delivers therapeutic genes and peptides to the brain via brain-targeted ligand modification, overcoming the BBB. PEGylated DGLs have been shown to reduce Aβ formation, neurofibrillary tangles, and memory loss, demonstrating its potential as a versatile platform for brain diseases in transgenic AD mice. In another study, a tau-targeted multifunctional nanoinhibitor using polymeric micelles decorated with tau-binding peptides effectively inhibits tau aggregation, blocks seeding in neural cells, and mitigates tau-mediated cytotoxicity. This nanoinhibitor-tau complex is relatively readily degradable compared to mature aggregates, enhancing therapeutic outcomes and offering a promising strategy for advancing anti-tau therapies in AD treatment (Zhu et al., 2021). Zhang et al. (2014) developed a dual-functional nanoparticle drug delivery system loaded with the β-sheet breaker peptide H102. Two peptides, TGN and QSH, were conjugated on the surface of the NPs to facilitate BBB penetration and target Aβ, respectively. This drug delivery system enhances the delivery of H102 peptide to the brain. In preclinical studies, the dual-functional NPs (TQNP/H102) significantly improved spatial memory and reduced neurodegenerative markers in the AD mouse model, suggesting a targeted approach to AD management (Zhang et al., 2014).

2.3.3 Theranostic Nanoparticles

The development of theranostic platforms to study and influence neuroinflammatory and neurodegenerative processes associated with AD is an innovative and promising strategy with immense potential. These platforms integrate diagnostic and therapeutic capabilities, enabling simultaneous disease tracking and treatment delivery. This dual capability is invaluable as it allows precise investigation of cellular responses including inflammation, protein aggregation, and cell death pathways, which are essential in AD pathology (La Barbera et al., 2022). Moreover, these approaches enhance the therapeutic efficacy of drugs by ensuring targeted delivery, minimizing off-target effects, and improving the bioavailability of treatments at the site of pathology. By bridging the gap between diagnostics and therapeutics, such nanovector systems pave the way for more personalized and effective interventions to combat neurodegenerative diseases like AD (La Barbera et al., 2022). The most widely used NPs with a notable role in AD diagnosis and treatment include polymeric, protein-based, gold, polysaccharide-based, selenium, and gadolinium NPs. Moreover, carbon-based nanomaterials such as carbon nanostructures, carbon dots, carbon nanotubes, graphite, graphene, and fullerene have gained significant attention in this field (Shabbir et al., 2020). Polymer-based NPs provide a novel approach to developing theranostic drugs for neurodegenerative disease imaging and probing. For example, the NPs formed by the coassembly of chitosan and hyaluronic acid, cross-linked with glutaraldehyde (CHG NPs), have shown effectiveness as theranostic agents. These NPs have dual functions both for imaging and probing and for inhibiting Aβ fibrillization *in vitro* and *in vivo*. The CHG NPs demonstrate selective binding to soluble Aβ oligomers, emitting enhanced red fluorescence upon interaction. They effectively regulate Aβ aggregation, inhibiting fibril formation at concentrations above 360 μg/mL. In *Caenorhabditis elegans* models, CHG NPs showed efficacy in imaging Aβ plaques and preventing deposition, highlighting their potential as diagnostic and therapeutic agents for AD (Wang et al., 2021).

Pure iron oxides including magnetite (Fe_3O_4) and maghemite (γ-Fe_2O_3), are widely recognized as biodegradable and biocompatible magnetic nanomaterials for a wide range of biomedical applications. These iron oxides are biologically tolerated, non-toxic, and can integrate into natural iron metabolism after administration, making them ideal for use as MRI contrast agents and drug delivery systems. Moreover, superparamagnetic iron oxide nanoparticles (SPIONs) are utilized in various biomedical fields, such as iron supplementation, protein separation, *in vivo* cellular and molecular labeling, and magnetic hyperthermia therapy (Ling and Hyeon, 2013; Soares et al., 2016; Chaparro et al., 2023). A novel magnetic resonance microimaging (μMRI) method detects Aβ plaques in transgenic mice using magnetically labeled Aβ1-40 peptide (with gadolinium or monocrystalline iron oxide nanoparticles) and mannitol to transiently open the BBB. *In vivo* imaging correlated well with immunohistochemistry results, enabling accurate Aβ plaque detection. This technique offers potential for diagnostic MRI applications in AD patients (Wadghiri et al., 2003). Cheng et al. (2015) reported that CUR-conjugated SPIONs (CUR-MNPs) crossed an *in vitro* BBB and successfully visualized amyloid plaques in Tg2576 mouse brains using T2*-weighted MRI, demonstrating their potential for early AD diagnosis.

2.3.4 Nanovaccine

Current immunotherapies such as Aβ vaccines, anti-Aβ monoclonal antibody therapy, and adoptive regulatory T (Treg) cell transfer are limited by their focus on single mechanisms, often resulting in suboptimal therapeutic efficacy. Nanovaccines represent a transformative strategy for tackling AD by combining the principles of nanotechnology and immunotherapy. Nanovaccines use NPs as carriers for antigens, adjuvants, or immunomodulatory agents. These nanoscale systems improve therapeutic drug stability, bioavailability, and targeted delivery, allowing more precise interaction with the immune system. Jung et al. (2023) developed a lipid nanoparticle-based nanovaccine loaded with Aβ peptides and rapamycin that targets multiple pathophysiological mechanisms of AD. It combines the effects of anti-Aβ antibody therapy and adoptive Aβ-specific Treg cell transfer, effectively reducing Aβ plaques, alleviating neuroinflammation, preventing Th1-mediated immune responses, and improving cognitive function in mice (Jung et al., 2023). The nanovaccine, which outperforms Aβ vaccines in efficacy, is cost-effective, easy to produce, and offers a promising new therapeutic approach for AD, effectively addressing the shortcomings of existing immunotherapies. In another study, a novel nanovaccine, lipid nanoparticle loaded with Aβ peptides and rapamycin (LNP-R/Aβ), was tested in 5XFAD AD mice. It generated anti-Aβ antibodies and induced Aβ-specific Treg cells, reducing Aβ plaques, neuroinflammation, and reactive glial cells. Treated mice showed cognitive improvement in the Morris water maze, a test of spatial learning. This approach synergistically combines anti-Aβ antibody and Treg cell therapies, offering promising potential for AD treatment (Lee et al., 2023).

2.4 GENE THERAPY

Since only about 1% of AD cases are familial (FAD) and linked to genetic mutations, the use of genome editing technologies like CRISPR/Cas9 in addressing sporadic Alzheimer's disease (SAD) may initially seem less relevant. However, FAD and SAD share a pathological hallmark such as dysregulated Aβ metabolism. This involves either increased production or decreased clearance of Aβ, which contributes to its accumulation and subsequent plaque formation in the brain, driving neurodegeneration and cognitive decline (Hanafy et al., 2020). CRISPR/Cas9 could be used as a therapeutic strategy to target and correct pathways that cause altered Aβ metabolism. For instance, editing genes involved in the production of amyloid precursor protein (APP) or the activity of β- or γ-secretases could reduce excessive Aβ production. CRISPR could improve the function of genes involved in Aβ clearance, such as those coding for microglial or astrocytic receptors that mediate the uptake and degradation of Aβ (Hanafy et al., 2020). György et al. (2018) reported that the selective disruption of the mutant APPswe (Swedish) allele using CRISPR/Cas9, achieving around 60% reduction in secreted Aβ in patient-derived fibroblasts and successful allele-specific indel formation in primary neurons and hippocampal tissue of APPswe transgenic mice. These findings provide proof-of-concept for using CRISPR/Cas9 as a potential gene therapy tool for AD caused by APPswe and similar mutations. Another study reported that targeting BACE1 using CRISPR-Cas9 nanocomplexes effectively reduced the Aβ-associated pathologies and cognitive deficits in two AD mouse models with minimal off-target effects, highlighting the potential of CRISPR-Cas9 systems for treating neurodegenerative diseases (Park et al., 2019).

Several studies have reported that the CRISPR-Cas9 system holds significant potential for advancing new therapeutic strategies to treat AD (György et al., 2018; Park et al., 2019; Hanafy et al., 2020; Thapar et al., 2024). However, this technology is safe and effective, but efficient delivery remains a significant challenge that must be addressed for its successful translation into practical applications. The

CRISPR-Cas9 system can be delivered through viral or non-viral methods. The choice of an appropriate delivery vehicle depends on the specific CRISPR strategy used and whether the delivery is intended for *in vitro* or *in vivo* applications (Hanafy et al., 2020). Viral vectors are more efficient for CRISPR-Cas9 delivery, but non-viral vectors offer more safety, cost-effectiveness, and flexibility, making them more suitable for AD applications. Park et al. (2019) developed amphiphilic nanocomplexes for CRISPR-Cas9 delivery to post-mitotic neurons *in vivo*. This study suggests that targeting *BACE1* with this system reduced Aβ levels, alleviated cognitive deficits, and mitigated AD phenotypes in two mouse models. The nanocomplexes showed efficient gene editing with minimal off-target effects and no significant toxicity. These results establish proof-of-concept for using CRISPR-Cas9 nanocomplexes as a therapeutic strategy for AD (Park et al., 2019). Several challenges must be addressed to successfully administer CRISPR-Cas9 non-virally for the treatment of AD. The delivery vector needs to be reliable and able to transport the cargo to the desired location efficiently. Once at the target cells, it must enable internalization, avoid lysosomal degradation, and confirm nuclear targeting. These hurdles become even more complex when dealing with CRISPR-Cas9 plasmids (Hanafy et al., 2020).

2.5 CONCLUSION AND FUTURE PERSPECTIVES

AD remains a significant issue for currently approved drugs. The currently available drugs provide symptomatic relief in AD patients but fail to address the fundamental causes of the disease. Several novel therapeutic approaches including disease-modifying drugs, gene therapy, and nanotechnology-based treatment strategies represent significant progress in the treatment and management of AD. Moreover, advances in the field of nanomedicine have facilitated targeted and efficient drug delivery, diagnostic advancements, and theranostic systems. Similarly, genome editing tools like CRISPR-Cas9 have great potential to identify and address the genetic factors that contribute to the pathophysiology of AD. There has been significant progress in the management of AD; however, numerous challenges still exist including the safety and off-target effects of advanced therapies, scalability, cost-effectiveness, effective drug delivery to BBB, and minimizing unwanted side effects. These challenges must be addressed in order to successfully translate scientific innovations into clinical applications. Future perspectives in AD research emphasize the need for an integrative approach that combines multiple treatment modalities such as precision medicine, nanotechnology, and advanced molecular therapies. Moreover, the use of artificial intelligence and big data analytics holds significant potential for enhancing our understanding of AD pathogenesis, identifying novel biomarkers, and developing personalized treatment strategies for AD patients.

ACKNOWLEDGMENT

The authors are thankful to the Director and Management of the Shriram Institute for Industrial Research, Delhi, for providing their support and encouragement in the preparation of this book chapter which has been assigned the number SRI-MS# 20250110-01.

REFERENCES

Alzheimer's Association (2024). Alzheimer's disease facts and figures. *Alzheimers Dement*, 2024; *20*(5). Available from: https://www.alz.org/media/Documents/alzheimers-facts-and-figures.pdf

Arndt, J. W., Qian, F., Smith, B. A., Quan, C., Kilambi, K. P., Bush, M. W., & Weinreb, P. H. (2018). Structural and kinetic basis for the selectivity of aducanumab for aggregated forms of amyloid-β. *Scientific Reports*, *8*(1), 6412. doi: 10.1038/s41598-018-24501-0.

Ashok, A., Andrabi, S. S., Mansoor, S., Kuang, Y., Kwon, B. K., & Labhasetwar, V. (2022). Antioxidant therapy in oxidative stress-induced neurodegenerative diseases: Role of nanoparticle-based drug delivery systems in clinical translation. *Antioxidants*, *11*(2), 408. doi: 10.3390/antiox11020408.

Avgerinos, K. I., Ferrucci, L., & Kapogiannis, D. (2021). Effects of monoclonal antibodies against amyloid-β on clinical and biomarker outcomes and adverse event risks: A systematic review and meta-analysis of phase III RCTs in Alzheimer's disease. *Ageing Research Reviews*, *68*, 101339. doi: 10.1016/j.arr.2021.101339.

Bautista-Aguilera, ÓM., Ismaili, L., Iriepa, I., Diez-Iriepa, D., Chabchoub, F., Marco-Contelles, J., & Pérez, M. (2021). Tacrines as therapeutic agents for Alzheimer's disease. V. Recent developments. *The Chemical Record*, *21*(1), 162–174. doi: 10.1002/tcr.202000107.

Birks, J. (2006). Cholinesterase inhibitors for Alzheimer's disease. *Cochrane Database Syst Rev*, *2006*, CD005593. doi: 10.1002/14651858.CD005593.

Butterfield, D. A., & Halliwell, B. (2019). Oxidative stress, dysfunctional glucose metabolism and Alzheimer disease. *Nature Reviews Neuroscience*, *20*(3), 148–160. doi: 10.1038/s41583-019-0132-6.

Chaparro, C. I., Simões, B. T., Borges, J. P., Castanho, M. A., Soares, P. I., & Neves, V. (2023). A promising approach: Magnetic nanosystems for Alzheimer's disease theranostics. *Pharmaceutics*, *15*(9), 2316. doi: 10.3390/pharmaceutics15092316.

Cheng, K. K., Chan, P. S., Fan, S., Kwan, S. M., Yeung, K. L., Wáng, Y. X. J., & Baum, L. (2015). Curcumin-conjugated magnetic nanoparticles for detecting amyloid plaques in Alzheimer's disease mice using magnetic resonance imaging (MRI). *Biomaterials*, *44*, 155–172. doi: 10.1016/j.biomaterials.2014.12.005.

Choonara, Y. E., Pillay, V., Du Toit, L. C., Modi, G., Naidoo, D., Ndesendo, V. M., & Sibambo, S. R. (2009). Trends in the molecular pathogenesis and clinical therapeutics of common neurodegenerative disorders. *International Journal of Molecular Sciences*, *10*(6), 2510–2557. doi: 10.3390/ijms10062510.

Coimbra, A., Williams, D. S., & Hostetler, E. D. (2006). The role of MRI and PET/SPECT in Alzheimer's disease. *Current Topics in Medicinal Chemistry*, *6*(6), 629–647. doi: 10.2174/156802606776743075.

Cummings, J., Zhou, Y., Lee, G., Zhong, K., Fonseca, J., & Cheng, F. (2023). Alzheimer's disease drug development pipeline: 2023. *Alzheimers Dement (NY)*, *9*(2), e12385. doi: 10.1002/trc2.12385.

Duan, L., Li, X., Ji, R., Hao, Z., Kong, M., Wen, X., & Ma, S. (2023). Nanoparticle-based drug delivery systems: An inspiring therapeutic strategy for neurodegenerative diseases. *Polymers*, *15*(9), 2196. https://doi.org/10.3390/polym15092196.

Eisenstein, M. (2024). 2021: Anti-amyloid antibodies take a bumpy road to the clinic. *Nature*. https://www.nature.com/articles/d41586-024-02952-y

Fang, E. F., Hou, Y., Palikaras, K., Adriaanse, B. A., Kerr, J. S., Yang, B., & Bohr, V. A. (2019). Mitophagy inhibits amyloid-β and tau pathology and reverses cognitive deficits in models of Alzheimer's disease. *Nature Neuroscience*, *22*(3), 401–412. doi: 10.1038/s41593-018-0332-9.

Grutzendler, J., & Morris, J. C. (2001). Cholinesterase inhibitors for Alzheimer's disease. *Drugs*, *61*, 41–52. doi: 10.2165/00003495-200161010-00005.

György, B., Lööv, C., Zaborowski, M. P., Takeda, S., Kleinstiver, B. P., Commins, C., & Ingelsson, M. (2018). CRISPR/Cas9 mediated disruption of the Swedish APP allele as a therapeutic approach for early-onset Alzheimer's disease. *Molecular Therapy-Nucleic Acids*, *11*, 429–440. doi: 10.1016/j.omtn.2018.03.007.

Hanafy, A. S., Schoch, S., & Lamprecht, A. (2020). CRISPR/Cas9 delivery potentials in Alzheimer's disease management: A mini review. *Pharmaceutics*, *12*(9), 801. doi: 10.3390/pharmaceutics12090801.

Heidebrink, J. L., & Paulson, H. L. (2024). Lessons learned from approval of aducanumab for Alzheimer's disease. *Annual Review of Medicine*, *75*(1), 99–111. doi: 10.1146/annurev-med-051022-043645.

Hippius, H., & Neundörfer, G. (2003). The discovery of Alzheimer's disease. *Dialogues in Clinical Neuroscience*, *5*(1), 101–108. doi: 10.31887/DCNS.2003.5.1/hhippius.

Johnson, J. W., & Kotermanski, S. E. (2006). Mechanism of action of memantine. *Current Opinion in Pharmacology*, *6*(1), 61–67. doi: 10.1016/j.coph.2005.09.007.

Jung, M., Lee, S., Park, S., Hong, J., Kim, C., Cho, I., & Kim, B. S. (2023). A therapeutic nanovaccine that generates anti-amyloid antibodies and amyloid-specific regulatory t cells for Alzheimer's disease. *Advanced Materials*, *35*(3), 2207719. doi: 10.1002/adma.202207719.

Kang, J., Lemaire, H. G., Unterbeck, A., Salbaum, J. M., Masters, C. L., Grzeschik, K. H., & Müller-Hill, B. (1987). The precursor of Alzheimer's disease amyloid A4 protein resembles a cell-surface receptor. *Nature*, *325*(6106), 733–736. doi: 10.1038/325733a0.

Kiani, L., & Hodson, R. (2024). The history of Alzheimer's disease, 1906–2024. Retrieved from https://www.nature.com/immersive/alzheimers-disease-history/index.html

Klunk, W. E., Engler, H., Nordberg, A., Wang, Y., Blomqvist, G., Holt, D. P., & Långström, B. (2004). Imaging brain amyloid in Alzheimer's disease with Pittsburgh compound-b. *Annals of Neurology: Official Journal of the American Neurological Association and the Child Neurology Society*, *55*(3), 306–319. doi: 10.1002/ana.20009.

La Barbera, L., Mauri, E., D'Amelio, M., & Gori, M. (2022). Functionalization strategies of polymeric nanoparticles for drug delivery in Alzheimer's disease: Current trends and future perspectives. *Frontiers in Neuroscience*, *16*, 939855. doi: 10.3389/fnins.2022.939855.

Lamptey, R. N., Chaulagain, B., Trivedi, R., Gothwal, A., Layek, B., & Singh, J. (2022). A review of the common neurodegenerative disorders: Current therapeutic approaches and the potential role of nanotherapeutics. *International Journal of Molecular Sciences*, *23*(3), 1851. doi: 10.3390/ijms23031851.

Lane, C. A., Hardy, J., & Schott, J. M. (2018). Alzheimer's disease. *European Journal of Neurology*, *25*(1), 59–70. doi: 10.1111/ene.13439.

Lee, S., Jung, M., Kim, B. S., & Kim, Y. (2023). The development of therapeutic nanovaccine that elicits anti-Aβ antibodies and aβ-specific regulatory t cells for the treatment of Alzheimer's disease. *Alzheimer's & Dementia*, *19*, e076411. doi: 10.1002/alz.076411.

Ling, D., & Hyeon, T. (2013). Chemical design of biocompatible iron oxide nanoparticles for medical applications. *Small*, *9*(9-10), 1450–1466. doi: 10.1002/smll.201202111.

Liu, Y., An, S., Li, J., Kuang, Y., He, X., Guo, Y., & Jiang, C. (2016). Brain-targeted co-delivery of therapeutic gene and peptide by multifunctional nanoparticles in Alzheimer's disease mice. *Biomaterials*, *80*, 33–45. doi: 10.1016/j.biomaterials.2015.11.060.

Marucci, G., Buccioni, M., Dal Ben, D., Lambertucci, C., Volpini, R., & Amenta, F. (2021). Efficacy of acetylcholinesterase inhibitors in Alzheimer's disease. *Neuropharmacology*, *190*, 108352. doi: 10.1016/j.neuropharm.2020.108352.

Mashal, Y., Abdelhady, H., & Iyer, A. K. (2022). Comparison of tau and amyloid-β targeted immunotherapy nanoparticles for Alzheimer's disease. *Biomolecules*, *12*(7), 1001. doi: 10.3390/biom12071001.

Mittal, P., Singh, N., Chaturvedi, S., Jyoti, A., Mishra, A. K., & Hazari, P. P. (2021). Comprehensive review on design perspective of PET ligands based on β-amyloids, tau and neuroinflammation for diagnostic intervention of Alzheimer's disease. *Clinical and Translational Imaging*, *9*, 153–175.

Muller, A. P., Ferreira, G. K., Pires, A. J., de Bem Silveira, G., de Souza, D. L., de Abreu Brandolfi, J., & Silveira, P. C. L. (2017). Gold nanoparticles prevent cognitive deficits, oxidative stress and inflammation in a rat model of sporadic dementia of Alzheimer's type. *Materials Science and Engineering: C*, *77*, 476–483. doi: 10.1016/j.msec.2017.03.283.

Park, H., Oh, J., Shim, G., Cho, B., Chang, Y., Kim, S., & Kim, J. (2019). In vivo neuronal gene editing via CRISPR–Cas9 amphiphilic nanocomplexes alleviates deficits in mouse models of Alzheimer's disease. *Nature Neuroscience*, *22*(4), 524–528. doi: 10.1038/s41593-019-0352-0.

Parums, D. V. (2021). Targets for disease-modifying therapies in Alzheimer's disease, including amyloid β and tau protein. *Medical Science Monitor: International Medical Journal of Experimental and Clinical Research*, *27*, e934077–1. doi: 10.12659/MSM.934077.

Parums, D. V. (2024). A review of the current status of disease-modifying therapies and prevention of Alzheimer's disease. *Medical Science Monitor: International Medical Journal of Experimental and Clinical Research*, *30*, e945091–1. doi: 10.12659/MSM.945091.

Qaseem, A., Snow, V., Cross, J. T. Jr, Forciea, M. A., Hopkins, R. Jr, & Shekelle, P. Joint American College of Physicians/American Academy of Family Physicians Panel on Dementia (2008). Current pharmacologic treatment of dementia: A clinical practice guideline from the American college of physicians and the American academy of family physicians. *Annals of Internal Medicine*, *148*(5), 370–378. doi: 10.7326/0003-4819-148-5-200803040-00008.

Reisberg, B., Doody, R., Stöffler, A., Schmitt, F., Ferris, S., & Möbius, H. J. (2003). Memantine in moderate-to-severe Alzheimer's disease. *New England Journal of Medicine*, *348*(14), 1333–1341. doi: 10.1056/NEJMoa013128.

Roghani, A. K., Garcia, R. I., Roghani, A., Reddy, A., Khemka, S., Reddy, R. P., & Sehar, U.. (2024). Treating Alzheimer's disease using nanoparticle-mediated drug delivery strategies/systems. *Ageing Research Reviews*, 102291. doi: 10.1016/j.arr.2024.102291.

Scheltens, P., Blennow, K., Breteler, M. M., De Strooper, B., Frisoni, G. B., Salloway, S., & Van der Flier, W. M. (2016). Alzheimer's disease. *The Lancet*, *388*(10043), 505–517. doi: 10.1016/S0140-6736(15)01124-1.

Sevigny, J., Chiao, P., Bussière, T., Weinreb, P. H., Williams, L., Maier, M., & Sandrock, A. (2016). The antibody aducanumab reduces aβ plaques in Alzheimer's disease. *Nature*, *537*(7618), 50–56.

Shabbir, U., Rubab, M., Tyagi, A., & Oh, D. H. (2020). Curcumin and its derivatives as theranostic agents in Alzheimer's disease: The implication of nanotechnology. *International Journal of Molecular Sciences*, *22*(1), 196.

Sharma, M., Tiwari, V., Chaturvedi, S., Wahajuddin, M., Shukla, S., & Panda, J. J. (2022). Self-fluorescent lone tryptophan nanoparticles as theranostic agents against Alzheimer's disease. *ACS Applied Materials & Interfaces*, *14*(11), 13079–13093.

Sims, J. R., Zimmer, J. A., Evans, C. D., Lu, M., Ardayfio, P., Sparks, J., & Kaul, S. (2023). Donanemab in early symptomatic Alzheimer disease: The TRAILBLAZER-ALZ 2 randomized clinical trial. *Jama*, *330*(6), 512–527.

Soares, P. I., Laia, C. A., Carvalho, A., Pereira, L. C., Coutinho, J. T., Ferreira, I. M., & Borges, J. P. (2016). Iron oxide nanoparticles stabilized with a bilayer of oleic acid for magnetic hyperthermia and MRI applications. *Applied Surface Science*, *383*, 240–247. https://doi.org/10.1016/j.apsusc.2016.04.181

Sperling, R. A., Aisen, P. S., Beckett, L. A., Bennett, D. A., Craft, S., Fagan, A. M., & Phelps, C. H. (2011). Toward defining the preclinical stages of Alzheimer's disease: Recommendations from the national institute on aging-Alzheimer's association workgroups on diagnostic guidelines for Alzheimer's disease. *Alzheimer's & Dementia*, *7*(3), 280–292. doi: 10.1016/j.jalz.2011.03.003.

Teleanu, D. M., Negut, I., Grumezescu, V., Grumezescu, A. M., & Teleanu, R. I. (2019). Nanomaterials for drug delivery to the central nervous system. *Nanomaterials*, *9*(3), 371. doi: 10.3390/nano9030371.

Thapar, N., Eid, M. A. F., Raj, N., Kantas, T., Billing, H. S., & Sadhu, D. (2024). Application of CRISPR/Cas9 in the management of Alzheimer's disease and Parkinson's disease: A review. *Annals of Medicine and Surgery*, *86*(1), 329–335.

Thomas, S. J., & Grossberg, G. T. (2009). Memantine: A review of studies into its safety and efficacy in treating Alzheimer's disease and other dementias. *Clinical Interventions in Aging*, *4*, 367–377. doi: 10.2147/cia.s6666.

Van Dyck, C. H., Swanson, C. J., Aisen, P., Bateman, R. J., Chen, C., Gee, M., & Iwatsubo, T. (2023). Lecanemab in early Alzheimer's disease. *New England Journal of Medicine*, *388*(1), 9–21. doi: 10.1056/NEJMoa2212948.

Wadghiri, Y. Z., Sigurdsson, E. M., Sadowski, M., Elliott, J. I., Li, Y., Scholtzova, H., & Turnbull, D. H. (2003). Detection of Alzheimer's amyloid in transgenic mice using magnetic resonance microimaging. *Magnetic Resonance in Medicine: An Official Journal of the International Society for Magnetic Resonance in Medicine*, *50*(2), 293–302. doi: 10.1002/mrm.10529.

Wang, W., Liu, M., Gao, W., Sun, Y., & Dong, X. (2021). Coassembled chitosan–hyaluronic acid nanoparticles as a theranostic agent targeting Alzheimer's β-amyloid. *ACS Applied Materials & Interfaces*, *13*(47), 55879–55889. doi: 10.1021/acsami.1c17267.

Wattmo, C., Blennow, K., & Hansson, O. (2020). Cerebro-spinal fluid biomarker levels: Phosphorylated tau (T) and total tau (N) as markers for rate of progression in Alzheimer's disease. *BMC Neurology*, *20*, 1–12. doi: 10.1186/s12883-019-1591-0.

Wilar, G., Suhandi, C., Wathoni, N., Fukunaga, K., & Kawahata, I. (2024). Nanoparticle-based drug delivery systems enhance treatment of cognitive defects. *International Journal of Nanomedicine*, 11357–11378. doi: 10.2147/IJN.S484838.

Yang, M., Jin, L., Wu, Z., Xie, Y., Zhang, P., Wang, Q., & Cui, W. (2021). PLGA-PEG nanoparticles facilitate in vivo anti-Alzheimer's effects of fucoxanthin, a marine carotenoid derived from edible brown algae. *Journal of Agricultural and Food Chemistry*, *69*(34), 9764–9777. doi: 10.1021/acs.jafc.1c00569.

Zeng, H. M., Han, H. B., Zhang, Q. F., & Bai, H. (2021). Application of modern neuroimaging technology in the diagnosis and study of Alzheimer's disease. *Neural Regeneration Research*, *16*(1), 73–79. doi: 10.4103/1673-5374.286957.

Zhang, C., Zheng, X., Wan, X., Shao, X., Liu, Q., Zhang, Z., & Zhang, Q. (2014). The potential use of H102 peptide-loaded dual-functional nanoparticles in the treatment of Alzheimer's disease. *Journal of Controlled Release*, *192*, 317–324. doi: 10.1016/j.jconrel.2014.07.050.

Zhang, J., Liu, R., Zhang, D., Zhang, Z., Zhu, J., Xu, L., & Guo, Y. (2021). Neuroprotective effects of maize tetrapeptide-anchored gold nanoparticles in Alzheimer's disease. *Colloids and Surfaces B: Biointerfaces*, *200*, 111584. doi: 10.1016/j.colsurfb.2021.111584.

Zhu, L., Xu, L., Wu, X., Deng, F., Ma, R., Liu, Y., & Shi, L. (2021). Tau-targeted multifunctional nanoinhibitor for Alzheimer's disease. *ACS Applied Materials & Interfaces*, *13*(20), 23328–23338. https://doi.org/10.1021/acsami.1c00257.

3 Pharmacological Approaches to Alleviate Neuroinflammation in Alzheimer's Disease

Deena Prakash, Divya Bisht, and Oshin Verma

3.1 INTRODUCTION

There are about 50 million people with Alzheimer's disease (AD) globally. AD is the most common cause of dementia in the aged population and is a neurodegenerative illness (Guo et al., 2022). Although the precise cause of the disease is still unknown, amyloid plaques and neurofibrillary tangles in the brain are signs of the condition (Dubois et al., 2021). The patients' quality of life and the disease's progression may be slowed by current drug treatments for AD; however, they are frequently only minimally effective and do not serve as cures. Recent data indicates that the pathophysiology of AD includes important interactions with the immune system of the brain in addition to neuronal dysfunction. The body's innate immunological responses and the production of inflammatory mediators are triggered by misfolded and aggregated proteins activating pattern recognition receptors (RRRs) on microglia and astrocytes, which further contributes to the severity and progression of the disease (Van Eldik et al., 2016). Numerous risk genes, many of which are involved in controlling glial activity, such as the removal of misfolded proteins and the control of inflammatory responses, have been connected to sporadic AD by genome-wide association studies (GWAS) (Andrade-Guerrero et al., 2023). Furthermore, external influences such as systemic inflammation and obesity can disrupt brain immune functions, potentially accelerating the progression of AD.

The accumulation of amyloid-β (Aβ) and tau pathology are thought to correlate with neuroinflammation, amplifying the processes that lead to neurodegeneration (Zhang et al., 2023). Apart from the pivotal functions of tau and Aβ, a number of other factors are believed to play a part in the pathophysiology of AD such as neuroinflammation, oxidative stress, imbalances in biometals, disruptions in glutamate regulation, insulin resistance, alterations in the gut microbiome, disturbances in cholesterol homeostasis, mitochondrial dysfunction, and impairments in autophagy processes (Tamagno et al., 2021; Fanlo-Ucar et al., 2024; Zhang et al., 2024a). This review explores investigational therapies designed to address neuroinflammation, with many of these treatments currently being evaluated in clinical trials. It

DOI: 10.1201/9781003543381-3

discusses the mechanisms by which these therapies function and their place within the broader pathological context of AD. Addressing these risk factors and targeting immune pathways offers promising prospects for developing therapeutic and preventive strategies for AD. Furthermore, the review highlights both the potential benefits and limitations of therapies targeting inflammation and examines recent patent submissions for novel anti-inflammatory strategies in the treatment of AD.

3.2 NEUROINFLAMMATION IN ALZHEIMER'S DISEASE

Neuroinflammation in AD is initiated by the innate immune response to Aβ aggregates and tau pathology along with chronic activation of glial cells, particularly microglia and astrocytes (Cai et al., 2022). Under normal conditions, microglia do not produce reactive oxygen species (ROS) or pro-inflammatory cytokines. However, pathological conditions or traumatic injury activate microglia, which then release pro-inflammatory chemicals that worsen neuronal dysfunction and death (Simpson and Oliver, 2020). PRRs on microglia, such as triggering receptors expressed on myeloid cells 2 (TREM2) and toll-like receptors (TLRs) recognize these abnormal proteins, activating microglia. ROS, chemokines, and pro-inflammatory cytokines (such as TNF-α, IL-1β, etc.) are released by activated microglia, which exacerbate synaptic dysfunction and neuronal injury (Gao et al., 2023). Various inflammatory cytokines in the brain such as interleukin-1α (IL-1α), IL-1β, IL-6, and tumor necrosis factor-α (TNF-α), along with the elevated level of cyclooxygenase-2 enzymes are reported in the AD (Domingues et al., 2017). According to reported research, AD patients' serum and brain tissue had higher concentrations of pro-inflammatory cytokines, such as interleukin 6 (IL-6) and tumor necrosis factor α (TNF-α), than control subjects (Rani et al., 2022).

3.2.1 Astrocytes in the Neuroinflammation in the AD

Astrocytes are the most abundant glial cells in the brain constituting approximately 20–50% part of the brain, and it plays a critical role in maintaining brain homeostasis in the CNS (Lee et al., 2022). They maintain the blood-brain barrier (BBB), control synaptic transmission, and give neurons structural and metabolic support. However, astrocytes exhibit morphological and functional alterations in pathological circumstances like-, changing into a reactive state known as reactive astrogliosis, which is an early clinical marker of AD (Preman et al., 2021). This reactivity, characterized by hypertrophy and altered gene expression, is a hallmark of neuroinflammation and contributes to disease progression (Price et al., 2021). In AD, astrocytes become reactive in response to various stimuli, including the buildup of plaques called Aβ, tau pathology, and signals from other immune cells such as microglia. Aβ deposits are particularly potent in inducing astrocytic activation (Stanca et al., 2023). TLRs and other PRRs are expressed by astrocytes in response to Aβ. These receptors identify the aggregates and start inflammatory signaling pathways. ROS, cytokines, and other chemokines are released as a result of this activation, which increases neuroinflammation and damages neurons. (Kraft and Harry, 2011).

Numerous pro-inflammatory mediators, such as complement proteins, tumor necrosis factor-α, interleukin-1β, and interleukins are produced by reactive astrocytes.

These molecules contribute to a chronic inflammatory environment that exacerbates neurodegeneration (Lawrence et al., 2023). Moreover, astrocytes can release glutamate and other toxic molecules during activation, leading to neuronal injury and synaptic dysfunction (Satarker et al., 2022). This pro-inflammatory response often works in conjunction with microglial activation, creating a feedback loop that sustains and amplifies inflammation (Gullotta et al., 2023). Under normal conditions, astrocytes play a role in clearing Aβ from the brain via phagocytosis and degradation (Rodríguez-Giraldo et al., 2022). However, in AD, this clearance capacity is impaired. Reactive astrocytes exhibit reduced efficiency in degrading Aβ, leading to its accumulation and the exacerbation of disease pathology. This impaired clearance is linked to alterations in astrocytic lysosomal function and the downregulation of key Aβ-degrading enzymes such as neprilysin (Liu et al., 2016). In addition to their interactions with Aβ, astrocytes are also implicated in tau pathology (González-Reyes et al., 2017). Reactive astrocytes contribute to tau hyperphosphorylation and aggregation through the release of inflammatory mediators. They may also promote the spread of tau pathology by secreting extracellular vesicles containing pathological tau species (Chen and Yu, 2023). Elevated levels of the astrocyte marker glial fibrillary acidic protein (GFAP) are another indicator of astrogliosis. This increase in GFAP expression is observed around amyloid deposits, both within the brain tissue and in the cerebral microvasculature (Kamphuis et al., 2014).

3.2.2 Microglia in the Activation of Neuroinflammation in the AD

The resident immune cells widely distributed throughout the brain are known as Microglia. These cells release substances that promote tissue preservation while also extending their highly mobile activities to identify pathogens and cellular debris. This allows them to specialize in monitoring their specified regions (Colonna and Butovsky, 2017; Prinz et al., 2019). Additionally, microglia play a role in protecting and remodeling synapses, contributing to the proper maintenance and plasticity of neuronal circuits. In a healthy brain, microglia exist in a quiescent or surveillance state, constantly monitoring the environment for cellular damage or pathogens (Andoh and Koyama, 2021). Their highly motile processes allow them to scan brain tissue and vasculature, ensuring the maintenance of brain function (Michell-Robinson et al., 2015). In addition, microglia release factors that support neuronal survival and tissue integrity. Microglia also play a crucial role in clearing Aβ from the brain through phagocytosis. These specialized cells engulf and degrade Aβ aggregates, preventing their accumulation and toxicity (Lee and Landreth, 2010).

Microglia play a pivotal role in neuroinflammation including the accumulation of tau tangles, Aβ plaques, and neuronal damage in AD (Cai et al., 2022). The impairment of phagocytic clearance process of Aβ by excessive inflammatory mediators and altered receptor expression, along with impaired lysosomal activity is thought to be the reason for the exacerbating neuroinflammation and driving further microglial activation (Doens and Fernández, 2014). Beyond Aβ-related inflammation, microglia are also implicated in tau pathology. Activated microglia contribute to tau hyperphosphorylation and its spread across the brain (Wang and Xie, 2022). They may also release factors that promote tau-related neurodegeneration (Gulisano et al., 2018).

Inflammatory pathways are triggered by Aβ aggregates interaction with PRRs on microglia. Upon activation, microglia transform by changing shape, migrating to the affected areas, and becoming pro-inflammatory (Mandrekar-Colucci and Landreth, 2010; Wang et al., 2015). These molecules are part of the immune response microglia use to defend against perceived threats. This inflammatory response becomes dysregulated, contributing to neuronal damage instead of protection. Chronic microglial activation leads to the continuous production of these mediators, fostering a persistent inflammatory environment that accelerates neurodegeneration (Muzio et al., 2021). In addition to cytokines, microglia also generate ROS which are the inducers of oxidative stress and damage key cellular components like lipids, proteins, and DNA. This oxidative damage worsens neuronal function, contributing to synaptic loss and cognitive decline—two hallmark symptoms of AD (Reynolds et al., 2007; Smith et al., 2022; Mohan Kumar et al., 2023). Furthermore, microglia play a role in synaptic loss, a critical feature of cognitive decline in AD. Once activated, activated microglia release pro-inflammatory cytokines, and ROS cause damage in synapses and disrupt neuronal communication and contributing to memory deficits (Woodburn et al., 2021).

3.3 MEDIATORS OF NEUROINFLAMMATION IN THE AD

Neuroinflammation contributes in AD disease progression and neuronal damage. It involves an intricate network of immune responses within the brain, primarily mediated by microglia and astrocytes, which act as the brain's resident immune cells (Adamu et al., 2024). These cells in AD become hyperactivated in reaction to pathogenic elements like tau tangles and Aβ plaques causing to release pro-inflammatory cytokines and initiating oxidative stress (Maccioni et al., 2018). Intracellular pro-inflammatory modulators are crucial players in the brain's immune response, contributing to the progression of neuroinflammation and neuronal damage. These molecules can exacerbate neuronal dysfunction, synaptic loss, and further promote amyloid-beta accumulation (Deng et al., 2023). Understanding the key mediators of neuroinflammation is essential for developing targeted therapies to mitigate their harmful effects and slow AD progression.

3.3.1 Intracellular Pro-Inflammatory Modulators

3.3.1.1 Cytokines

The primary cytokine sources in AD are astrocytes and microglia contributing nearly every aspect of inflammation in the body, including neuroinflammation. Microglia produce more pro-inflammatory cytokines as well as macrophage inflammatory peptide (MIP-1α) and macrophage colony-stimulating factor (M-CSF) when exposed to pre-aggregated Aβ. (Heneka et al., 2015; Miao et al., 2023). It has been shown that the brains of people with mild cognitive impairment (MCI) and AD have higher levels of caspase-1, which is necessary for transforming IL-1β from its inactive pro-form to its mature version (Heneka et al., 2013). Serum, cerebrospinal fluid, and brain tissue from people with AD or other types of dementia have been found to contain higher amounts of IL-1 (Medeiros and LaFerla, 2013). A crucial downstream signaling kinase, p38, is necessary for glial cells to generate inflammatory cytokines including TNF-α and IL-1β (Shaftel et al., 2008; Bachstetter and Van Eldik, 2010).

Moreover, IL-1β stimulates the release of other cytokines, including IL-1β, IL-6, and IL-18, and increases the activity of inducible nitric oxide synthase, which leads to neurotoxicity, by activating other cell types, such as astrocytes and microglia (Akama and Van Eldik, 2000; Tjalkens et al., 2017). Increased IL-1β production results in the activation of the NF-κB signaling pathway in glial cells, further stimulating the MAPK-p38 signaling cascade, which promotes the cleavage of APP by BACE1- a β-secretase, resulting in the production of Aβ (Srinivasan et al., 2004; Solito and Sastre, 2012). Notably, IL-1β is overexpressed in regions of neuroinflammation in the AD brain and induces the MAPK-p38 pathway, further contributing to disease progression (Shaftel et al., 2008).

3.3.1.2 Chemokines

In AD, chemokines are believed to contribute to the localization of inflammatory reactions by guiding microglial migration to areas of neuroinflammation (Savarin-Vuaillat and Ransohoff, 2007). Studies have reported the upregulation of chemokine ligand 2 (CCL2), chemokine receptor 3, and chemokine receptor 5 in reactive microglia, while reactive astrocytes near Aβ plaques have been shown to express chemokine ligand 4 (CCL4) (Ishizuka et al., 1997; Hwang et al., 2016).

3.3.1.3 Caspases

A class of intracellular proteases known as caspases is essential for mediating inflammation and apoptosis (Abdelghany et al., 2024). Signal-dependent auto-activation within multiprotein complexes called "inflammasomes" regulates the enzymatic activity of caspase-1, one of the inflammatory caspases' functions (Martinon and Tschopp, 2007). Inflammasomes facilitate the activation of caspase-1, which cleaves the precursors of IL-1β and IL-18 into their physiologically active cytokine forms and causes further brain neuroinflammation (Kelley et al., 2019; Van Opdenbosch and Lamkanfi, 2019).

3.3.2 Reactive Oxygen Species

ROS play a significant role in the pathophysiology of AD, contributing to both neuronal damage and the progression of neuroinflammation (Manoharan et al., 2016). The buildup of tau tangles and amyloid-beta in AD can exacerbate oxidative stress, resulting in an imbalance between the brain's capacity to eliminate ROS with antioxidants and the generation of ROS (Roy et al., 2023). This increased oxidative stress impairs neuronal function and sets off inflammatory reactions by destroying cellular components such as proteins, lipids, and DNA. Additionally, microglia and astrocytes, the brain's immune cells, generate ROS during their activation in response to neurotoxic stimuli, further exacerbating neuroinflammation (Lull and Block, 2010). This vicious cycle of oxidative damage and inflammation accelerates neurodegeneration, leading to synaptic loss and cognitive decline (Kim et al., 2015). Targeting ROS and enhancing the brain's antioxidant defenses are potential therapeutic strategies being explored to slow the progression of AD and mitigate its damaging effects.

3.3.3 Environmental Influences

3.3.3.1 Obesity and Metabolic Disorders

Elevations in circulating inflammatory markers and C-reactive protein (CRP) are linked to obesity, diabetes, and metabolic syndrome. These factors enhance neuroinflammatory responses and increase the risk of AD. Insulin resistance in diabetes can also impair energy metabolism in neurons, exacerbating neurodegeneration (Maldonado-Ruiz et al., 2017).

3.3.3.2 Diet and Nutrition

Saturated fat and refined sugar diets are associated with elevated systemic inflammation and oxidative stress, contributing to AD risk. Conversely, anti-inflammatory diets rich in polyphenols, antioxidants, and omega-3 fatty acids can lower neuroinflammation and enhance cognitive function. (van Zonneveld et al., 2024).

3.3.3.3 Infections and Microbiome Dysbiosis

Chronic infections, such as periodontal disease or viral infections (e.g., herpes simplex virus), may trigger systemic inflammation that indirectly influences neuroinflammation in AD (Butler and Walker, 2021). Additionally, emerging evidence emphasizes on how the gut-brain axis regulates brain inflammation through the gut bacteria. Dysbiosis in the gut microbiome can lead to increased production of pro-inflammatory molecules that exacerbate neuroinflammatory responses (Suganya and Koo, 2020).

3.3.3.4 Stress and Lifestyle Factors

Psychological stress and sleep disturbances are associated with elevated cortisol levels, which can exacerbate neuroinflammation. Chronic stress also disrupts immune homeostasis, further promoting glial activation and cytokine release in the brain (Knezevic et al., 2023).

3.3.3.5 Environmental Toxins

Exposure to pollutants found in the environment, or heavy metals like lead or mercury, can induce oxidative stress and neuroinflammation, contributing to neuronal damage and increasing AD risk (Chin-Chan et al., 2015; Olloquequi et al., 2024).

3.3.4 Genetic Influences

The onset and course of AD are significantly influenced by genetic predisposition, especially in relation to neuroinflammation. Numerous genetic variations linked to the risk of AD have been found by GWAS, many of which are connected to immunological control and neuroinflammatory pathways (Karch and Goate, 2015; Andrade-Guerrero et al., 2023).

APOE (Apolipoprotein E): The most potent genetic risk factor for sporadic AD is the APOE ε4 allele. Beyond its role in amyloid-beta (Aβ) metabolism, *APOE* is involved in modulating glial responses (Serrano-Pozo et al., 2021).

Carriers of the ε4 allele exhibit heightened neuroinflammatory responses, characterized by excessive microglial activation and increased cytokine production, which accelerate disease progression (Filippini et al., 2009; Parhizkar and Holtzman, 2022).

TREM2 (Triggering Receptor Expressed on Myeloid Cells 2): Microglia express TREM2, which controls their activation and phagocytic potential. Mutations in TREM2 impair the clearance of Aβ and other debris, leading to a pro-inflammatory state that exacerbates neuronal damage (Liu et al., 2020).

CD33: This gene encodes a receptor involved in the suppression of microglial activity. Variants of CD33 that increase its expression are linked to reduced clearance of Aβ and enhanced inflammatory responses, increasing AD risk (Griciuc et al., 2013).

Other Genes: Variants in genes such as CR1 (complement receptor 1), CLU (clusterin), and INPP5D also influence immune regulation, glial function, and neuroinflammatory processes, contributing to AD susceptibility (Cao et al., 2024).

3.4 PHARMACOLOGICAL INTERVENTION TO TREAT NEUROINFLAMMATION

Pharmacological interventions aimed at treating AD neuroinflammation are a promising area. Inflammation is thought to play a major role in the disease's progression. These treatments focus on modulating the brain's immune response, specifically targeting overactive microglia and astrocytes, which become dysfunctional in AD and exacerbate neuronal damage (Al-Ghraiybah et al., 2022). Numerous approaches have been investigated, such as immune-modulating medicines, non-steroidal anti-inflammatory drugs (NSAIDs), and specific inhibitors of pro-inflammatory signaling pathways, including those involving p38 mitogen-activated protein kinase (MAPK) and nuclear factor-kappa B (NF-κB) (Guo et al., 2024; Detka et al., 2024). By targeting the molecules and pathways involved in neuroinflammation, these therapies aim to reduce the pro-inflammatory cytokines-induced inflammation, potentially slowing disease progression and improving cognitive function (Kölliker-Frers et al., 2021). However, challenges remain in identifying effective treatments, as the complexity of AD pathology requires a multifaceted approach to address both neuroinflammation and other key factors such as amyloid-beta accumulation and tau aggregation.

3.4.1 Non-Steroidal Anti-Inflammatory Drugs

NSAIDs are over-the-counter drugs that are used to treat pain, fever, and other types of inflammation. Epidemiological studies have shown that NSAIDs can reduce AD pathology in the aging population. As a result, NSAIDs have become one of the first anti-inflammatory drug types explored for developing new AD treatments (Rivers-Auty et al., 2020; Kaduševičius, 2021). The primary mechanism of action of these medications is believed to be the inhibition of cyclooxygenase (COX) enzyme activity, which lowers the production of prostaglandins, which are important mediators of inflammation (Zarghi and Arfaei, 2011). Various studies have shown that NSAIDs can reduce microglial activation and cytokine production in animal models of AD (Krause and Müller, 2010). Prostaglandins, thromboxanes, and leukotriene B4 are examples of eicosanoid lipid mediators that are produced when arachidonic acid is oxidized by cyclooxygenase enzymes like COX-1 and 2 (Wang et al., 2021). These mediators play key roles in regulating immune and inflammatory responses and are significantly involved in the progression of various neurodegenerative diseases. In a COX-independent mechanism, several NSAIDs, such as ibuprofen and indomethacin, reduce the production of Aβ42 by activating the peroxisome proliferator-activated receptor-γ (PPARγ) and modifying the activity of γ secretases (Sastre et al., 2003). Ongoing research has shown that combining ibuprofen with cromolyn (ALZT-OP1) can target the early stages of AD by improving neuroinflammatory responses and disrupting plaque formation (Lozupone et al., 2022). Currently, Phase III clinical studies for AD are now being conducted on ALZT-OP1. The Alzheimer's Disease Anti-inflammatory Prevention Trial (ADAPT) and other randomized controlled trials have shown conflicting findings, with little benefit for people who already have AD (Meinert et al., 2009; McDade et al., 2021). Timing of intervention may be critical, as NSAIDs appear more effective in preclinical stages.

3.4.1.1 Limitations

The chronic use of anti-inflammatory drugs is linked to serious adverse effects, such as cardiovascular risks and gastrointestinal bleeding, which restricts their applicability for long-term care in elderly patients (Marcum and Hanlon, 2010).

3.4.2 Cytokine and Chemokine Inhibitors

A number of NSAIDs have shown anti-inflammatory properties by preventing immune cells from secreting or expressing pro-inflammatory cytokines. Nuclear factor κB (NF-κB), p38 MAPK, c-Jun NH2-terminal kinase, and other signaling pathways are activated when TNF-α binds to TNF receptor-1, mediating the inflammatory response (Dinarello, 2010; Subedi et al., 2020). Notably, thalidomide has been shown to suppress the release of TNF-α in monocytes (Tramontana et al., 1995). Thalidomide has been shown to have neuroprotective effects in the hippocampus in addition to inhibiting the generation of TNF-α by astrocytes and microglia in an inflammatory AD mice model (Ryu and McLarnon, 2008). Neflamapimod has been demonstrated to decrease p38 signaling, which is another method of preventing the production of cytokines in AD patients. Additionally, in a mouse model of AD, it dramatically decreased the buildup of Aβ (Gee et al., 2020). Additionally, this medication showed beneficial effects on synaptic activity, enhancing the expression of synaptic proteins like postsynaptic density protein and enhancing the performance of older rats in behavioral tests like the Morris water maze. (Colavitta and Barrantes, 2023). Neflamapimod is presently being studied in Phase II clinical trials for AD (Alam et al., 2017). Another medication called Etanercept, is a biopharmaceutical composed of two copies of the human TNF-α receptor's extracellular ligand-binding domain bound to the Fc region of human immunoglobulin G (IgG) (Pontejo et al., 2019). It binds to TNF-α as a decoy receptor to stop its signaling. Unfortunately, etanercept's phase II clinical trials for AD have not revealed any appreciable behavioral or cognitive benefits (Butchart et al., 2015; Torres-Acosta et al., 2020). IL-1β is another key pro-inflammatory cytokine that has been implicated in promoting neurotoxicity and synaptic dysfunction (Lindblad et al., 2023).

3.4.2.1 Limitations

Targeting individual cytokines may not fully address the complex inflammatory milieu in AD. Moreover, systemic inhibition of cytokines carries risks of impairing immune responses to infections.

3.4.3 Granulocyte Macrophage Colony-Stimulating Factor (GM-CSF) Modulator

A cytokine and hematopoietic growth factor called granulocyte-macrophage colony-stimulating factor (GM-CSF) encourages myeloid progenitor cells to differentiate and proliferate into either granulocytes or macrophages (Shi et al., 2006). In an AD animal model, GM-CSF has been demonstrated to have neuroprotective benefits by promoting microglia migration to Aβ plaques and modifying microglia activation state (Kiyota et al., 2018). A synthetic version of GM-CSF called Sargramostim has been used to treat leukemia (Lazarus et al., 2021). Additionally, it reduces the pro-inflammatory cytokines production and enhances microglial phagocytosis of Aβ; it is being explored as a potential treatment for AD (Van Eldik et al., 2016). It was reported that GM-CSF resulted in a 50% decrease in amyloid load, expansion of the synaptic area, and restoration of spatial memory to normal levels (Potter et al., 2021). Sargramostim is presently being studied in Phase II clinical studies for AD (Uddin et al., 2020).

3.4.3.1 Limitations

GM-CSF can cause side effects like flu-like symptoms, myalgias, and fever. High doses can cause a generalized capillary leak syndrome. Rare side effects of GMCSF include autoimmune reactions, cutaneous vasculitis, and accelerated hemolysis (Root and Dale, 1999)

3.4.4 Modulator of Angiotensin Type 1 Receptor

AD treatment may focus on the renin-angiotensin system (RAS), which is vital for heart function. Elderly people with high blood pressure are known to have a higher chance of AD (Noureddine et al., 2020; Santisteban et al., 2023). The RAS's active peptide, angiotensin II, attaches itself to the angiotensin type 1 receptor (AT1R) and the angiotensin type 2 receptor (AT2R) on microglia, neurons, and astrocytes (Jackson et al., 2018). It has various effects in the brain like induction of oxidative stress and neuronal cellular necrosis. Two AT1R antagonists used as hypertension medicines, telmisartan, and candesartan, are presently undergoing Phase II clinical trials for AD (Ababei et al., 2023).

3.4.4.1 Limitations

Inconsistent clinical efficacy, blood pressure-related concerns, and the interference of the RAD have been observed in AD patients with ATR1 therapy. Further research and more targeted drug development are needed to optimize AT1R modulation as a therapeutic approach for AD (Kehoe and Passmore, 2012).

3.4.5 Amyloid Beta Removal Therapy

Microglia performs immune surveillance through a vast array of surface receptors, and these receptors are involved in enhancing microglial phagocytosis of Aβ, which helps increase Aβ clearance and improve AD (Long et al., 2022). Microglia express the purinergic receptor P2Y6, which aids in mediating the inflammatory response and controlling the activation and phagocytosis of microglia (Zhang et al., 2024b). Anti-amyloid drugs are designed to reduce the levels of beta-amyloid in the brain, with the goal of preserving brain cell function for a longer period by clearing plaques (Zhao et al., 2023). These drugs function as a form of immunotherapy, utilizing monoclonal antibodies that target the harmful protein. Donanemab (Kisunla) and lecanemab (Leqembi) are two anti-amyloid drugs. In 2023, lecanemab received accelerated approval from the U.S. Food and Drug Administration (FDA) due to the release of the Phase III Clarity AD trial's final results (Cummings, 2023). These developments have reinforced the hypothesis that Aβ plays a causative role in AD pathogenesis. However, the modest clinical benefits observed with these drugs suggest that additional factors likely contribute to the disease process.

3.4.5.1 Limitations

While amyloid-beta removal therapies represent a promising approach to treating AD, they face several limitations. These include inconsistent efficacy in improving cognitive function, side effects such as brain swelling, challenges in identifying the right patient population, and the high cost of treatment (Li et al., 2024). Moreover, the exact role of amyloid-beta in AD is still not fully understood, and targeting amyloid alone may not be sufficient to halt disease progression. More research is needed to refine these therapies and develop complementary strategies that address the broader neurodegenerative processes in AD.

3.4.6 Anti-RAGE Therapy

Microglia and astrocytes both express RAGE, which has been demonstrated to cause cytotoxic or pro-inflammatory reactions (Fang et al., 2010). People with AD have higher levels of RAGE expression in their hippocampal microglia and astrocytes (Yan et al., 2009). Blocking the interaction between RAGE and Aβ was reported to suppress microglial inflammatory responses and decrease the transcytotic influx of circulating Aβ into the brain in a transgenic AD mice model (Deane et al., 2012). However, in 2018, azeliragon's Phase III clinical studies were unsuccessful and failed to demonstrate efficacy.

3.4.7 Insulin Resistance Therapy

AD and type 2 diabetes both occur as a result of chronic inflammation. The brain's insulin-degrading enzyme's synthesis and activity have been demonstrated to decrease with impaired insulin signaling, which results in inefficient Aβ clearance (Sędzikowska and Szablewski, 2021). Furthermore, high levels of pro-inflammatory cytokinesare strongly associated with insulin resistance (Shoelson et al., 2006). Consequently, antidiabetic drugs have been proposed as possible AD treatments. PPARγ agonists pioglitazone and rosiglitazone are used to treat diabetes, specifically to address the pathophysiology of insulin resistance and hyperglycemia (Pérez and Quintanilla, 2015). Pioglitazone was shown to exhibit anti-inflammatory and neuroprotective properties in a diabetic mice model. The NLR family pyrin domain containing 3 (NLRP3) inflammasome, a crucial microglial sensor that mediates the Aβ-induced release of IL-1β, was similarly attenuated (Wang et al., 2017). However, both the drugs were found failure in phase III trials. NLRP3 Inflammasome inhibitors targeting this pathway, such as MCC950, have shown efficacy in reducing neuroinflammation and protecting neurons in animal models (Md et al., 2021).

3.4.8 Targeting Microglial Receptors

Drugs that modulate microglial activity by targeting receptors such as TREM2 have shown promise in preclinical studies. TREM2 agonists enhance microglial phagocytosis of Aβ while reducing inflammatory cytokine production (Biber et al., 2019).

3.4.9 Other Therapies Including Antibiotics and Immunoglobulin Therapy

Minocycline, a type of tetracycline antibiotic, can penetrate the BBB. It also exhibits neuroprotective and anti-inflammatory properties by reducing the production of IL-6, IL-1β, and TNF by microglia (Kielian et al., 2007). Notably, minocycline decreased neuronal loss, suppressed microglial activation, and enhanced cognitive performance in transgenic mouse models of AD (Choi et al., 2007). Phase II clinical trials are being conducted on the antiviral medication valaciclovir to treat early-stage AD due to its potential to target herpes simplex virus (HSV) infections, which have been linked to the development of AD (Devanand et al., 2020). Research suggests that HSV infections, particularly HSV-1, may contribute to the accumulation of amyloid-beta plaques and neuroinflammation, key factors in AD progression. In the early stages of AD, valaciclovir may help lower these factors by blocking viral replication, which could slow or stop cognitive loss (Iqbal et al., 2020). A mixture of polyclonal IgG antibodies from thousands of healthy human donors makes up intravenous immunoglobulin (Ig). Remarkably, intravenous Ig formulations like Octagam, Flebogamma, and Gammagard have been utilized for many years to treat a variety of autoimmune and infectious diseases (Hooper, 2008).

3.4.10 Combination Therapies

Considering the complexity of AD, combination therapies that simultaneously target amyloid pathology, tau aggregation, and neuroinflammation are being developed. For example, anti-amyloid monoclonal antibodies combined with anti-inflammatory agents may provide synergistic benefits (Cummings et al., 2024).

3.5 CHALLENGES IN TARGETING NEUROINFLAMMATION

Neuroinflammation occurs early in AD pathogenesis, suggesting that treatments must be initiated in preclinical or early symptomatic stages to be effective. The overlapping and redundant nature of inflammatory pathways complicates the identification of specific targets. Systemic inhibition of inflammation risks impairing physiological immune functions. Addressing both genetic and environmental factors provides a comprehensive approach to reducing neuroinflammation and its detrimental effects in AD.

3.6 CONCLUSION

Given the increasing understanding of the role inflammation plays in the development of AD, pharmaceutical strategies that target neuroinflammation have drawn a lot of attention. These therapies aim to modulate the immune response in the brain, focusing on microglial activation, pro-inflammatory cytokines, and related pathways that contribute to neurodegeneration. Several strategies have been explored, including the use of monoclonal antibodies and NSAIDs targeting Aβ, and agents that modulate specific receptors involved in inflammation, such as RAGE and PPAR-γ. Despite promising preclinical results, many of these treatments have shown limited success in clinical trials. NSAIDs, for instance, have had mixed results, with some drugs demonstrating reduced inflammation without significant cognitive improvement. Similarly, targeting amyloid-beta has not consistently translated into meaningful benefits for patients, and safety concerns, such as brain swelling and microhemorrhages, have been noted with some monoclonal antibodies. Other approaches, like targeting microglial receptors (e.g., TREM2) and the RAS, are still under investigation and show potential for selectively modulating neuroinflammation. However, the complexity of AD's pathophysiology, which involves amyloid, tau, metabolic dysfunction, and genetic factors, makes it difficult for anti-inflammatory therapies to fully reverse or halt disease progression. In conclusion, while pharmaceutical approaches targeting neuroinflammation offer hope for AD treatment, challenges remain in achieving sustained efficacy. Future research should focus on refining these therapies, identifying the most suitable patient populations, and combining anti-inflammatory agents with other strategies that address the broader spectrum of AD pathology.

REFERENCES

Ababei, D. C., Bild, V., Macadan, I., Vasincu, A., Rusu, R. N., Blaj, M., Stanciu, G. D., Lefter, R. M., & Bild, W. (2023). Therapeutic Implications of Renin-Angiotensin System Modulators in Alzheimer's Dementia. Pharmaceutics, 15(9), 2290. https://doi.org/10.3390/pharmaceutics15092290

Abdelghany, L., Sillapachaiyaporn, C., & Zhivotovsky, B. (2024). The Concealed Side of Caspases: Beyond a Killer of Cells. Cellular and Molecular LifeSciences: CMLS, 81(1), 474. https://doi.org/10.1007/s00018-024-05495-7

Adamu, A., Li, S., Gao, F., & Xue, G. (2024). The Role of Neuroinflammation in Neurodegenerative Diseases: Current Understanding and Future Therapeutic Targets. Frontiers in Aging Neuroscience, 16, 1347987. https://doi.org/10.3389/fnagi.2024.1347987

Akama, K. T., & Van Eldik, L. J. (2000). Beta-Amyloid Stimulation of Inducible Nitric-Oxide Synthase in AstrocytesIsInterleukin-1beta- and Tumor Necrosis Factor-Alpha (TNF alpha)-Dependent, and Involves a TNF alpha Receptor-Associated Factor- and NF kappaB-Inducing Kinase-Dependent Signaling Mechanism. The Journal of Biological Chemistry, 275(11), 7918–7924. https://doi.org/10.1074/jbc.275.11.7918

Alam, J., Blackburn, K., & Patrick, D. (2017). Neflamapimod: Clinical Phase 2b-Ready Oral Small Molecule Inhibitor of p38α to Reverse Synaptic Dysfunction in Early Alzheimer's Disease. The Journal of Prevention of Alzheimer's Disease, 4(4), 273–278. https://doi.org/10.14283/jpad.2017.41

Al-Ghraiybah, N. F., Wang, J., Alkhalifa, A. E., Roberts, A. B., Raj, R., Yang, E., & Kaddoumi, A. (2022). Glial Cell-Mediated Neuroinflammation in Alzheimer's Disease. International Journal of Molecular Sciences, 23(18), 10572. https://doi.org/10.3390/ijms231810572

Andoh, M., & Koyama, R. (2021). Microglia Regulate Synaptic Development and Plasticity. Developmental Neurobiology, 81(5), 568–590. https://doi.org/10.1002/dneu.22814

Andrade-Guerrero, J., Santiago-Balmaseda, A., Jeronimo-Aguilar, P., Vargas-Rodríguez, I., Cadena-Suárez, A. R., Sánchez-Garibay, C., Pozo-Molina, G., Méndez-Catalá, C. F., Cardenas-Aguayo, M. D., Diaz-Cintra, S., Pacheco-Herrero, M., Luna-Muñoz, J., & Soto-Rojas, L. O. (2023). Alzheimer's Disease: An Updated Overview of Its Genetics. International Journal of Molecular Sciences, 24(4), 3754. https://doi.org/10.3390/ijms24043754

Bachstetter, A. D., & Van Eldik, L. J. (2010). The p38 MAP Kinase Family as Regulators of Proinflammatory Cytokine Production in Degenerative Diseases of the CNS. Aging and Disease, 1(3), 199–211.

Biber, K., Bhattacharya, A., Campbell, B. M., Piro, J. R., Rohe, M., Staal, R. G. W., Talanian, R. V., & Möller, T. (2019). Microglial Drug Targets in AD: Opportunities and Challenges in Drug Discovery and Development. Frontiers in Pharmacology, 10, 840. https://doi.org/10.3389/fphar.2019.00840

Butchart, J., Brook, L., Hopkins, V., Teeling, J., Püntener, U., Culliford, D., Sharples, R., Sharif, S., McFarlane, B., Raybould, R., Thomas, R., Passmore, P., Perry, V. H., & Holmes, C. (2015). Etanercept in Alzheimer Disease: A Randomized, Placebo-Controlled, Double-Blind, Phase 2 Trial. Neurology, 84(21), 2161–2168. https://doi.org/10.1212/WNL.0000000000001617

Butler, L., & Walker, K. A. (2021). The Role of Chronic Infection in Alzheimer's Disease: Instigators, Co-Conspirators, or Bystanders? Current Clinical Microbiology Reports, 8(4), 199–212. https://doi.org/10.1007/s40588-021-00168-6

Cai, Y., Liu, J., Wang, B., Sun, M., & Yang, H. (2022). Microglia in the Neuroinflammatory Pathogenesis of Alzheimer's Disease and Related Therapeutic Targets. Frontiers in Immunology, 13, 856376. https://doi.org/10.3389/fimmu.2022.856376

Cao, C., Fu, G., Xu, R., & Li, N. (2024). Coupling of Alzheimer's Disease Genetic Risk Factors with Viral Susceptibility and Inflammation. Aging and Disease, 15(5), 2028–2050. https://doi.org/10.14336/AD.2023.1017

Chen, Y., & Yu, Y. (2023). Tau and Neuroinflammation in Alzheimer's Disease: Interplay Mechanisms and Clinical Translation. Journal of Neuroinflammation, 20(1), 165. https://doi.org/10.1186/s12974-023-02853-3

Chin-Chan, M., Navarro-Yepes, J., & Quintanilla-Vega, B. (2015). Environmental Pollutants as Risk Factors for Neurodegenerative Disorders: Alzheimer and Parkinson Diseases. Frontiers in Cellular Neuroscience, 9, 124. https://doi.org/10.3389/fncel.2015.00124

Choi, Y., Kim, H. S., Shin, K. Y., Kim, E. M., Kim, M., Kim, H. S., Park, C. H., Jeong, Y. H., Yoo, J., Lee, J. P., Chang, K. A., Kim, S., & Suh, Y. H. (2007). Minocycline Attenuates Neuronal Cell Death and Improves Cognitive Impairment in Alzheimer's Disease Models. Neuropsychopharmacology: Official Publication of the American College of Neuropsychopharmacology, 32(11), 2393–2404. https://doi.org/10.1038/sj.npp.1301377

Colavitta, M. F., & Barrantes, F. J. (2023). Therapeutic Strategies Aimed at Improving Neuroplasticity in Alzheimer Disease. Pharmaceutics, 15(8), 2052. https://doi.org/10.3390/pharmaceutics15082052

Colonna, M., & Butovsky, O. (2017). Microglia Function in the Central Nervous System During Health and Neurodegeneration. Annual Review of Immunology, 35, 441–468. https://doi.org/10.1146/annurev-immunol-051116-052358

Cummings, J. (2023). Anti-Amyloid Monoclonal Antibodies Are Transformative Treatments That Redefine Alzheimer's Disease Therapeutics. Drugs, 83(7), 569–576. https://doi.org/10.1007/s40265-023-01858-9

Cummings, J. L., Osse, A. M. L., Kinney, J. W., Cammann, D., & Chen, J. (2024). Alzheimer's Disease: Combination Therapies and Clinical Trials for Combination Therapy Development. CNS Drugs, 38(8), 613–624. https://doi.org/10.1007/s40263-024-01103-1

Deane, R., Singh, I., Sagare, A. P., Bell, R. D., Ross, N. T., LaRue, B., Love, R., Perry, S., Paquette, N., Deane, R. J., Thiyagarajan, M., Zarcone, T., Fritz, G., Friedman, A. E., Miller, B. L., & Zlokovic, B. V. (2012). A Multimodal RAGE-Specific Inhibitor Reduces Amyloid β-Mediated Brain Disorder in a Mouse Model of Alzheimer Disease. The Journal of Clinical Investigation, 122(4), 1377–1392. https://doi.org/10.1172/JCI58642

Deng, M., Yan, W., Gu, Z., Li, Y., Chen, L., & He, B. (2023). Anti-Neuroinflammatory Potential of Natural Products in the Treatment of Alzheimer's Disease. Molecules (Basel, Switzerland), 28(3), 1486. https://doi.org/10.3390/molecules28031486

Detka, J., Płachtij, N., Strzelec, M., Manik, A., & Sałat, K. (2024). p38α Mitogen-Activated Protein Kinase-An Emerging Drug Target for the Treatment of Alzheimer's Disease. Molecules (Basel, Switzerland), 29(18), 4354. https://doi.org/10.3390/molecules29184354

Devanand, D. P., Andrews, H., Kreisl, W. C., Razlighi, Q., Gershon, A., Stern, Y., Mintz, A., Wisniewski, T., Acosta, E., Pollina, J., Katsikoumbas, M., Bell, K. L., Pelton, G. H., Deliyannides, D., Prasad, K. M., & Huey, E. D. (2020). Antiviral Therapy: Valacyclovir Treatment of Alzheimer's Disease (VALAD) Trial: Protocol for a Randomised, Double-Blind, Placebo-Controlled, Treatment Trial. BMJ Open, 10(2), e032112. https://doi.org/10.1136/bmjopen-2019-032112

Dinarello, C. A. (2010). Anti-Inflammatory Agents: Present and Future. Cell, 140(6), 935–950. https://doi.org/10.1016/j.cell.2010.02.043

Doens, D., & Fernández, P. L. (2014). Microglia Receptors and Their Implications in the Response to Amyloid β for Alzheimer's Disease Pathogenesis. Journal of Neuroinflammation, 11, 48. https://doi.org/10.1186/1742-2094-11-48

Domingues, C., da Cruz E Silva, O. A. B., & Henriques, A. G. (2017). Impact of Cytokines and Chemokines on Alzheimer's Disease Neuropathological Hallmarks. Current Alzheimer Research, 14(8), 870–882. https://doi.org/10.2174/1567205014666170317113606

Dubois, B., Villain, N., Frisoni, G. B., Rabinovici, G. D., Sabbagh, M., Cappa, S., Bejanin, A., Bombois, S., Epelbaum, S., Teichmann, M., Habert, M. O., Nordberg, A., Blennow, K., Galasko, D., Stern, Y., Rowe, C. C., Salloway, S., Schneider, L. S., Cummings, J. L., & Feldman, H. H. (2021). Clinical Diagnosis of Alzheimer's Disease: Recommendations of the International Working Group. The Lancet. Neurology, 20(6), 484–496. https://doi.org/10.1016/S1474-4422(21)00066-1

Fang, F., Lue, L. F., Yan, S., Xu, H., Luddy, J. S., Chen, D., Walker, D. G., Stern, D. M., Yan, S., Schmidt, A. M., Chen, J. X., & Yan, S. S. (2010). RAGE-Dependent Signaling in Microglia Contributes to Neuroinflammation, A beta Accumulation, and Impaired learning/memory in a Mouse Model of Alzheimer's Disease. FASEB Journal: Official Publication of the Federation of American Societies for Experimental Biology, 24(4), 1043–1055. https://doi.org/10.1096/fj.09-139634

Fanlo-Ucar, H., Picón-Pagès, P., Herrera-Fernández, V., ILL-Raga, G., & Muñoz, F. J. (2024). The Dual Role of Amyloid Beta-Peptide in Oxidative Stress and Inflammation: Unveiling Their Connections in Alzheimer's Disease Etiopathology. Antioxidants, 13(10), 1208. https://doi.org/10.3390/antiox13101208

Filippini, N., MacIntosh, B. J., Hough, M. G., Goodwin, G. M., Frisoni, G. B., Smith, S. M., Matthews, P. M., Beckmann, C. F., & Mackay, C. E. (2009). Distinct Patterns of Brain Activity in Young Carriers of the APOE-epsilon4 Allele. Proceedings of the National Academy of Sciences of the United States of America, 106(17), 7209–7214. https://doi.org/10.1073/pnas.0811879106

Gao, C., Jiang, J., Tan, Y., & Chen, S. (2023). Microglia in Neurodegenerative Diseases: Mechanism and Potential Therapeutic Targets. Signal Transduction and Targeted Therapy, 8(1), 359. https://doi.org/10.1038/s41392-023-01588-0

Gee, M. S., Son, S. H., Jeon, S. H., Do, J., Kim, N., Ju, Y. J., Lee, S. J., Chung, E. K., Inn, K. S., Kim, N. J., & Lee, J. K. (2020). A Selective p38α/β MAPK Inhibitor Alleviates Neuropathology and Cognitive Impairment, and Modulates Microglia Function in 5XFAD Mouse. Alzheimer's Research & Therapy, 12(1), 45. https://doi.org/10.1186/s13195-020-00617-2

González-Reyes, R. E., Nava-Mesa, M. O., Vargas-Sánchez, K., Ariza-Salamanca, D., & Mora-Muñoz, L. (2017). Involvement of Astrocytes in Alzheimer's Disease from a Neuroinflammatory and Oxidative Stress Perspective. Frontiers in Molecular Neuroscience, 10, 427. https://doi.org/10.3389/fnmol.2017.00427

Griciuc, A., Serrano-Pozo, A., Parrado, A. R., Lesinski, A. N., Asselin, C. N., Mullin, K., Hooli, B., Choi, S. H., Hyman, B. T., & Tanzi, R. E. (2013). Alzheimer's Disease Risk Gene CD33 Inhibits Microglial Uptake of Amyloid Beta. Neuron, 78(4), 631–643. https://doi.org/10.1016/j.neuron.2013.04.014

Gulisano, W., Maugeri, D., Baltrons, M. A., Fà, M., Amato, A., Palmeri, A., D'Adamio, L., Grassi, C., Devanand, D. P., Honig, L. S., Puzzo, D., & Arancio, O. (2018). Role of Amyloid-β and Tau Proteins in Alzheimer's Disease: Confuting the Amyloid Cascade. Journal of Alzheimer's Disease: JAD, 64(s1), S611–S631. https://doi.org/10.3233/JAD-179935

Gullotta, G. S., Costantino, G., Sortino, M. A., & Spampinato, S. F. (2023). Microglia and the Blood-Brain Barrier: An External Player in Acute and Chronic Neuroinflammatory Conditions. International Journal of Molecular Sciences, 24(11), 9144. https://doi.org/10.3390/ijms24119144

Guo, F., Li, Q., Zhang, X., Liu, Y., Jiang, J., Cheng, S., Yu, S., Zhang, X., Liu, F., Li, Y., Rose, G., & Zhang, H. (2022). Applications of Carbon Dots for the Treatment of Alzheimer's Disease. International Journal of Nanomedicine, 17, 6621–6638. https://doi.org/10.2147/IJN.S388030

Guo, Q., Jin, Y., Chen, X., Ye, X., Shen, X., Lin, M., Zeng, C., Zhou, T., & Zhang, J. (2024). NF-κB in Biology and Targeted Therapy: New Insights and Translational Implications. Signal Transduction and Targeted Therapy, 9(1), 53. https://doi.org/10.1038/s41392-024-01757-9

Heneka, M. T., Carson, M. J., El Khoury, J., Landreth, G. E., Brosseron, F., Feinstein, D. L., Jacobs, A. H., Wyss-Coray, T., Vitorica, J., Ransohoff, R. M., Herrup, K., Frautschy, S. A., Finsen, B., Brown, G. C., Verkhratsky, A., Yamanaka, K., Koistinaho, J., Latz, E., Halle, A., Petzold, G. C., & Kummer, M. P. (2015). Neuroinflammation in Alzheimer's Disease. The Lancet. Neurology, 14(4), 388–405. https://doi.org/10.1016/S1474-4422(15)70016-5

Heneka, M. T., Kummer, M. P., Stutz, A., Delekate, A., Schwartz, S., Vieira-Saecker, A., Griep, A., Axt, D., Remus, A., Tzeng, T. C., Gelpi, E., Halle, A., Korte, M., Latz, E., & Golenbock, D. T. (2013). NLRP3 Is Activated in Alzheimer's Disease and Contributes to Pathology in APP/PS1 Mice. Nature, 493(7434), 674–678. https://doi.org/10.1038/nature11729

Hooper, J. A. (2008). Intravenous Immunoglobulins: Evolution of Commercial IVIG Preparations. Immunology and Allergy Clinics of North America, 28(4), 765–viii. https://doi.org/10.1016/j.iac.2008.06.002

Hwang, C. J., Park, M. H., Hwang, J. Y., Kim, J. H., Yun, N. Y., Oh, S. Y., Song, J. K., Seo, H. O., Kim, Y. B., Hwang, D. Y., Oh, K. W., Han, S. B., & Hong, J. T. (2016). CCR5 Deficiency Accelerates Lipopolysaccharide-Induced Astrogliosis, Amyloid-Beta Deposit and Impaired Memory Function. Oncotarget, 7(11), 11984–11999. https://doi.org/10.18632/oncotarget.7453

Iqbal, U. H., Zeng, E., & Pasinetti, G. M. (2020). The Use of Antimicrobial and Antiviral Drugs in Alzheimer's Disease. International Journal of Molecular Sciences, 21(14), 4920. https://doi.org/10.3390/ijms21144920

Ishizuka, K., Kimura, T., Igata-yi, R., Katsuragi, S., Takamatsu, J., & Miyakawa, T. (1997). Identification of MonocyteChemoattractantProtein-1 in senile Plaques and Reactive Microglia of Alzheimer's Disease. Psychiatry and Clinical Neurosciences, 51(3), 135–138. https://doi.org/10.1111/j.1440-1819.1997.tb02375.x

Jackson, L., Eldahshan, W., Fagan, S. C., & Ergul, A. (2018). Within the Brain: The Renin Angiotensin System. International Journal of Molecular Sciences, 19(3), 876. https://doi.org/10.3390/ijms19030876

Kaduševičius, E. (2021). Novel Applications of NSAIDs: Insight and Future Perspectives in Cardiovascular, Neurodegenerative, Diabetes and Cancer Disease Therapy. International Journal of Molecular Sciences, 22(12), 6637. https://doi.org/10.3390/ijms22126637

Kamphuis, W., Middeldorp, J., Kooijman, L., Sluijs, J. A., Kooi, E. J., Moeton, M., Freriks, M., Mizee, M. R., & Hol, E. M. (2014). Glial Fibrillary Acidic Protein Isoform Expression in Plaque Related Astrogliosis in Alzheimer's Disease. Neurobiology of Aging, 35(3), 492–510. https://doi.org/10.1016/j.neurobiolaging.2013.09.035

Karch, C. M., & Goate, A. M. (2015). Alzheimer's Disease Risk Genes and Mechanisms of Disease Pathogenesis. Biological Psychiatry, 77(1), 43–51. https://doi.org/10.1016/j.biopsych.2014.05.006

Kehoe, P. G., & Passmore, P. A. (2012). The Renin-Angiotensin System and Antihypertensive Drugs in Alzheimer's Disease: Current Standing of the Angiotensin Hypothesis? Journal of Alzheimer's Disease: JAD, 30 Suppl 2, S251–S268. https://doi.org/10.3233/JAD-2012-111376

Kelley, N., Jeltema, D., Duan, Y., & He, Y. (2019). The NLRP3 Inflammasome: An Overview of Mechanisms of Activation and Regulation. International Journal of Molecular Sciences, 20(13), 3328. https://doi.org/10.3390/ijms20133328

Kielian, T., Esen, N., Liu, S., Phulwani, N. K., Syed, M. M., Phillips, N., Nishina, K., Cheung, A. L., Schwartzman, J. D., & Ruhe, J. J. (2007). Minocycline Modulates Neuroinflammation Independently of Its Antimicrobial Activity in *Staphylococcus aureus*-Induced Brain Abscess. The American Journal of Pathology, 171(4), 1199–1214. https://doi.org/10.2353/ajpath.2007.070231

Kim, G. H., Kim, J. E., Rhie, S. J., & Yoon, S. (2015). The Role of Oxidative Stress in Neurodegenerative Diseases. Experimental Neurobiology, 24(4), 325–340. https://doi.org/10.5607/en.2015.24.4.325

Kiyota, T., Machhi, J., Lu, Y., Dyavarshetty, B., Nemati, M., Yokoyama, I., Mosley, R. L., & Gendelman, H. E. (2018). Granulocyte-Macrophage Colony-Stimulating Factor Neuroprotective Activities in Alzheimer's Disease Mice. Journal of Neuroimmunology, 319, 80–92. https://doi.org/10.1016/j.jneuroim.2018.03.009

Knezevic, E., Nenic, K., Milanovic, V., & Knezevic, N. N. (2023). The Role of Cortisol in Chronic Stress, Neurodegenerative Diseases, and Psychological Disorders. Cells, 12(23), 2726. https://doi.org/10.3390/cells12232726

Kölliker-Frers, R., Udovin, L., Otero-Losada, M., Kobiec, T., Herrera, M. I., Palacios, J., Razzitte, G., & Capani, F. (2021). Neuroinflammation: An Integrating Overview of Reactive-Neuroimmune Cell Interactions in Health and Disease. Mediators of Inflammation, 2021, 9999146. https://doi.org/10.1155/2021/9999146

Kraft, A. D., & Harry, G. J. (2011). Features of Microglia and Neuroinflammation Relevant to Environmental Exposure and Neurotoxicity. International Journal of Environmental Research and Public Health, 8(7), 2980–3018. https://doi.org/10.3390/ijerph8072980

Krause, D. L., & Müller, N. (2010). Neuroinflammation, Microglia and Implications for Anti-Inflammatory Treatment in Alzheimer's Disease. International Journal of Alzheimer's Disease, 2010, 732806. https://doi.org/10.4061/2010/732806

Lawrence, J. M., Schardien, K., Wigdahl, B., & Nonnemacher, M. R. (2023). Roles of Neuropathology-Associated Reactive Astrocytes: a Systematic Review. Acta Neuropathologica Communications, 11(1), 42. https://doi.org/10.1186/s40478-023-01526-9

Lazarus, H. M., Ragsdale, C. E., Gale, R. P., & Lyman, G. H. (2021). Sargramostim (Rhu GM-CSF) as Cancer Therapy (Systematic Review) and An Immunomodulator. A Drug Before Its Time? Frontiers in Immunology, 12, 706186. https://doi.org/10.3389/fimmu.2021.706186

Lee, C. Y., & Landreth, G. E. (2010). The Role of Microglia in Amyloid Clearance from the AD Brain. Journal of Neural Transmission (Vienna, Austria: 1996), 117(8), 949–960. https://doi.org/10.1007/s00702-010-0433-4

Lee, H. G., Wheeler, M. A., & Quintana, F. J. (2022). Function and Therapeutic Value of Astrocytes in Neurological Diseases. Nature Reviews. Drug Discovery, 21(5), 339–358. https://doi.org/10.1038/s41573-022-00390-x

Li, J., Haj Ebrahimi, A., & Ali, A. B. (2024). Advances in Therapeutics to Alleviate Cognitive Decline and Neuropsychiatric Symptoms of Alzheimer's Disease. International Journal of Molecular Sciences, 25(10), 5169. https://doi.org/10.3390/ijms25105169

Lindblad, C., Rostami, E., & Helmy, A. (2023). Interleukin-1 Receptor Antagonist as Therapy for Traumatic Brain Injury. Neurotherapeutics: the Journal of the American Society for Experimental Neurotherapeutics, 20(6), 1508–1528. https://doi.org/10.1007/s13311-023-01421-0

Liu, R. X., Huang, C., Bennett, D. A., Li, H., & Wang, R. (2016). The Characteristics of Astrocyte on Aβ Clearance Altered in Alzheimer's Disease Were Reversed by Anti-Inflammatory Agent (+)-2-(1-Hydroxyl-4-Oxocyclohexyl) Ethyl Caffeate. American Journal of Translational Research, 8(10), 4082–4094.

Liu, W., Taso, O., Wang, R., Bayram, S., Graham, A. C., Garcia-Reitboeck, P., Mallach, A., Andrews, W. D., Piers, T. M., Botia, J. A., Pocock, J. M., Cummings, D. M., Hardy, J., Edwards, F. A., & Salih, D. A. (2020). Trem2 Promotes Anti-Inflammatory Responses in Microglia and Is Suppressed Under Pro-Inflammatory Conditions. Human Molecular Genetics, 29(19), 3224–3248. https://doi.org/10.1093/hmg/ddaa209

Long, H. Z., Zhou, Z. W., Cheng, Y., Luo, H. Y., Li, F. J., Xu, S. G., & Gao, L. C. (2022). The Role of Microglia in Alzheimer's Disease from the Perspective of Immune Inflammation and Iron Metabolism. Frontiers in Aging Neuroscience, 14, 888989. https://doi.org/10.3389/fnagi.2022.888989

Lozupone, M., Berardino, G., Mollica, A., Sardone, R., Dibello, V., Zupo, R., Lampignano, L., Castellana, F., Bortone, I., Stallone, R., Daniele, A., Altamura, M., Bellomo, A., Solfrizzi, V., & Panza, F. (2022). ALZT-OP1: an Experimental Combination Regimen for the Treatment of Alzheimer's Disease. Expert Opinion on Investigational Drugs, 31(8), 759–771. https://doi.org/10.1080/13543784.2022.2095261

Lull, M. E., & Block, M. L. (2010). Microglial Activation and Chronic Neurodegeneration. Neurotherapeutics: The Journal of the American Society for Experimental Neuro Therapeutics, 7(4), 354–365. https://doi.org/10.1016/j.nurt.2010.05.014

Maccioni, R. B., González, A., Andrade, V., Cortés, N., Tapia, J. P., & Guzmán-Martínez, L. (2018). Alzheimer's Disease in the Perspective of Neuroimmunology. The Open Neurology Journal, 12, 50–56. https://doi.org/10.2174/1874205X01812010050

Maldonado-Ruiz, R., Montalvo-Martínez, L., Fuentes-Mera, L., & Camacho, A. (2017). Microglia Activation Due to Obesity Programs Metabolic Failure Leading to Type Two Diabetes. Nutrition & Diabetes, 7(3), e254. https://doi.org/10.1038/nutd.2017.10

Mandrekar-Colucci, S., & Landreth, G. E. (2010). Microglia and Inflammation in Alzheimer's Disease. CNS & Neurological Disorders Drug Targets, 9(2), 156–167. https://doi.org/10.2174/187152710791012071

Manoharan, S., Guillemin, G. J., Abiramasundari, R. S., Essa, M. M., Akbar, M., & Akbar, M. D. (2016). The Role of Reactive Oxygen Species in the Pathogenesis of Alzheimer's Disease, Parkinson's Disease, and Huntington's Disease: A Mini Review. Oxidative Medicine and Cellular Longevity, 2016, 8590578. https://doi.org/10.1155/2016/8590578

Marcum, Z. A., & Hanlon, J. T. (2010). Recognizing the Risks of Chronic Nonsteroidal Anti-Inflammatory Drug Use in Older Adults. The Annals of Long-Term Care: the Official Journal of the American Medical Directors Association, 18(9), 24–27.

Martinon, F., & Tschopp, J. (2007). Inflammatory Caspases and Inflammasomes: Master Switches of Inflammation. Cell Death and Differentiation, 14(1), 10–22. https://doi.org/10.1038/sj.cdd.4402038

McDade, E., Llibre-Guerra, J. J., Holtzman, D. M., Morris, J. C., & Bateman, R. J. (2021). The Informed Road Map to Prevention of Alzheimer Disease: A Call to Arms. Molecular Neurodegeneration, 16(1), 49. https://doi.org/10.1186/s13024-021-00467-y

Md, S., Alhakamy, N. A., Alfaleh, M. A., Afzal, O., Altamimi, A. S. A., Iqubal, A., & Shaik, R. A. (2021). Mechanisms Involved in Microglial-Interceded Alzheimer's Disease and Nanocarrier-Based Treatment Approaches. Journal of Personalized Medicine, 11(11), 1116. https://doi.org/10.3390/jpm11111116

Medeiros, R., & LaFerla, F. M. (2013). Astrocytes: Conductors of the Alzheimer Disease Neuroinflammatory Symphony. Experimental Neurology, 239, 133–138. https://doi.org/10.1016/j.expneurol.2012.10.007

Meinert, C. L., McCaffrey, L. D., & Breitner, J. C. (2009). Alzheimer's Disease Anti-Inflammatory Prevention Trial: Design, Methods, and Baseline Results. Alzheimer's & Dementia: the Journal of the Alzheimer's Association, 5(2), 93–104. https://doi.org/10.1016/j.jalz.2008.09.004

Miao, J., Ma, H., Yang, Y., Liao, Y., Lin, C., Zheng, J., Yu, M., & Lan, J. (2023). Microglia in Alzheimer's Disease: Pathogenesis, Mechanisms, and Therapeutic Potentials. Frontiers in Aging Neuroscience, 15, 1201982. https://doi.org/10.3389/fnagi.2023.1201982

Michell-Robinson, M. A., Touil, H., Healy, L. M., Owen, D. R., Durafourt, B. A., Bar-Or, A., Antel, J. P., & Moore, C. S. (2015). Roles of Microglia in Brain Development, Tissue Maintenance and Repair. Brain: a Journal of Neurology, 138(Pt 5), 1138–1159. https://doi.org/10.1093/brain/awv066

Mohan Kumar, S. M. J., Murugan, A., Palaniyappan, A., & Mohan Kumar, P. S. (2023). Role of Cytokines and Reactive Oxygen Species in Brain Aging. Mechanisms of Ageing and Development, 214, 111855. https://doi.org/10.1016/j.mad.2023.111855

Muzio, L., Viotti, A., & Martino, G. (2021). Microglia in Neuroinflammation and Neurodegeneration: From Understanding to Therapy. Frontiers in Neuroscience, 15, 742065. https://doi.org/10.3389/fnins.2021.742065

Noureddine, F. Y., Altara, R., Fan, F., Yabluchanskiy, A., Booz, G. W., & Zouein, F. A. (2020). Impact of the Renin-Angiotensin System on the Endothelium in Vascular Dementia: Unresolved Issues and Future Perspectives. International Journal of Molecular Sciences, 21(12), 4268. https://doi.org/10.3390/ijms21124268

Olloquequi, J., Díaz-Peña, R., Verdaguer, E., Ettcheto, M., Auladell, C., & Camins, A. (2024). From Inhalation to Neurodegeneration: Air Pollution as a Modifiable Risk Factor for Alzheimer's Disease. International Journal of Molecular Sciences, 25(13), 6928. https://doi.org/10.3390/ijms25136928

Parhizkar, S., & Holtzman, D. M. (2022). APOE Mediated Neuroinflammation and Neurodegeneration in Alzheimer's Disease. Seminars in Immunology, 59, 101594. https://doi.org/10.1016/j.smim.2022.101594

Pérez, M. J., & Quintanilla, R. A. (2015). Therapeutic Actions of the Thiazolidinediones in Alzheimer's Disease. PPAR Research, 2015, 957248. https://doi.org/10.1155/2015/957248

Pontejo, S. M., Sanchez, C., Ruiz-Argüello, B., & Alcami, A. (2019). Insights into Ligand Binding by a Viral Tumor Necrosis Factor (TNF) Decoy Receptor Yield a Selective Soluble Human Type 2 TNF Receptor. The Journal of Biological Chemistry, 294(13), 5214–5227. https://doi.org/10.1074/jbc.RA118.005828

Potter, H., Woodcock, J. H., Boyd, T. D., Coughlan, C. M., Shaughnessy, J. R., Borges, M. T., Thaker, A. A., Raj, B. A., Adamszuk, Scott, Adame, Anton, Chial, H. J., Gray, Daniels, Stocker, M. E., & Sillau, S. H. (2021). Safety and Efficacy of Sargramostim (GM-CSF) in the Treatment of Alzheimer's Disease. Alzheimer's & Dementia (New York, N. Y.), 7(1), e12158. https://doi.org/10.1002/trc2.12158

Preman, P., Alfonso-Triguero, M., Alberdi, E., Verkhratsky, A., & Arranz, A. M. (2021). Astrocytes in Alzheimer's Disease: Pathological Significance and Molecular Pathways. Cells, 10(3), 540. https://doi.org/10.3390/cells10030540

Price, B. R., Johnson, L. A., & Norris, C. M. (2021). Reactive Astrocytes: The Nexus of Pathological and Clinical Hallmarks of Alzheimer's Disease. Ageing Research Reviews, 68, 101335. https://doi.org/10.1016/j.arr.2021.101335

Prinz, M., Jung, S., & Priller, J. (2019). Microglia Biology: One Century of Evolving Concepts. Cell, 179(2), 292–311. https://doi.org/10.1016/j.cell.2019.08.053

Rani, V., Verma, R., Kumar, K., & Chawla, R. (2022). Role of Pro-Inflammatory Cytokines in Alzheimer's Disease and Neuroprotective Effects of Pegylated Self-Assembled Nanoscaffolds. Current Research in Pharmacology and Drug Discovery, 4, 100149. https://doi.org/10.1016/j.crphar.2022.100149

Reynolds, A., Laurie, C., Mosley, R. L., & Gendelman, H. E. (2007). Oxidative stress and the pathogenesis of neurodegenerative disorders. International Review of Neurobiology, 82, 297–325. https://doi.org/10.1016/S0074-7742(07)82016-2

Rivers-Auty, J., Mather, A. E., Peters, R., Lawrence, C. B., & Brough, D. (2020). Anti-Inflammatories in Alzheimer's Disease-Potential Therapy or Spurious Correlate? Brain Communications, 2(2), fcaa109. https://doi.org/10.1093/braincomms/fcaa109

Rodríguez-Giraldo, M., González-Reyes, R. E., Ramírez-Guerrero, S., Bonilla-Trilleras, C. E., Guardo-Maya, S., & Nava-Mesa, M. O. (2022). Astrocytes as a Therapeutic Target in Alzheimer's Disease-Comprehensive Review and Recent Developments. International Journal of Molecular Sciences, 23(21), 13630. https://doi.org/10.3390/ijms232113630

Root, R. K., & Dale, D. C. (1999). Granulocyte Colony-Stimulating Factor and Granulocyte-Macrophage Colony-Stimulating Factor: Comparisons and Potential for Use in the Treatment of Infections in Nonneutropenic Patients. The Journal of Infectious Diseases, 179(Suppl 2), S342–S352. https://doi.org/10.1086/513857

Roy, R. G., Mandal, P. K., & Maroon, J. C. (2023). Oxidative Stress Occurs Prior to Amyloid Aβ Plaque Formation and Tau Phosphorylation in Alzheimer's Disease: Role of Glutathione and Metal Ions. ACS Chemical Neuroscience, 14(17), 2944–2954. https://doi.org/10.1021/acschemneuro.3c00486

Ryu, J. K., & McLarnon, J. G. (2008). Thalidomide Inhibition of Perturbed Vasculature and Glial-Derived Tumor Necrosis Factor-Alpha in an Animal Model of Inflamed Alzheimer's Disease Brain. Neurobiology of Disease, 29(2), 254–266. https://doi.org/10.1016/j.nbd.2007.08.019

Santisteban, M. M., Iadecola, C., & Carnevale, D. (2023). Hypertension, Neurovascular Dysfunction, and Cognitive Impairment. Hypertension (Dallas, Tex.: 1979), 80(1), 22–34. https://doi.org/10.1161/HYPERTENSIONAHA.122.18085

Sastre, M., Dewachter, I., Landreth, G. E., Willson, T. M., Klockgether, T., van Leuven, F., & Heneka, M. T. (2003). Nonsteroidal Anti-Inflammatory Drugs and Peroxisome Proliferator-Activated Receptor-gamma Agonists Modulate Immunostimulated Processing of Amyloid Precursor Protein Through Regulation of Beta-Secretase. The Journal of Neuroscience: the Official Journal of the Society for Neuroscience, 23(30), 9796–9804. https://doi.org/10.1523/JNEUROSCI.23-30-09796.2003

Satarker, S., Bojja, S. L., Gurram, P. C., Mudgal, J., Arora, D., & Nampoothiri, M. (2022). Astrocytic Glutamatergic Transmission and Its Implications in Neurodegenerative Disorders. Cells, 11(7), 1139. https://doi.org/10.3390/cells11071139

Savarin-Vuaillat, C., & Ransohoff, R. M. (2007). Chemokines and Chemokine Receptors in Neurological Disease: Raise, Retain, or Reduce? Neurotherapeutics: the Journal of the American Society for Experimental Neuro Therapeutics, 4(4), 590–601. https://doi.org/10.1016/j.nurt.2007.07.004

Sędzikowska, A., & Szablewski, L. (2021). Insulin and Insulin Resistance in Alzheimer's Disease. International Journal of Molecular Sciences, 22(18), 9987. https://doi.org/10.3390/ijms22189987

Serrano-Pozo, A., Das, S., & Hyman, B. T. (2021). APOE and Alzheimer's Disease: Advances in Genetics, Pathophysiology, and Therapeutic Approaches. The Lancet. Neurology, 20(1), 68–80. https://doi.org/10.1016/S1474-4422(20)30412-9

Shaftel, S. S., Griffin, W. S., & O'Banion, M. K. (2008). The Role of Interleukin-1 in Neuroinflammation and Alzheimer Disease: an Evolving Perspective. Journal of Neuroinflammation, 5, 7. https://doi.org/10.1186/1742-2094-5-7

Shi, Y., Liu, C. H., Roberts, A. I., Das, J., Xu, G., Ren, G., Zhang, Y., Zhang, L., Yuan, Z. R., Tan, H. S., Das, G., & Devadas, S. (2006). Granulocyte-Macrophage Colony-Stimulating Factor (GM-CSF) and T-Cell Responses: What We Do and Don't Know. Cell Research, 16(2), 126–133. https://doi.org/10.1038/sj.cr.7310017

Shoelson, S. E., Lee, J., & Goldfine, A. B. (2006). Inflammation and Insulin Resistance. The Journal of Clinical Investigation, 116(7), 1793–1801. https://doi.org/10.1172/JCI29069

Simpson, D. S. A., & Oliver, P. L. (2020). ROS Generation in Microglia: Understanding Oxidative Stress and Inflammation in Neurodegenerative Disease. Antioxidants (Basel, Switzerland), 9(8), 743. https://doi.org/10.3390/antiox9080743

Smith, A. N., Shaughness, M., Collier, S., Hopkins, D., & Byrnes, K. R. (2022). Therapeutic Targeting of Microglia Mediated Oxidative Stress after Neurotrauma. Frontiers in Medicine, 9, 1034692. https://doi.org/10.3389/fmed.2022.1034692

Solito, E., & Sastre, M. (2012). Microglia Function in Alzheimer's Disease. Frontiers in Pharmacology, 3, 14. https://doi.org/10.3389/fphar.2012.00014

Srinivasan, D., Yen, J. H., Joseph, D. J., & Friedman, W. (2004). Cell Type-Specific Inter leukin-1beta Signaling in the CNS. The Journal of Neuroscience: the Official Journal of the Society for Neuroscience, 24(29), 6482–6488. https://doi.org/10.1523/JNEUROSCI.5712-03.2004

Stanca, S., Rossetti, M., & Bongioanni, P. (2023). Astrocytes as Neuroimmunocytes in Alzheimer's Disease: A Biochemical Tool in the Neuron-Glia Crosstalk Along the Pathogenetic Pathways. International Journal of MolecularSciences, 24(18), 13880. https://doi.org/10.3390/ijms241813880

Subedi, L., Lee, S. E., Madiha, S., Gaire, B. P., Jin, M., Yumnam, S., & Kim, S. Y. (2020). Phytochemicals Against TNFα-Mediated Neuroinflammatory Diseases. International Journal of Molecular Sciences, 21(3), 764. https://doi.org/10.3390/ijms21030764

Suganya, K., & Koo, B. S. (2020). Gut-Brain Axis: Role of Gut Microbiota on Neurological Disorders and How Probiotics/Prebiotics Beneficially Modulate Microbial and Immune Pathways to Improve Brain Functions. International Journal of Molecular Sciences, 21(20), 7551. https://doi.org/10.3390/ijms21207551

Tamagno, E., Guglielmotto, M., Vasciaveo, V., & Tabaton, M. (2021). Oxidative Stress and Beta Amyloid in Alzheimer's Disease. Which Comes First: The Chicken or the Egg? Antioxidants (Basel, Switzerland, 10(9), 1479. https://doi.org/10.3390/antiox10091479

Tjalkens, R. B., Popichak, K. A., & Kirkley, K. A. (2017). Inflammatory activation of microglia and astrocytes in manganese neurotoxicity. Advances in Neurobiology, 18, 159–181. https://doi.org/10.1007/978-3-319-60189-2_8

Torres-Acosta, N., O'Keefe, J. H., O'Keefe, E. L., Isaacson, R., & Small, G. (2020). Therapeutic Potential of TNF-α Inhibition for Alzheimer's Disease Prevention. Journal of Alzheimer's Disease: JAD, 78(2), 619–626. https://doi.org/10.3233/JAD-200711

Tramontana, J. M., Utaipat, U., Molloy, A., Akarasewi, P., Burroughs, M., Makonkawkeyoon, S., Johnson, B., Klausner, J. D., Rom, W., & Kaplan, G. (1995). Thalidomide Treatment Reduces Tumor Necrosis Factor Alpha Production and Enhances Weight Gain in Patients With Pulmonary Tuberculosis. Molecular Medicine (Cambridge, Mass.), 1(4), 384–397.

Uddin, M. S., Kabir, M. T., Mamun, A. A., Barreto, G. E., Rashid, M., Perveen, A., & Ashraf, G. M. (2020). Pharmacological Approaches to Mitigate Neuroinflammation in Alzheimer's Disease. International Immunopharmacology, 84, 106479. https://doi.org/10.1016/j.intimp.2020.106479

Van Eldik, L. J., Carrillo, M. C., Cole, P. E., Feuerbach, D., Greenberg, B. D., Hendrix, J. A., Kennedy, M., Kozauer, N., Margolin, R. A., Molinuevo, J. L., Mueller, R., Ransohoff, R. M., Wilcock, D. M., Bain, L., & Bales, K. (2016). The Roles of Inflammation and Immune Mechanisms in Alzheimer's Disease. Alzheimer's & Dementia (New York, N. Y.), 2(2), 99–109. https://doi.org/10.1016/j.trci.2016.05.001

Van Opdenbosch, N., & Lamkanfi, M. (2019). Caspases in Cell Death, Inflammation, and Disease. Immunity, 50(6), 1352–1364. https://doi.org/10.1016/j.immuni.2019.05.020

van Zonneveld, S. M., van den Oever, E. J., Haarman, B. C. M., Grandjean, E. L., Nuninga, J. O., van de Rest, O., & Sommer, I. E. C. (2024). An Anti-Inflammatory Diet and Its Potential Benefit for Individuals with Mental Disorders and Neurodegenerative Diseases-A Narrative Review. Nutrients, 16(16), 2646. https://doi.org/10.3390/nu16162646

Wang, B., Wu, L., Chen, J., Dong, L., Chen, C., Wen, Z., Hu, J., Fleming, I., & Wang, D. W. (2021). Metabolism Pathways of Arachidonic Acids: Mechanisms and Potential Therapeutic Targets. Signal Transduction and Targeted Therapy, 6(1), 94. https://doi.org/10.1038/s41392-020-00443-w

Wang, Q., & Xie, C. (2022). Microglia Activation Linking Amyloid-β Drive Tau Spatial Propagation in Alzheimer's Disease. Frontiers in Neuroscience, 16, 951128. https://doi.org/10.3389/fnins.2022.951128

Wang, W. Y., Tan, M. S., Yu, J. T., & Tan, L. (2015). Role of Pro-Inflammatory Cytokines Released from Microglia in Alzheimer's Disease. Annals of Translational Medicine, 3(10), 136. https://doi.org/10.3978/j.issn.2305-5839.2015.03.49

Wang, Y., Yu, B., Wang, L., Yang, M., Xia, Z., Wei, W., Zhang, F., & Yuan, X. (2017). Pioglitazone Ameliorates Glomerular NLRP3 Inflammasome Activation in Apolipoprotein E Knockout Mice With Diabetes mellitus. PloS One, 12(7), e0181248. https://doi.org/10.1371/journal.pone.0181248

Woodburn, S. C., Bollinger, J. L., & Wohleb, E. S. (2021). The Semantics of Microglia Activation: Neuroinflammation, Homeostasis, and Stress. Journal of Neuroinflammation, 18(1), 258. https://doi.org/10.1186/s12974-021-02309-6

Yan, S. D., Bierhaus, A., Nawroth, P. P., & Stern, D. M. (2009). RAGE and Alzheimer's Disease: a Progression Factor for Amyloid-Beta-Induced Cellular Perturbation?Journal of Alzheimer's Disease: JAD, 16(4), 833–843. https://doi.org/10.3233/JAD-2009-1030

Zarghi, A., & Arfaei, S. (2011). Selective COX-2 Inhibitors: A Review of Their Structure-Activity Relationships. Iranian Journal of Pharmaceutical Research: IJPR, 10(4), 655–683.

Zhang, J., Zhang, Y., Wang, J., Xia, Y., Zhang, J., & Chen, L. (2024a). Recent Advances in Alzheimer's Disease: Mechanisms, Clinical Trials and New Drug Development Strategies. Signal Transduction and Targeted Therapy, 9(1), 211. https://doi.org/10.1038/s41392-024-01911-3

Zhang, W., Xiao, D., Mao, Q., & Xia, H. (2023). Role of Neuroinflammation in Neurodegeneration Development. Signal Transduction and Targeted Therapy, 8(1), 267. https://doi.org/10.1038/s41392-023-01486-5

Zhang, Y., Tang, Y., & Illes, P. (2024b). Modification of Neural Circuit Functions by Microglial P2Y6 Receptors in Health and Neurodegeneration. Molecular Neurobiology, 10.1007/s12035-024-04531-8. Advance online publication. https://doi.org/10.1007/s12035-024-04531-8

Zhao, Z., Liu, Y., Ruan, S., & Hu, Y. (2023). Current Anti-Amyloid-β Therapy for Alzheimer's Disease Treatment: From Clinical Research to Nanomedicine. International Journal of Nanomedicine, 18, 7825–7845. https://doi.org/10.2147/IJN.S444115

4 Nanotechnological Advances in the Delivery of CNS Therapeutics

Anushri Sharma and Ankita Lakra

4.1 INTRODUCTION

Nanotechnology, within nanomedicine, is described as methodologies for developing therapeutic and imaging agent nanocarriers, tiny electronic sensors, small devices, and miniaturized devices using structures at the nanoscale [1]. Progress in nanotechnology has been notable in creating new methods for delivering drugs, especially for the central nervous system (CNS), which present challenges for therapeutic delivery due to the blood–brain barrier (BBB) and other physiological constraints. Progress in nanotechnology has offered hopeful solutions to improve how drugs are delivered, absorbed, and released for treating CNS disorders like Alzheimer's, Parkinson's, glioblastoma, and multiple sclerosis. Fundamental science and technologies provide the basis of both nanomedicine and nanotechnology. The content within the text should be rephrased using the same language and maintaining the word count, not exceeding it techniques used to analyze nanostructured materials, particles. The dimensions and surface characteristics of nanoparticles can also be utilized for the characterization of nanocarriers [2].

Researching medications that target the CNS is difficult because of the intricate nature of the brain, potential side effects, as well as the challenge of passing through the BBB [3]. The blood brain barrier safeguards the cognitive process, which is the most delicate and complex system. It serves as a barrier that shields the brain's neurons from harmful substances in the blood, yet it hinders the transportation of medications to the CNS [4].

4.2 NANOTECHNOLOGY AND BLOOD BRAIN BARRIER

The BBB has its own unique structure and involves the interaction of the brain's cellular and acellular parts. The primary role of the BBB is to create a conducive environment for neuron function, crucial for maintaining balance and regulating the movement of substances in and out of the brain, while also protecting it from harmful toxins [5]. The BBB is made up of a continuous layer of endothelial cells that are connected through gap junctions (GJs), adherents' junctions, and tight junctions (TJs). TJs seem to be the main BBB physical element that increases trans-endothelial permeability [6]. The intersections help to control the movement of drugs through the

DOI: 10.1201/9781003543381-4

barrier by securely connecting to nearby cells, blocking the space between them [7]. There are hardly any intercellular interstitial spaces present within brain capillaries. Hence, the transit probably takes place through every cell. Therefore, lipid-soluble molecules may be able to easily pass through the endothelial membrane, potentially allowing them to cross the BBB without difficulty [8]. Since brain abnormalities are the most resistant to treatment, the therapeutic benefits of pushing prescription medications have been undermined.

Drugs can cross the BBB either through active targeting that requires energy, or through passive targeting based on gradients. Due to the presence of TJs connecting to neighboring cells, water solutes passively flow through them. This activity has no significance in normal bodily conditions. Another option is to use transcellular transport, where the nanoparticles are transported through the endothelial cells. Nanoparticles weighing 500 Da are appropriate for transporting across cells [9]. Medication can be delivered to the CNS through transcytosis or receptor-mediated transport across the barrier. To achieve this the nanoparticle must be transported by a vector to the center of the polarized cells' apical and basolateral surfaces [10].

Advancements in nanotechnology could bring about greater understanding of brain pathways and new approaches for diagnosing and treating brain disorders [11]. This appears to be especially important considering the built-in constraints of current methods for delivering medication through the BBB to the CNS. The unique properties of nanomaterials like reduced size, biocompatibility, extended circulation time, and lack of toxicity have been harnessed to develop an innovative delivery system for carrying therapeutic drugs to the brain [12,13].

4.3 TYPE OF NANOPARTICLES DURING DRUG DELIVERY

Nanotechnology provides an efficient method for transporting medications to address CNS conditions. Because of their small size, these specially made biodegradable and bio-friendly nanoparticles are able to cross the BBB. To ensure optimal compatibility between the drug and nanoparticles, the nanoparticles' surface can be easily altered [14]. The nanoparticle is made up of two sections: One section protects the drug from enzymatic degradation, targets specific brain cells, crosses the barrier and releases the drug at specific pH. The nano-engineered complex makes up the other portion. Nanoparticles have a specific drug delivery system at a certain site to breach the BBB, giving them an edge [15]. There are various types of nanoparticles, each having unique compositions and functions. Figure 4.1 shows types of nanoparticles, and a list of nanocarriers used for drug delivery is presented in Table 4.1.

4.3.1 Liposomes

They are tiny spherical colloidal vesicles of the first generation. These consist of hydrophilic parts and contain one or more lipid bilayers at the core, giving them a similar appearance to cell membranes and allowing them to be utilized for delivering drugs [16,17]. Due to their extensive history of research, low toxicity, and

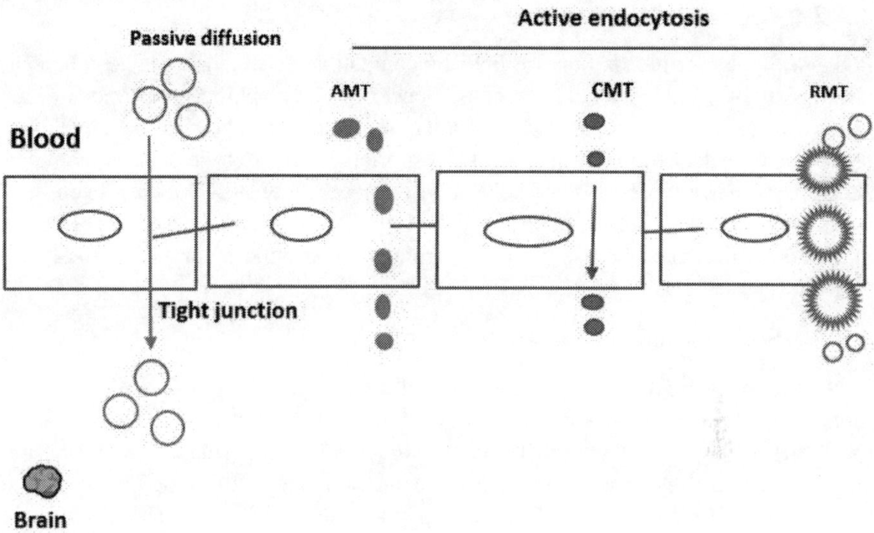

FIGURE 4.1 Types of nanomedicine.

effectiveness in delivering various compounds, liposomes are likely the most studied and clinically acknowledged nanocarriers [18].

Liposomes have the potential to target brain tumors by being capable of successfully delivering medications across the BBB to the desired location. Multiple research studies have documented the utilization of liposomes for transporting anticancer medications such as methotrexate [19]. The primary advantage includes the ease of surface modification to produce complex liposomal formulations, such as immunoliposomes, for accurate delivery is known as CNS delivery [20].

The newer generation of liposomes are also characterized by increased stability [20]. Indeed, the recently introduced liposomal forms usually last for a few months before expiring. More liposomal formulations are expected to be utilized for delivering drugs to the CNS.

TABLE 4.1
Summary of Nanocarrier and Drug Delivered

S. No.	Carrier Type	Drug Delivered
1.	Liposomes	Cisplatin, Stavudine
2.	Polymeric nanoparticle	Methotrexate, Dalargin, Lamivudine, Superoxide dimutase
3.	Solid-liquid nanoparticle	Melatonin, Paclitaxel, Baclofen
4.	Emulsion	Saquinavir, Paclitaxel, Ceramide
5.	Micelle	Amphotericin, Biphalin, Doxurubicin, Vinblastin
6.	Dendrimer	Lamivudine
7.	Nanogel	Antisense-oligonucleotide

4.3.2 Polymeric Nanoparticles

PNP's are polymer blends that are both biocompatible and biodegradable. The center consists of a compact polymer matrix enclosing a lipophilic medication, which offers stabilizing the nanoparticles sterically. Medication can be absorbed, enclosed, or chemically attached to the surface of transportation [21]. Acrylic polymer nanoparticles, particularly those made of poly(butyl cyanoacrylate) (PBCA), have been thoroughly researched for delivering drugs to the CNS [22,23]. Rapid breakdown of PBCA in the body can reduce the risk of toxicity from polymer build-up in the CNS [24].

4.3.3 Solid Liquid Nanoparticle

SLNs consist of lipids like triglycerides and fatty acids in aqueous colloidal mixtures. Once these nanoparticles are dispersed in a liquid, they acquire the capability to solidify as they cool down [5]. They are evaluated for delivering drugs to the brain because they are physically steady, prevent medications from being changed, and have less toxicity to cells. [25]. Both nanocarriers need surfactants, either non-ionic or ionic, to remain stable. These tiny carriers help to continuously release therapeutic agents in a controlled manner possess a mild level of toxicity [26]. Moreover, lipophilic particles can effectively penetrate the BBB and enter the CNS compartment without any surface alterations. Indeed, SLN were discovered to also attach to apolipoproteins and localize in brain tissues similar to PCBA nanoparticles [27,28]. They show great promise for delivering drugs to the CNS.

SLNs are capable of containing hydrophilic and lipophilic medications, and these enclosed medications remain more stable within SLNs when compared to PNPs, allowing for a potential release timeline lasting month to years. In contrast to PNPs, SLNs prevent leaks and safeguard the active drug ingredient against degradation (photochemical, oxidative, and chemical degradation) by containing it inside, leading to a stable formula [29]. The presence of SLNs in the formulation is said to enhance the bioavailability of hydrophobic drugs [30].

4.3.4 Nanoemulsion

NEs are typically made up of edible/cooking oils, surfactant, and water, creating a colloidal system. Their span spans from 100 to 500 nanometers [31]. They are being recommended for use as drug delivery systems to address various issues such as poor targeting and BBB penetration [32]. NEs have lower solubility in water and reduced stability across different pH levels, temperatures, and salinity levels. Their action also begins slowly. Because of this factor, nasal delivery of drugs is typically done using NEs.

4.4 MECHANISM OF NANOPARTICLE IN ACTION

Characteristics such as small dimensions, surface charge, hydrophilicity, and nanocarrier ligand targeting enable nanoparticles to penetrate the brain endothelial tissue. Due to electrostatic interactions, the positive charge on the nanoparticle's surface

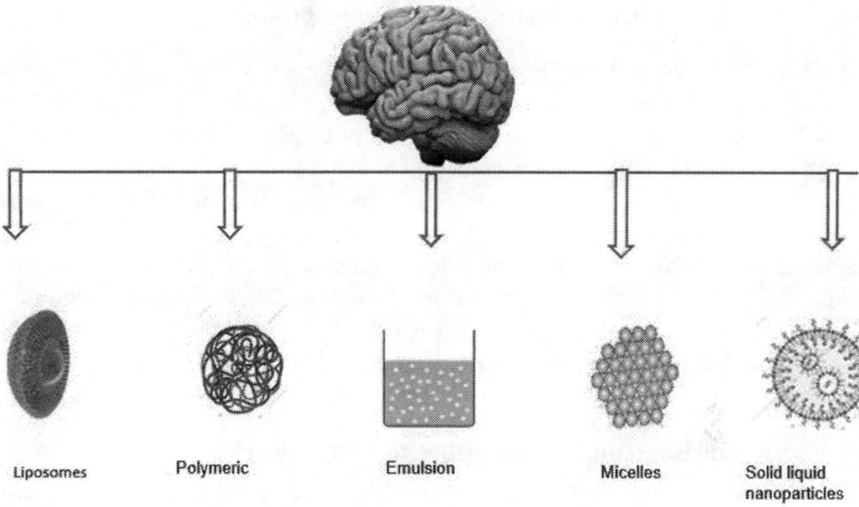

FIGURE 4.2 Nanoparticles based blood-brain barrier for drug delivery. *Abbreviations:* AMT, adsorption-mediated transcytosis; CMT, carrier-mediated transport; RMT, receptor-mediated transcytosis.

interacts with the weak charge on the brain's endothelial cells. Hydrophobic characteristics of the nanomaterials boost their qualities and speed up the absorption procedure by interacting with the compound's solubility and permeability [33,34]. The nanoparticle is taken in by the brain endothelial cells through endocytosis and transcytosis, which have low-density lipoprotein receptors, and then released [35]. The particles return to the bloodstream as a result of this desorption, where they release the drug contained within them at the upper part of the BBB, diffusing through the brain's parenchyma. The average diameter of human blood capillaries is 6–9 micrometer, while the 20-micrometer cell diameter allows nanoparticles to flow easily by endocytosis and transcytosis due to their small size [36]. These nanoparticles carrying drugs are taken up by endocytosis and penetrate deeper into the cell or brain parenchyma. Even though researchers have not fully investigated how nanoparticles deliver drugs, it is thought that they function through multiple mechanisms [37,38]. Figure 4.2 shows nanoparticle based on BBB for drug delivery.

4.5 STIMULI-RESPONSIVE NANOCARRIERS

Stimuli-sensitive nanocarriers are a type of drug delivery systems that release their therapeutic contents in reaction to particular internal or external triggers. Their capacity to detect and react to modifications in the surroundings makes them very appealing for precise and regulated drug transportation, particularly for difficult situations such as CNS treatments [39]. These systems can be customized to deliver medications at precise locations in the body, like tumors or inflamed tissues, or in reaction to specific environmental factors such as pH, temperature, light, or magnetic fields.

4.5.1 Varieties of Nanocarriers that React to Stimuli

4.5.1.1 pH-Sensitive Nanocarriers

Method: These nanocarriers take advantage of the variations in pH levels among various sections of the body (such as blood, healthy tissues, tumor tissues, or inflamed regions). As an illustration, tumor microenvironment tends to be more acidic (pH 6.0–6.5) in contrast to tissues that are normal (pH 7.4), likewise inflamed regions may also exhibit decreased pH levels [40].

Nanomaterials like polymeric nanoparticles, liposomes, and micelles are commonly utilized as pH-sensitive materials. These materials contain functional groups (such as amines, carboxylates) that react to pH variations, resulting in a structural transformation or degradation, leading to drug release at the desired location [39].

4.5.1.2 Nanocarriers that Are Sensitive to Temperature

Method: These transporters react to temperature variations by using materials that have thermo-responsive characteristics. These substances change from being water-loving to water-repellent, or vice versa, at certain temperatures, causing the drug to be released. Nanomaterials like poly(N-isopropylacrylamide) (PNIPAM) and polyethylene glycol (PEG) are commonly used as temperature-sensitive nanocarriers [41]. These polymers experience a transition in phase at approximately body temperature (37°C) or slightly above, causing variations in their solubility or structure and allowing for the release of drugs.

4.5.1.3 Light-Sensitive Nanocarriers

Method: Nanocarriers sensitive to light are formulated to release their contents when they are illuminated with a particular wavelength of light, often ultraviolet (UV) or near-infrared (NIR) light. Light has the ability to initiate a photochemical response that changes the composition of the nanocarrier, leading to the liberation of the enclosed medication [42].

Nanomaterials: Nanocarriers are frequently modified with light-responsive molecules such as azobenzenes or photoisomerizable groups that experience a change in shape when illuminated.

4.5.1.4 Magnetic-Field-Responsive Nanocarriers

Method: These nanocarriers are equipped with magnetic nanoparticles (such as iron oxide nanoparticles) that react to magnetic fields outside the system. Magnetic nanoparticles are usually embedded in bigger nanocarriers, allowing the magnetic field to guide particles to certain areas in the body and activate drug release through heat or mechanical stress [43].

The use of magnetic targeting is specifically beneficial in tumor treatment, as it involves directing nanocarriers to tumor locations using magnetic fields. Furthermore, the use of magnetic fields can also activate hyperthermic drug release, which can be beneficial when used alongside magnetic hyperthermia therapies [44].

4.5.1.5 Enzyme-Sensitive Nanocarriers

These nanocarriers release their cargo when encountering particular enzymes that are highly expressed in specific tissues or conditions such as tumors, inflammation, or bacterial infections. The release of the drug is triggered by the enzymatic breaking of peptide bonds or other chemical bonds within the structure of the nanocarrier [45]. Nanomaterials frequently consist of polymers, liposomes, or micelles that are attached to peptide linkers which react to proteases such as matrix metalloproteinases (MMPs), cathepsins, or other enzymes related to disease.

4.6 MAIN BENEFITS OF RESPONSIVE NANOCARRIER IN CNS THERAPEUTICS

Smart nanocarriers, known as responsive nanocarriers, are a type of drug delivery systems that are created to release their therapeutic contents based on particular stimuli from the surrounding conditions. These stimuli may consist of alterations in pH, temperature, light, magnetic fields, enzymes, or other biological cues. In the realm of CNS therapeutics, utilizing responsive nanocarriers presents numerous benefits that could greatly improve treatment results for neurological conditions. Listed below are the primary advantages of employing responsive nanocarriers for delivering drugs to the CNS.

Targeted Drug Delivery: After passing through the BBB, nanocarriers can be programmed to release the medication directly at the desired location, such as a tumor, inflamed area, or specific region of the brain, in reaction to local circumstances. This decreases overall side effects and improves the effectiveness of treatment [46].

Controlled Release: Responsive nanocarriers regulate the release of treatment to ensure ideal drug concentrations in the brain, decreasing toxicity. This decreases the chance of toxicity linked to elevated drug levels in the body while maintaining the drug's efficacy for an extended duration [47].

Many medications experience quick metabolism or breakdown in the bloodstream, leading to reduced drug loss. Responsive nanocarriers can shield drugs from early breakdown or elimination, guaranteeing a greater concentration of the therapeutic substance reaches the brain [48].

4.6.1 Improved Drug Stability

- **Preservation of Vulnerable Medications**: A large number of CNS medications, especially biologics (such as proteins and peptides), are extremely fragile when in the blood system. Responsive nanocarriers are able to shield these drugs from enzymatic degradation, physical instability, or oxidation, ensuring that their therapeutic efficacy remains intact until they reach their intended destination [49].
- **Encapsulation of Numerous Agents**: Nanocarriers have the ability to encapsulate various drugs, such as hydrophobic molecules, that might be difficult to transport to the CNS. This permits the simultaneous administration of several therapeutic substances, which is especially beneficial for addressing complicated CNS conditions such as neurodegenerative disorders or brain tumors [49].

4.6.2 Reduced Negative Reactions

- **Decreased Off-target Effects**: The accuracy of drug delivery, activated by environmental conditions (such as pH or enzyme levels), leads to better targeting and reduces off-target effects. This is especially important for CNS treatments, since the brain is responsive to alterations in its surroundings [50].
- **Reduced Systemic Exposure**: Responsive nanocarriers release drugs specifically at the desired site, decreasing exposure of surrounding organs and tissues to the medication and ultimately minimizing systemic side effects.

4.7 ADMINISTRATION WITHOUT THE NEED FOR PENETRATION OR INVASIVE PROCEDURE

- **Possibility for Non-invasive Options**: Nanocarriers can be designed for non-invasive methods of administration, like oral, nasal, or transdermal delivery. This is especially crucial for treatments of the CNS, as invasive methods such as intracerebral injection may be expensive, dangerous, and not suitable for prolonged therapy [50,51].
- **Decreased Requirement for Invasive Methods**: The capacity to efficiently administer medications through the BBB with limited side effects and no need for invasive methods is a significant advantage for patient adherence and safety [51].

Utilizing combination therapy, nanocarriers can be engineered to deliver multiple therapeutic agents at the same time. One possibility is for them to transport a mix of medications, like small compounds, biologics, or nucleic acids, that complement each other in order to address disorders of the CNS. This makes them perfect for treating neurodegenerative disorder, brain tumors, and stroke.

4.8 NANOTECHNOLOGY IN IMAGING AND DIAGNOSIS

Nanotechnology has transformed imaging and diagnosis by providing improved abilities for detecting diseases early, producing precise images, and monitoring diseases in real-time. Nanomaterials have made important advancements in diagnostic imaging in different medical areas because of their tiny size, adjustable characteristics, and ability to interact molecularly with biological systems.

Nanoparticles such as gold nanoparticles, quantum dots, silica nanoparticles, and iron oxide particles have the potential to serve as contrast agents in different imaging techniques, such as MRI, CT, ultrasound, and optical imaging [52]. These nanoparticles offer increased sensitivity and resolution when compared to conventional contrast agents. Nanoparticles provide greater sensitivity and resolution than traditional contrast agents due to their unique optical, magnetic, or acoustic properties. For example, gold nanoparticles enhance X-ray and CT imaging by improving signal contrast through superior scattering capabilities, enabling the detection of subtle tissue abnormalities.

Gold Nanoparticles have the ability to improve the contrast in X-ray and CT imaging due to their enhanced scattering properties [53].

Iron oxide nanoparticles, such as magnetic nanoparticles, are utilized in MRI to improve tissue contrast [54].

Quantum Dots, semiconductor nanoparticles, offer bright and stable fluorescence, making them perfect for high-resolution imaging in optical methods [55].

4.9 APPLICATION IN CNS DRUG DELIVERY

- **Parkinson's Disease**: Nanocarriers have the potential to transport neuroprotective substances or gene therapies directly into the brain, providing targeted and prolonged therapy in reaction to particular cues.
- **Alzheimer's Disease**: Responsive carriers can be employed to deliver drugs targeting amyloid plaque or anti-inflammatory agents to brain areas with disease-related alterations in pH, temperature, or enzyme levels.
- **Brain Tumors**: Nanocarriers may be created to selectively discharge chemotherapy drugs at tumor locations, activated by the tumor's acidic surroundings or specific enzymes overly produced by cancer cells.
- **Stroke and Neuroprotection**: Temperature-sensitive carriers could be utilized for administering neuroprotective agents or anti-inflammatory medications that react to the temperature fluctuations linked to ischemia.

4.9.1 Gene and RNA-Based Therapy Delivery

Gene therapy shows great potential in the treatment of various CNS disorders, especially those resulting from genetic mutations like Huntington's disease, spinal muscular atrophy (SMA), and certain brain cancers. Nanoparticles are ready to have a crucial impact on gene therapy to the brain [56]. Upcoming advancements in this field encompass:

- **siRNA Delivery**: Nanoparticles may be designed to shield siRNA from enzymatic breakdown and effectively transport it to the brain to treat genetic CNS conditions such as Huntington's disease or Alzheimer's [57].
- **CRISPR-based Delivery**: Nanoparticles will be used more and more to transport gene-editing tools such as CRISPR/Cas9 to address genetic mutations in the CNS. This has the potential to completely change the way genetic neurological disorders are treated through allowing for precise gene modification. Similarly, nanocarriers will be necessary for RNA-based therapies like antisense oligonucleotides or small interfering RNAs that target gene expression in the brain [58].
- **Tailored Gene Therapy**: Nanoparticles created to transport individualized genetic material could support personalized gene therapy methods, minimizing unintended impacts. This may be especially beneficial for managing uncommon or intricate CNS conditions with distinct genetic patterns [59].

4.9.2 Neuroprotection and Regenerative Medicine

Nanotechnology is progressing the growth of neuroprotective agents and treatments focused on renewing brain tissue. Nanoparticles have the potential to transport growth factors, antioxidants, or neuroprotective compounds for the treatment of ailments such as stroke, Parkinson's disease, or traumatic brain injury.

Neurotrophic Factors: Nanoparticles have the ability to trap and discharge neurotrophic factors (like brain-derived neurotrophic factor, BDNF) in order to boost the development and longevity of neurons [60].

Stem Cell Therapy: Nanomaterials have the ability to aid in delivering stem cells or cell-based therapies that help in the regeneration of injured brain tissues [60].

4.10 MAJOR CHALLENGES

Significant progress has been achieved in CNS drug delivery for therapeutics with the help of nanotechnology. There is much optimism about the potential of nanotechnology in treating neurological disorders due to its ability to surpass barriers like BBB, improve drug solubility and target particular areas of the brain. Although nanotechnology holds great potential, it also encounters various obstacles that need to be resolved before widespread clinical use can be realized. Understanding these challenges and the future directions of nanotechnology in the delivery of medications to the CNS is crucial to maximizing its advantages. Some advantages and disadvantages are mentioned in Table 4.2.

BBB Penetration: The BBB is a significant barrier to supplying the brain with therapeutic medications. Most medications are unable to get through due to selective permeability, particularly bigger compounds or those with low lipid solubility [61].

Current Solutions: Liposomes, polymeric nanoparticles, dendrimers, and solid lipid nanoparticles (SLNs) have been engineered to increase BBB permeability by mechanisms including as receptor-mediated transcytosis, adsorptive-mediated endocytosis, and tight junction regulation [61].

Challenge for the Future: Developing techniques that enable adequate BBB penetration and specific targeting of CNS areas while maintaining safety remains a key problem. Many nanoparticles that cross the BBB may not effectively target specific brain regions or cell types, resulting in nonspecific accumulation and potential negative effects [61].

TABLE 4.2
Advantages and Disadvantages of Nanotechnology

S. No.	Advantages	Disadvantages
1	Increase stability	Inadequate stability
2	Biocompatible and biodegradable	Low solubility
3	Increase efficacy	Leakage of drug
4	Ease of penetration	Osmotically sensitive
5	Site avoidance effect	High production cost

4.10.1 Toxicity and Compatibility of Nanoparticles

We do not have a complete understanding of the long-term toxicity of nanoparticles in the CNS. Possible adverse effects over time can result from problems such as neurotoxicity, immune system activation and the ongoing build-up of nanoparticles in the brain.

Current efforts are concentrated on creating nanoparticles that are both compatible with living organisms and capable of breaking down naturally, such as PEGylated liposomes, hydrogels, and polymeric nanoparticles. The application of PEG to surfaces is frequently done to decrease the immune reaction and enhance circulation durations [62].

Future Challenge: More research is required to assess the extended destiny of nanoparticles in the brain and to create techniques for their regulated breakdown and removal. It is essential for patient safety to make sure that nanoparticles do not build up in the CNS or other organs [62].

Transport of Large Biomolecules (Proteins, mRNA, Genes): Difficulty arises in delivering bulky, delicate biomolecules like proteins, mRNA, and gene-editing tools (e.g., CRISPR-Cas9) to the CNS because of their size, fragility, and limited capability to penetrate the BBB.

Existing Options: Various nanocarrier systems, such as LNPs, polymeric nanoparticles, and exosomes, are under development for transporting these sizable biomolecules to the brain. LNPs have displayed significant potential in transporting mRNA to the CNS, as evidenced by their application in COVID-19 vaccinations [63].

Future Challenge: Successfully delivering gene therapies and mRNA vaccines to specific areas of the CNS without degradation still poses a major hurdle. Moreover, overcoming immune responses and toxicity to ensure safe delivery of genetic material is a crucial challenge [63].

4.10.2 Challenges in Scalability and Production

- **Challenge**: The creation of nanoparticles with uniform size, shape, and surface properties on a large scale for medical purposes is still difficult. Quality assurance of nanomedicines is crucial to guarantee that every set of nanoparticles meets the necessary safety and effectiveness criteria [64].
- **Existing Methods**: Nano particles have been produced in a controlled fashion using microfluidic systems and solvent evaporation techniques. Scientists are also developing methods to automate the production process in order to improve reproducibility and increase production capacity [64].
- **Future Challenge**: Successfully producing nanomedicines on a large scale at a low cost while meeting strict regulatory criteria remains a major hurdle. In order to facilitate commercial production, it is necessary to tackle the diversity of nanoparticle formulations and the intricacy of synthesis processes [64].

4.11 FUTURE PERSPECTIVE AND POTENTIAL SOLUTION

Nanotechnology has become a revolutionary force in creating new drug delivery methods, especially for complex medical areas). Nanotechnology is set to revolutionize treatment of neurological diseases with improved drug delivery, the capability to surpass the barrier, and is potential for customized therapies. In the future, the role of nanotechnology in CNS therapeutics is being influenced by various important trends and perspectives, presenting both promising chances and the requirement for more innovation.

4.11.1 Improvements in Crossing the Blood-Brain Barrier and Focusing on Specific Areas

Emerging technologies such as focused ultrasound (FUS) paired with nanoparticles could potentially facilitate the controlled opening of the BBB, improving the transport of drugs or genes to the brain. Furthermore, advanced nanocarriers that react to changes in the environment, such as pH or temperature, could be created to enable precise and regulated release. Future studies will concentrate on creating nanocarriers that are able to pinpoint certain types of cells within the CNS (such as neurons and glial cells) or particular areas of the brain (like the basal ganglia in Parkinson's disease) with great accuracy through the use of advanced targeting techniques [65].

4.11.2 Tailored Nanotechnology for Medical Treatment

With advancements in our knowledge of genetic, molecular, and environmental aspects in CNS diseases, customized nanomedicine could be created to cater treatment according to each patient's distinct characteristics. This may entail choosing the optimal nanocarrier and drug pairing by considering genetic or biomarker profiling [66].

By utilizing genetic engineering, nanotechnology, and artificial intelligence, we can potentially monitor the brain in real-time and deliver drugs tailored to disease progression more precisely, ultimately leading to better outcomes for patients with complex CNS conditions.

4.11.3 The Collaboration between Gene Therapy and Nanomedicine

Nanotechnology is expected to have a key role in bringing gene therapy for CNS diseases to clinical fruition. The creation of versatile nanoparticles that can transport CRISPR-Cas9 systems, RNA treatments, and gene-editing instruments is expected to create fresh possibilities for treating genetic disorders, neurodegenerative illnesses, and brain tumors.

Advancements in non-invasive drug delivery methods, like intranasal delivery of nanoparticles or gene therapies, could simplify the process of administering treatments to the brain without invasive procedures. The firm's financial performance has improved significantly over the past quarter. Continued monitoring over a prolonged period and ensuring safety, utilizing nanoparticle imaging could enable the monitoring of drug delivery in the CNS in real-time, offering information about how therapeutics are distributed, accumulated, and released in the brain [67].

4.12 CONCLUSION

Nanotechnology has become a revolutionary instrument in the realm of drug delivery, providing fresh opportunities to address the enduring obstacles in treating CNS illnesses. The BBB, a strong protective barrier surrounding the brain, has always been a significant challenge in creating successful treatments for the CNS. Nevertheless, nanotechnology has displayed remarkable potential in addressing this challenge by leveraging its distinct capability to control materials on a nanoscale, enabling precise drug delivery, enhancing drug absorption, and improving treatment results with reduced side effects.

Nanotechnology enables the customization of nanoparticles in size, surface properties, and functional groups, allowing for precise drug delivery to specific areas of the brain. Nanoparticles can be modified to pass through the BBB using different techniques like receptor-mediated transcytosis, or can be fashioned to release their therapeutic cargo in a regulated fashion upon arrival at the desired location. Being able to target drugs precisely to the desired location is a significant improvement compared to conventional systemic drug delivery approaches, which can result in inadequate treatment levels and higher chances of toxicity.

Nanotechnology shows great promise in treating neurodegenerative diseases, brain tumors, and psychiatric disorders due to the limitations of conventional drugs in achieving effectiveness or avoiding serious side effects. Nanocarriers have demonstrated the ability to enhance drug solubility and stability, prolong circulation in the bloodstream, and decrease off-target effects. Furthermore, these carriers can be modified with special ligands or antibodies to improve the specificity of targeting for distinct cell types or brain areas, ultimately improving therapeutic results.

Although the potential of nanotech in delivering drugs to the CNS is great, there are still major obstacles that must be overcome before these advancements can be effectively utilized in medical treatment. Challenges like the ability to increase production, ensuring safety over time, possible immune responses, and getting regulatory approval for nanoparticle formulations are still major obstacles. To completely comprehend the harmful effects, more research is required of nanoparticles accumulating in the brain and other organs, as well as the impacts of prolonged exposure, in order to guarantee the safety and effectiveness of these systems in humans.

In spite of these obstacles, continued research and trials are getting us closer to fully utilizing nanotechnology for treating CNS disorders. As nanomedicines continue to advance, there is potential to combine them with gene editing and immunotherapy, leading to new possibilities in treating genetic CNS disorders and cancers. Additionally, the advancement of instant monitoring devices like imaging agents based on nanoparticles will enable more individualized treatment methods. This will empower healthcare providers to monitor the real-time distribution and impact of drug delivery systems.

In summary, progress in nanotechnology shows great potential in transforming the delivery of drugs to the CNS, providing fresh optimism for individuals with various neurological ailments. Nanotechnology improves the effectiveness and safety of current medications by overcoming the downsides of traditional therapies and enables the creation of new treatments customized for individual patient requirements. The advancement of the field is expected to make nanomedicine a key player in shaping the future of CNS therapeutics, providing improved, precise, and personalized treatment for neurological disorders.

REFERENCES

1. Wong HL, Wu XY, Bendayan R. Nanotechnological advances for the delivery of CNS therapeutics. Advanced Drug Delivery Reviews. 2012 May 15;64(7):686–700.
2. Bowman DM. More than a decade on: Mapping today's regulatory and policy landscapes following the publication of nanoscience and nanotechnologies: Opportunities and uncertainties. NanoEthics. 2017;11:169–86.
3. Mittal KR, Pharasi N, Sarna B, Singh M, Rachana, Haider S, Singh SK, Dua K, Jha SK, Dey A, Ojha S. Nanotechnology-based drug delivery for the treatment of CNS disorders. Translational Neuroscience. 2022 Dec 31;13(1):527–46.
4. Teleanu RI, Preda MD, Niculescu AG, Vladâcenco O, Radu CI, Grumezescu AM, Teleanu DM. Current strategies to enhance delivery of drugs across the blood–brain barrier. Pharmaceutics. 2022;14(5):987.
5. Barchet TM, Amiji MM. Challenges and opportunities in CNS delivery of therapeutics for neurodegenerative diseases. Expert Opinion on Drug Delivery. 2009;6(3):211–25.
6. Zhou Y, Peng Z, Seven ES, Leblanc RM. Crossing the blood-brain barrier with nanoparticles. Journal of Controlled Release. 2018 Jan 28;270:290–303.
7. Habgood M, Ek J. Delivering drugs into the brain: Barriers and possibilities. Therapeutic Delivery. 2010;1(4):483–8.
8. Engelhardt B, Sorokin L. The blood–brain and the blood–cerebrospinal fluid barriers: Function and dysfunction. In Seminars in Immunopathology 2009 Nov (Vol. 31, pp. 497–511). Springer-Verlag.
9. Georgieva JV, Hoekstra D, Zuhorn IS. Smuggling drugs into the brain: An overview of ligands targeting transcytosis for drug delivery across the blood–brain barrier. Pharmaceutics. 2014 Nov 17;6(4):557–83.
10. Rappoport JZ. Focusing on clathrin-mediated endocytosis. Biochemical Journal. 2008 Jun 15;412(3):415–23.
11. Ali IU, Chen X. Penetrating the blood–brain barrier: Promise of novel nanoplatforms and delivery vehicles. ACS Nano. 2015 Oct 27;9(10):9470–4.
12. Mangas-Sanjuan V, González-Alvarez M, Gonzalez-Alvarez I, Bermejo M. Drug penetration across the blood–brain barrier: An overview. Therapeutic Delivery. 2010;1(4):535–62.
13. Fakhoury M, Takechi R, Al-Salami H. Drug permeation across the blood-brain barrier: Applications of nanotechnology. British Journal of Medicine and Medical Research. 2015;6(6):547–56.
14. Kaur IP, Bhandari R, Bhandari S, Kakkar V. Potential of solid lipid nanoparticles in brain targeting. Journal of Controlled Release. 2008 Apr 21;127(2):97–109.
15. Fang Z, Chen S, Qin J, Chen B, Ni G, Chen Z, Zhou J, Li Z, Ning Y, Wu C, Zhou L. Pluronic P85-coated poly (butylcyanoacrylate) nanoparticles overcome phenytoin resistance in p-glycoprotein overexpressing rats with lithium-pilocarpine-induced chronic temporal lobe epilepsy. Biomaterials. 2016;97:110–21.
16. Ozkizilcik A, Davidson P, Turgut H, Sharma HS, Sharma A, Tian ZR. Nanocarriers as CNS drug delivery systems for enhanced neuroprotection. Drug and Gene Delivery to the Central Nervous System for Neuroprotection: Nanotechnological Advances. 2017;33–55.
17. Martins S, Sarmento B, Ferreira DC, Souto EB. Lipid-based colloidal carriers for peptide and protein delivery–liposomes versus lipid nanoparticles. International Journal of Nanomedicine. 2007;2(4):595–607.

18. Costantino L, Tosi G, Ruozi B, Bondioli L, Vandelli MA, Forni F. Colloidal systems for CNS drug delivery. Progress in Brain Research. 2009;180:35–69.
19. Hu Y, Rip J, Gaillard PJ, de Lange EC, Hammarlund-Udenaes M. The impact of liposomal formulations on the release And brain delivery of methotrexate: An in vivo microdialysis study. Journal of Pharmaceutical Sciences. 2017;106(9):2606–13.
20. Webb MS, Rebstein P, Lamson W, Bally MB. Liposomal drug delivery: Recent patents and emerging opportunities. Recent Patents on Drug Delivery & Formulation. 2007;1(3):185–94.
21. Parveen S, Misra R, Sahoo SK. Nanoparticles: A Boon to drug delivery, therapeutics, diagnostics and imaging. Nanomedicine in Cancer. 2017;47–98.
22. Alyaudtin RN, Reichel A, Löbenberg R, Ramge P, Kreuter J, Begley DJ. Interaction of poly (butylcyanoacrylate) nanoparticles with the blood-brain barrier in vivo and in vitro. Journal of Drug Targeting. 2001;9(3):209–21.
23. Rempe R, Cramer S, Hüwel S, Galla HJ. Transport of poly (n-butylcyano-acrylate) nanoparticles across the blood–brain barrier in vitro and their influence on barrier integrity. Biochemical and Biophysical Research Communications. 2011;406(1):64–9.
24. Gao K, Jiang X. Influence of particle size on transport of methotrexate across blood brain barrier by polysorbate 80-coated polybutylcyanoacrylate nanoparticles. International Journal of Pharmaceutics. 2006;310(1-2):213–9.
25. Huynh NT, Passirani C, Saulnier P, Benoît JP. Lipid nanocapsules: A new platform for nanomedicine. International Journal of Pharmaceutics. 2009 Sep 11;379(2):201–9.
26. Müller RH, Rühl D, Runge S, Schulze-Forster K, Mehnert W. Cytotoxicity of solid lipid nanoparticles as a function of the lipid matrix and the surfactant. Pharmaceutical Research. 1997;14:458–62.
27. Göppert TM, Müller RH. Polysorbate-stabilized solid lipid nanoparticles as colloidal carriers for intravenous targeting of drugs to the brain: Comparison of plasma protein adsorption patterns. Journal of Drug Targeting. 2005;13(3):179–87.
28. Kerwin BA. Polysorbates 20 and 80 used in the formulation of protein biotherapeutics: Structure and degradation pathways. Journal of Pharmaceutical Sciences. 2008;97(8):2924–35.
29. Freitas C, Müller RH. Correlation between long-term stability of solid lipid nanoparticles (SLN™) and crystallinity of the lipid phase. European Journal of Pharmaceutics and Biopharmaceutics. 1999;47(2):125–32.
30. Baek JS, Cho CW. Surface modification of solid lipid nanoparticles for oral delivery of curcumin: Improvement of bioavailability through enhanced cellular uptake, and lymphatic uptake. European Journal of Pharmaceutics and Biopharmaceutics. 2017;117:132–40.
31. Sarker DK. Engineering of nanoemulsions for drug delivery. Current Drug Delivery. 2005;2(4):297–310.
32. Lovelyn C, Attama AA. Current state of nanoemulsions in drug delivery. Journal of Biomaterials and Nanobiotechnology. 2011;2(05):626.
33. Markoutsa E, Pampalakis G, Niarakis A, Romero IA, Weksler B, Couraud PO, Antimisiaris SG. Uptake and permeability studies of BBB-targeting immunoliposomes using the hCMEC/D3 cell line. European Journal of Pharmaceutics and Biopharmaceutics. 2011;77(2):265–74.
34. Lien CF, Molnár E, Toman P, Tsibouklis J, Pilkington GJ, Górecki DC, Barbu E. In vitro assessment of alkylglyceryl-functionalized chitosan nanoparticles as permeating vectors for the blood–brain barrier. Biomacromolecules. 2012;13(4):1067–73.
35. Kim HR, Andrieux K, Delomenie C, Chacun H, Appel M, Desmaële D, Taran F, Georgin D, Couvreur P, Taverna M. Analysis of plasma protein adsorption onto PEGylated nanoparticles by complementary methods: 2-DE, CE and protein lab-on-chip® system. Electrophoresis. 2007;28(13):2252–61.

36. Vilella A, Tosi G, Grabrucker AM, Ruozi B, Belletti D, Vandelli MA, Boeckers TM, Forni F, Zoli M. Insight on the fate of CNS-targeted nanoparticles. Part i: Rab5-dependent cell-specific uptake and distribution. Journal of Controlled Release. 2014 Jan 28;174:195–201.
37. Kreuter J. Nanoparticulate systems for brain delivery of drugs. Advanced Drug Delivery Reviews. 2001 Mar 23;47(1):65–81.
38. Kreuter J. Mechanism of polymeric nanoparticle-based drug transport across the blood-brain barrier (BBB). Journal of Microencapsulation. 2013;30(1):49–54.
39. Liu X, Yang Y, Urban MW. Stimuli-responsive polymeric nanoparticles. Macromolecular Rapid Communications. 2017;38(13):1700030.
40. Cheng R, Meng F, Deng C, Klok HA, Zhong Z. Dual and multi-stimuli responsive polymeric nanoparticles for programmed site-specific drug delivery. Biomaterials. 2013;34(14):3647–57.
41. Karimi M, Sahandi Zangabad P, Ghasemi A, Amiri M, Bahrami M, Malekzad H, Ghahramanzadeh Asl H, Mahdieh Z, Bozorgomid M, Ghasemi A, Rahmani Taji Boyuk MR. Temperature-responsive smart nanocarriers for delivery of therapeutic agents: Applications and recent advances. ACS Applied Materials & Interfaces. 2016 Aug 24;8(33):21107–33.
42. Alvarez-Lorenzo C, Bromberg L, Concheiro A. Light-sensitive intelligent drug delivery systems. Photochemistry and Photobiology. 2009;85(4):848–60.
43. Jhaveri A. Magnetic field-responsive nanocarriers. Smart Pharmaceutical Nanocarriers. 2015;31:267–308.
44. Gong B, Sanford AR, Ferguson JS, Filipcsei G, Csetneki I, Szilágyi A, Zrínyi M. Magnetic field-responsive smart polymer composites. Oligomers-Polymer Composites-Molecular Imprinting. 2007;137–89.
45. Li N, Cai H, Jiang L, Hu J, Bains A, Hu J, Gong Q, Luo K, Gu Z. Enzyme-sensitive and amphiphilic PEGylated dendrimer-paclitaxel prodrug-based nanoparticles for enhanced stability and anticancer efficacy. ACS Applied Materials & Interfaces. 2017;9(8):6865–77.
46. Shah A, Aftab S, Nisar J, Ashiq MN, Iftikhar FJ. Nanocarriers for targeted drug delivery. Journal of Drug Delivery Science and Technology. 2021;62:102426.
47. Chamundeeswari M, Jeslin J, Verma ML. Nanocarriers for drug delivery applications. Environmental Chemistry Letters. 2019 Jun 15;17:849–65.
48. Gullotti E, Yeo Y. Extracellularly activated nanocarriers: A new paradigm of tumor targeted drug delivery. Molecular Pharmaceutics. 2009;6(4):1041–51.
49. Sundar S, Kundu J, Kundu SC. Biopolymeric nanoparticles. Science and Technology of Advanced Materials. 2010 Feb 26;11(1):014104.
50. Kreuter J. Drug delivery to the central nervous system by polymeric nanoparticles: What do we know? Advanced Drug Delivery Reviews. 2014;71:2–14.
51. Vergoni AV, Tosi G, Tacchi R, Vandelli MA, Bertolini A, Costantino L. Nanoparticles as drug delivery agents specific for CNS: In vivo biodistribution. Nanomedicine: Nanotechnology, Biology and Medicine. 2009;5(4):369–77.
52. Zhang X, Zhou J, Gu Z, Zhang H, Gong Q, Luo K. Advances in nanomedicines for diagnosis of central nervous system disorders. Biomaterials. 2021;269:120492.
53. Mieszawska AJ, Mulder WJ, Fayad ZA, Cormode DP. Multifunctional gold nanoparticles for diagnosis and therapy of disease. Molecular Pharmaceutics. 2013;10(3):831–47.
54. Farrell BT, Hamilton BE, Dósa E, Rimely E, Nasseri M, Gahramanov S, Lacy CA, Frenkel EP, Doolittle ND, Jacobs PM, Neuwelt EA. Using iron oxide nanoparticles to diagnose CNS inflammatory diseases and PCNSL. Neurology. 2013 Jul 16;81(3):256–63.
55. Hanif S, Muhammad P, Niu Z, Ismail M, Morsch M, Zhang X, Li M, Shi B. Nanotechnology-based strategies for early diagnosis of central nervous system disorders. Advanced NanoBiomed Research. 2021;1(10):2100008.

56. Ferdows BE, Patel DN, Chen W, Huang X, Kong N, Tao W. RNA cancer nanomedicine: Nanotechnology-mediated RNA therapy. Nanoscale. 2022;14(12):4448–55.
57. Di Francesco V, Chua AJ, Huang D, D'Souza A, Yang A, Bleier BS, Amiji MM. RNA therapies for CNS diseases. Advanced Drug Delivery Reviews. 2024; Mar 16:115283.
58. Padmakumar S, D'Souza A, Parayath NN, Bleier BS, Amiji MM. Nucleic acid therapies for CNS diseases: Pathophysiology, targets, barriers, and delivery strategies. Journal of Controlled Release. 2022;352:121–45.
59. Perez-Martinez FC, Carrion B, Cena V. The use of nanoparticles for gene therapy in the nervous system. Journal of Alzheimer's Disease. 2012;31(4):697–710.
60. Silva GA. Nanotechnology approaches for the regeneration and neuroprotection of the central nervous system. Surgical Neurology. 2005;63(4):301–6.
61. Barua S, Mitragotri S. Challenges associated with penetration of nanoparticles across cell and tissue barriers: A review of current status and future prospects. Nano Today. 2014;9(2):223–43.
62. Dobrovolskaia MA. Nanoparticle toxicity: General overview and insights into immunological compatibility. Pharmaceutical Nanotechnology. 2017; Volumes: Innovation and Production. 2.19.
63. Borrajo ML, Alonso MJ. Using nanotechnology to deliver biomolecules from nose to brain—Peptides, proteins, monoclonal antibodies and RNA. Drug Delivery and Translational Research. 2022;1:1–9.
64. Paliwal R, Babu RJ, Palakurthi S. Nanomedicine scale-up technologies: Feasibilities and challenges. Aaps Pharmscitech. 2014;15(6):1527–34.
65. Mittal D, Ali A, Md S, Baboota S, Sahni JK, Ali J. Insights into direct nose to brain delivery: Current status and future perspective. Drug Delivery. 2014;21(2):75–86.
66. Alghamdi MA, Fallica AN, Virzì N, Kesharwani P, Pittalà V, Greish K. The promise of nanotechnology in personalized medicine. Journal of Personalized Medicine. 2022 Apr 22;12(5):673.
67. Alqawlaq S, Huzil JT, Ivanova MV, Foldvari M. Challenges in neuroprotective nanomedicine development: Progress towards noninvasive Gene therapy of glaucoma. Nanomedicine. 2012;7(7):1067–83.

5 Nanomedicine

A Promising Way to Manage Alzheimer's Disease

Saish Pawar, Pawan Ganesh Nayak, Sarika Sharma, Surabhi Singh, Nidhi Puranik, and Arun Sharma

5.1 INTRODUCTION

Alzheimer's disease (AD) is a neurological illness that worsens with time and has a substantial effect on cognitive function. It causes behavioral abnormalities, language impairment, and impaired memory and cognitive abilities [1,2]. As AD is the most frequent cause of dementia in older persons, its rising incidence and lack of effective treatment choices present a major challenge to global health systems [3]. Millions of individuals worldwide are afflicted by AD, and as the population ages, it is predicted that the prevalence will increase significantly. Over 55 million individuals worldwide, with AD accounting for 60–70% of cases, are estimated to have dementia, according to the World Health Organization [4,5]. Due to the enormous socioeconomic burden of AD, hundreds of billions of dollars are spent each year on healthcare, lost productivity, and caring [6]. The incidences of AD are expected to double every 20 years as life expectancy rises, and more effective therapy approaches are desperately needed.

During AD pathology, tau protein tangles and amyloid-beta (Aβ) plaques accumulate in the brain, leading to neurodegeneration and cognitive decline [7,8]. Aβ plaques are extracellular deposits resulting from abnormal processing of amyloid precursor protein (APP), while tau tangles are intracellular aggregates composed of hyperphosphorylated tau proteins [9,10]. Due to the disruption of synaptic function and interference with neural communication, these aberrant traits result in substantial shrinking of the brain [8,11]. Even though the molecular mechanisms behind AD, developing effective therapies is still difficult due to the complex interplay of genetic, environmental, and lifestyle factors [2].

Innovative therapies that address the multifactorial character of AD are desperately needed, especially with the shortcomings of existing therapeutics. To treat AD effectively, methods that can alter disease processes at the molecular level, enhance medication transport to the brain, and minimize side effects are needed. Nanomedicine represents a solution to these problems with its ability to transform therapeutic targeting and drug delivery [12–14]. Figure 5.1 is providing a complete overview of AD therapeutics target, biomarkers and nanotechnological approaches used in AD treatment.

Applying the concepts of nanotechnology to the diagnosis, treatment, and prevention of diseases at the molecular and cellular levels is known as nanomedicine [15,16].

DOI: 10.1201/9781003543381-5

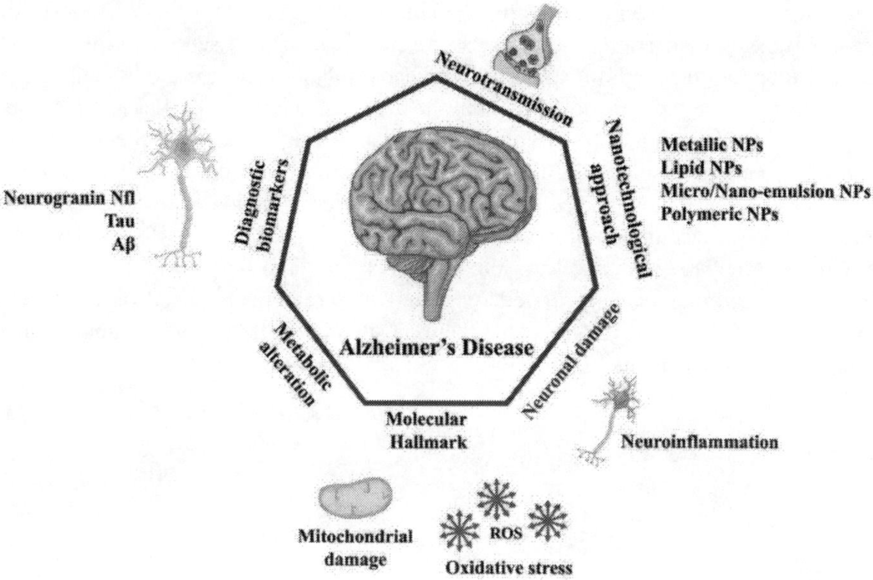

FIGURE 5.1 Schematic representation of therapeutic agents for Alzheimer's disease (AD), and use of various nanoparticles in the management of AD. (Reproduced from Ref. [12] [CC BY-NC 3.0].)

Targeted therapy, better imaging methods, and improved drug delivery are all made possible by the application of nanoscale materials and devices, such as liposomes, dendrimers, and nanoparticles [17–19]. Because of their small size and huge surface area, nanomaterials can precisely interact with biological systems, which makes them excellent choices for treating complicated disorders like AD [20].

Nanotechnology significantly changes the management of AD due to its ability to provide answers to persistent problems with drug distribution and efficacy. To help in the transport of therapeutic substances straight to the brain, for example, nanoparticles can be designed to penetrate the blood-brain barrier (BBB), which is a significant barrier in the treatment of neurological illnesses [21,22]. Personalized medicine in AD may also be made possible by nanomedicine through the creation of multifunctional platforms that integrate therapeutic and diagnostic functions. With the advancement of research in this field, nanomedicine comes as a more effective and focused approach for treating AD [23,24]. This chapter explores how nanomedicine, which is developing at the nexus of nanotechnology and medicine, may be able to solve the shortcomings of existing Alzheimer's therapies and provide encouraging new approaches to this illness.

5.2 NANOMEDICINE IN THE CONTEXT OF AD

Nanomedicine provides new pathways for the delivery of treatment agents, diagnosis, and AD monitoring by utilizing the special qualities of nanoscale materials [13,25]. Operating at the nanoscale, nanomedicine usually deals with objects that have a diameter of 1 to 100 nanometers [26,27]. These materials at the nanoscale consist of nanoparticles, nanocarriers, and nanosystems, all of which are essential for therapeutic intervention and drug administration. Drug encapsulation, surface modification, and controlled release are functions that may be achieved with nanoparticles, which are minuscule particles made of different materials including metals, polymers, or lipids [28,29]. Common nanocarriers used in drug delivery are represented in Figure 5.2.

A subclass of nanoparticles known as nanocarriers is made expressly to deliver medications to certain locations in the body, increasing treatment effectiveness and minimizing negative effects. Liposomes, dendrimers, and polymeric nanoparticles are a few examples of nanocarriers; each has unique benefits based on the therapeutic needs [30]. However, to enable theragnostic applications in AD, nanosystems relate to several elements, such as therapeutic and diagnostic agents [31].

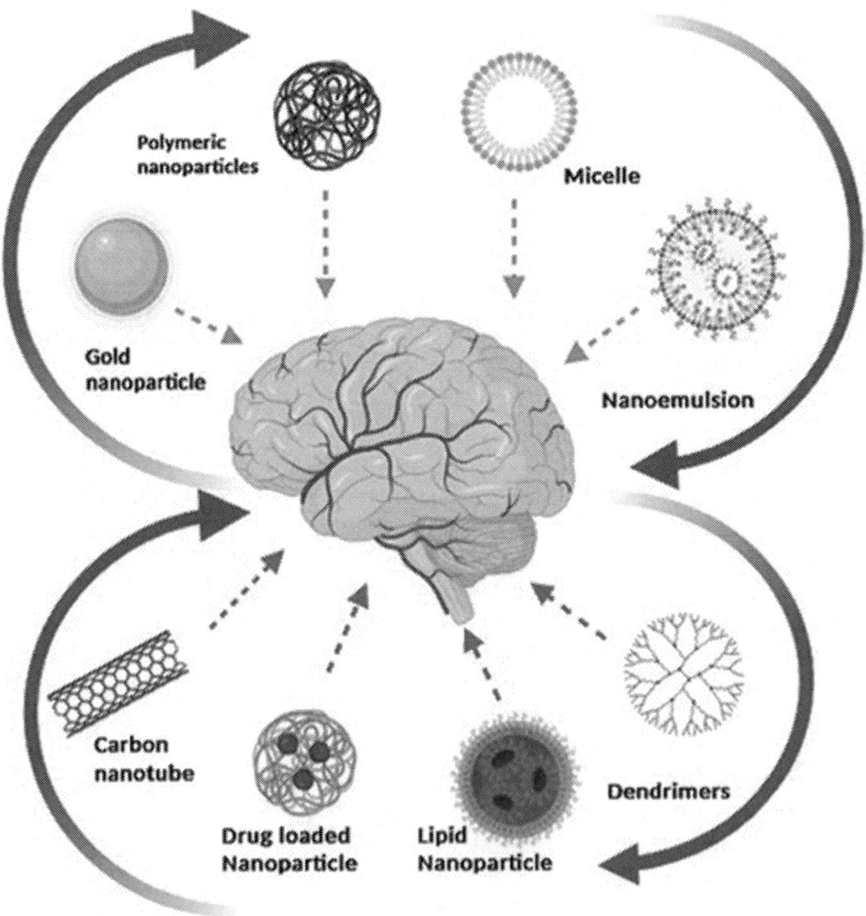

FIGURE 5.2 Nanomaterials for development of different novel drug carriers for brain targeting of therapeutics.

These systems' nanoscale design offers several benefits over conventional drug delivery techniques, especially when it comes to neurological conditions like AD. Delivering therapeutic agents across the BBB, a highly selective membrane that protects the brain but also blocks the passage of most medications is one of the biggest obstacles in the treatment of AD [32,33]. By exploiting processes like receptor-mediated endocytosis or momentarily rupturing the barrier with external stimuli like ultrasound or magnetic fields, nanoparticles can be designed to evade the BBB [34].

Targeting the molecular elements that drive the disease's progression is one of the main ways that nanomedicine interacts with AD pathogenesis. The main pathological characteristics of AD are tau protein tangles and Aβ plaques, which build up and cause neurodegeneration and cognitive loss [9]. Functionalizing nanoparticles with ligands or antibodies that bind to tau or Aβ selectively allows for targeted medicine administration or elimination of these harmful aggregates from the brain [35–37].

The ability of gold nanoparticles (AuNPs) to bind to Aβ plaques, for example, has been investigated as a potential delivery system for therapeutic drugs or as a diagnostic tool for imaging plaques using methods such as magnetic resonance imaging (MRI) or positron emission tomography (PET) scans [38,39]. As a potential therapeutic approach to reduce or stop the course of AD, nanocarriers loaded with siRNA or antisense oligonucleotides can be utilized to downregulate the expression of genes implicated in the generation or aggregation of tau and Aβ [40–42].

Nanomedicine offers potential not only for therapeutic uses but also for early AD diagnosis. Because substantial neuronal damage frequently occurs before the manifestation of clinical symptoms, early diagnosis is essential for effective treatment.

5.3 TYPES OF NANOMATERIALS USED IN AD MANAGEMENT

There is a wide range of nanomaterials available in nanomedicine, each with special qualities and uses in the treatment of AD. These materials are intended to increase the delivery of medications to the brain, improve imaging for diagnostic purposes, and offer novel therapeutic alternatives. This chapter examines several kinds of nanomaterials, such as lipid-based, polymer-based, metallic, carbon-based, and emerging nanomaterials that are employed in AD management.

5.3.1 Lipid-Based Nanoparticles: Liposomes and Solid Lipid Nanoparticles

The most researched nanocarriers for medication delivery in AD are lipid-based nanoparticles, such as liposomes and solid lipid nanoparticles (SLNs). The liposomes are spherical vesicles made of lipid bilayers that can encapsulate both hydrophilic and hydrophobic medicines, shielding them from degradation and enabling targeted delivery to the brain [43]. Liposomes are an effective way to transfer therapeutic compounds across the BBB because of their biocompatibility and ability to merge with cell membranes [44,45].

Similar benefits are provided by SLNs, which are made up of a solid lipid core stabilized by surfactants. SLNs are well-known for their stability, controlled drug release capabilities, and capacity to increase the bioavailability of medications with low solubility [46,47]. Preclinical research on SLNs' potential for delivering neuroprotective and anti-amyloid medications in the context of AD has produced encouraging findings [48].

Lipid-based nanoparticles have demonstrated a great deal of promise in administering a variety of therapeutic drugs directly to the brain [48]. They include small molecule medications, peptides, and nucleic acids that target tau protein aggregation, Aβ plaques, and other pathological characteristics of AD. Drugs like donepezil and curcumin have been encapsulated in liposomes to improve their therapeutic efficacy and brain transport [49–51]. In a similar vein, medications with neuroprotective and anti-amyloidogenic qualities as quercetin and resveratrol have been administered via SLNs [52–56].

5.3.2 Polymer-Based Nanoparticles: Dendrimers and Polymeric Micelles

Polymer-based nanoparticles, including as polymeric micelles and dendrimers, are another significant class of nanomaterials in the control of AD. Dendrimers are polymers that resemble trees and have many branches. They can be specifically designed to deliver drugs. High drug loading capacity and multivalent interactions with biological targets are made possible by their special structure [57]. Targeting ligands can be used to functionalize dendrimers, allowing them to pass across the BBB and deliver medications only to areas of the brain affected by AD [57–59].

Amphiphilic block copolymers self-assemble to generate polymeric micelles, which are another adaptable drug delivery platform. These micelles can encapsulate hydrophobic medicines within their core, shielding them from degradation and enabling regulated release [60]. Polymeric micelles have been investigated as a means of delivering medications such as galantamine and tacrine, which are used to treat cognitive symptoms in AD [61,62].

The capacity of polymer-based nanoparticles to deliver regulated and prolonged medication release is one of their main benefits [63,64]. For example, dendrimers can be engineered to release medications in response to particular stimuli, including pH changes or changes in enzyme activity, guaranteeing that the medication is delivered exactly where and when it is required [57]. Because polymeric micelles release medications gradually over time, they can assist in maintaining therapeutic concentrations in the brain, which lowers dosage frequency and increases patient compliance [65].

5.3.3 Metallic Nanoparticles: Gold, Silver, and Iron Oxide Nanoparticles

The distinct optical, magnetic, and chemical characteristics of metallic nanoparticles, such as gold, silver, and iron oxide nanoparticles, have attracted a lot of attention in AD research. Because of their biocompatibility and simplicity of functionalization, AuNPs are particularly well-known for being suitable for both therapeutic and diagnostic applications. To target tau proteins and Aβ plaques, AuNPs can be coupled with medicines, antibodies, or peptides. This allows for their removal from the brain or the delivery of therapeutic agents right to the pathological region [66].

Although silver nanoparticles (AgNPs) are most recognized for their antibacterial capabilities [67], they have also demonstrated promise in reducing inflammation [68] and oxidative stress in the brain, two major factors in the advancement of AD [69].

Conversely, iron oxide nanoparticles (IONPs) are frequently employed as contrast agents in MRI because of their superparamagnetic characteristics. It is possible to functionalize IONPs to target Aβ plaques, which will allow for the monitoring of disease development and early identification of AD [70].

5.3.3.1 Use of Metallic Nanoparticles in Imaging, Diagnostics, and Therapy

There are numerous applications for metallic nanoparticles in AD imaging, diagnosis, and treatment. For example, AuNPs have been used in a variety of imaging modalities, including computed tomography (CT) and surface-enhanced Raman scattering (SERS), to find AD biomarkers early on [71]. Due to the high magnetic characteristics of iron oxide nanoparticles, MRI contrast is improved, making it possible to see brain structures and pathological abnormalities such Aβ plaques in detail [70,72].

Metallic nanoparticles are being investigated for their possible applications in medicine in addition to imaging [73]. Using photothermal treatment, which involves converting light into heat to dissolve Aβ aggregates specifically, AuNPs have the potential to lower the brain's amyloid burden [74]. Comparably, iron oxide nanoparticles provide a non-invasive method of treating AD in magnetic hyperthermia, a condition in which an alternating magnetic field causes localized warmth [75].

5.3.4 Carbon-Based Nanomaterials: Carbon Nanotubes and Fullerenes

Carbon-based nanomaterials have great promise for managing AD through medication delivery and neuroprotection [76]. The distinctive structural and electrical characteristics of carbon-based nanomaterials like carbon nanotubes (CNTs) and fullerenes are receiving more interest in nanomedicine. These nanomaterials are well-known for their exceptional strength, electrical conductivity, and huge surface area. CNTs are cylindrical structures made of rolled-up graphene sheets [77]. Therapeutic compounds can be functionalized into CNTs to deliver drugs to specific brain regions. They are appealing for neuro-regenerative uses in AD because they can also serve as scaffolding for neuronal development [78,79]. CNTs may pass through cell membranes and the BBB; they can carry medications directly to AD-affected neurons, which may lessen the disease's neurodegenerative consequences [80,81]. Because of their conductive qualities, they can also be used to connect with neural tissues, opening up the potential for neuroprosthetics and brain–computer interfaces [82].

Fullerenes are spherical molecules with antioxidant qualities that help shield neurons from oxidative stress, a major component in AD pathogenesis. Fullerenes are carbon atoms grouped in a form like a football [83]. Additionally, fullerenes can be altered to target particular brain regions with medications or imaging agents, which have potential use in both therapy and diagnostics [83].

Due to the strong antioxidant properties of fullerenes, fullerenes can reduce oxidative damage in the brain, which in turn lessens the risk of neuronal death in AD [84]. It is well reported that fullerenes possess the ability to transport several therapeutic drugs, hence offering a versatile platform for combination therapies that address distinct facets of AD pathogenesis.

5.3.5 Emerging Nanomaterials: Quantum Dots, Nanogels, and Other Innovative Materials

Apart from conventional nanomaterials, novel materials including nanogels and quantum dots (QDs) are also being investigated for their possible application in AD treatment. The QDs are semiconductor nanoparticles with special optical characteristics that make them perfect for imaging applications [85]. QDs can be utilized to identify and monitor tau tangles and amyloid plaques in AD, offering real-time information on the course of the illness and the effectiveness of treatment [86,87].

Three-dimensional networks of polymer chains, or nanogels, are incredibly adaptable and can encapsulate a broad variety of medications, proteins, or nucleic acids. They are especially well suited for medication delivery across the BBB due to their high-water content and biocompatibility [88]. Additionally, nano-gels can react to changes in temperature or pH, which allows for the regulated release of therapeutic drugs into the brain [89].

The possibility of other cutting-edge nanomaterials, like hybrid nanoparticles and metal-organic frameworks (MOFs), in AD treatment is also being studied [90]. These materials can provide special benefits like large surface area, adjustable pore sizes, and the capacity to mix organic and inorganic elements, opening up new possibilities for therapeutic intervention and drug administration [91].

5.4 NANOMEDICINE FOR TARGETED DRUG DELIVERY IN AD

When it comes to addressing the major obstacles related to medication delivery in AD, nanomedicine offers great promise. Getting therapeutic agents beyond the BBB, which strictly controls how drugs enter the brain, is one of the biggest challenges in creating successful treatments for AD. Due to their special qualities, nanoparticles provide novel approaches to this issue by allowing the targeted delivery of medications to particular diseased brain locations, such as tau protein clumps and Aβ plaques.

5.4.1 Challenges of Blood–Brain Barrier in AD Drug Delivery

Nanomedicine has significant potential in overcoming the main challenges associated with the delivery of medication in AD. Getting therapeutic agents beyond the BBB, which tightly regulates drug entry into the brain, is one of the most difficult tasks in developing effective AD treatments [92]. Unique properties of nanoparticles provide innovative solutions to this problem by enabling the targeted delivery of drugs to specific diseased brain regions. This chapter further explores the use of nanomedicine for targeted medication delivery in AD, with a focus on strategies to pass the BBB, target Aβ aggregates, and prevent tau protein aggregation.

5.4.2 Nanoparticle Strategies to Cross the BBB

There are multiple ways that nanoparticles can get past the BBB and get medications into the brain. One method entails coating the surface of nanoparticles with ligands that bind to particular BBB receptors on endothelial cells, such as low-density lipoprotein receptors, transferrin, or insulin receptors. Through endocytosis, the nanoparticles can pass the BBB thanks to receptor-mediated transport [93,94]. For instance, it has been demonstrated that transferrin-functionalized nanoparticles may effectively pass the BBB and transport therapeutic drugs to the brain, providing a potential therapy option for AD [95].

Another strategy involves the use of nanoparticles that can transiently disrupt the BBB to enhance drug delivery. This can be achieved through the application of external stimuli, such as ultrasound or magnetic fields, which can temporarily open the tight junctions of the BBB and allow nanoparticles to pass through [96,97]. Additionally, nanoparticles can be engineered to release their drug payload in response to specific stimuli within the brain, such as changes in pH or the presence of certain enzymes, ensuring that the drug is released precisely at the target site [98–100].

5.4.3 Targeting Amyloid-Beta Aggregates: Nanoparticles Designed to Bind and Clear Amyloid Plaques

Aβ plaques are one of the hallmark pathological features of AD, and their accumulation in the brain is closely associated with neurodegeneration and cognitive decline. Nanoparticles can be designed to specifically target and bind to Aβ aggregates, facilitating their clearance from the brain or delivering therapeutic agents directly to the plaques. For example, AuNPs functionalized with Aβ-specific peptides or antibodies have been shown to selectively bind to Aβ plaques, potentially preventing their aggregation and promoting their removal from the brain [38,101,102].

In addition to targeting Aβ plaques, nanoparticles can also deliver therapeutic agents that inhibit Aβ aggregation or enhance its clearance via the immune system. For instance, polymeric nanoparticles loaded with Aβ-degrading enzymes, such as neprilysin, have demonstrated the ability to reduce Aβ levels in the brain, offering a potential therapeutic strategy for AD. Similarly, nanoparticles carrying siRNA or antisense oligonucleotides can downregulate the expression of APP or β-secretase, key proteins involved in Aβ production, thereby reducing Aβ accumulation [103–105].

Preclinical studies have provided promising evidence for the therapeutic efficacy of nanoparticles targeting Aβ aggregates. For example, in animal models of AD, AuNPs conjugated with Aβ-specific antibodies have been shown to reduce Aβ plaque burden and improve cognitive function [106]. Additionally, lipid-based nanoparticles delivering curcumin, a natural compound with anti-amyloidogenic properties, have demonstrated the ability to inhibit Aβ aggregation and reduce oxidative stress in the brain [107,108].

While clinical studies on nanoparticle-based therapies for AD are still in the early stages, initial results are encouraging. Clinical trials investigating the safety and efficacy of liposomal formulations and polymeric nanoparticles in AD patients have shown favorable outcomes, with some studies reporting improvements in cognitive function and reductions in Aβ levels [109,110].

5.4.4 Tau Protein Targeting: Approaches to Prevent Tau Aggregation Using Nanomedicine

Another significant pathogenic aspect of AD is the formation of neurofibrillary tangles by tau proteins, which impair neuronal function and promote neurodegeneration. In the treatment of AD, preventing tau aggregation is thus a key therapeutic objective. There are multiple ways to target tau proteins and prevent their aggregation with nanomedicine. Toxic tangles can be avoided by tau-specific peptides or antibodies binding to tau, which can be used to functionalize nanoparticles [111].

Nanoparticles can be utilized to deliver therapeutic drugs that control tau phosphorylation, a process that is crucial to the creation of tau tangles, in addition to directly inhibiting tau aggregation. For example, tau hyperphosphorylation can be decreased by nanoparticles containing kinase inhibitors or phosphatase activators, which will stop neurofibrillary tangles from forming. Additionally, tau or related protein expression can be downregulated using siRNA-loaded nanoparticles, providing a gene-silencing strategy to stop tau pathology in AD.

Numerous preclinical investigations have shown that nanomedicine has the ability to reduce tau pathology and prevent the formation of neurofibrillary tangles. In animal models of AD, for instance, it has been demonstrated that dendrimer-based nanoparticles functionalized with tau-specific antibodies decrease tau aggregation and enhance neuronal function [112]. In a similar vein, preclinical models have shown that polymeric nanoparticles containing small-molecule inhibitors of tau aggregation might lessen tau pathology and enhance cognitive results [113].

5.5 DIAGNOSTIC APPLICATIONS OF NANOMEDICINE IN ALZHEIMER'S DISEASE

AD is a neurological illness that causes thinking difficulties, memory loss, and cognitive decline. Due to its complexity, AD requires sophisticated diagnostic methods to be detected early and treated effectively. The field of nanomedicine, which uses nanotechnology for medical purposes, has demonstrated great promise in improving AD diagnosis.

5.5.1 Role of Nanotechnology in Improving Diagnostic Imaging (MRI, PET Scans)

With its improved resolution and specificity for identifying AD-related degenerative alterations in the brain, nanotechnology has completely transformed the diagnostic imaging area. Particularly in the early stages of AD, traditional imaging modalities such as PET and MRI have limitations in terms of sensitivity and specificity. By serving as contrast agents, nanoparticles can be designed to improve these imaging modalities [114].

For example, amyloid plaques, a defining feature of D, can be more easily seen in MRI scans when the contrast is improved by using superparamagnetic iron oxide nanoparticles (SPIONs). By improving the magnetic resonance signals, these nanoparticles enable more accurate imaging of the anatomy of the brain and the identification of early degenerative alterations linked to AD [115,116].

Nanoparticles coupled with radioisotopes can target particular AD biomarkers in PET imaging. By using a tailored technique, PET scans become more accurate and can identify tau protein tangles and Aβ plaques earlier than with traditional methods [117,118]. Nanotechnology helps in early AD diagnosis, which is important for prompt intervention and disease management. This is achieved by increasing the quality of imaging.

It is essential to identify AD early to manage the condition before serious neuronal damage happens. Because of their special qualities, which include a large surface area and the capacity to be functionalized with certain ligands, nanoparticles present a promising option as biomarkers for early detection. These functionalized nanoparticles can attach to biomarkers associated with AD, such as tau proteins, Aβ plaques, and neuroinflammatory markers [119].

For instance, Aβ plaques can be found in blood samples and cerebrospinal fluid (CSF) using AuNPs functionalized with antibodies against Aβ [120]. This non-invasive technique offers a useful tool for early management by detecting AD at the molecular level before the onset of clinical symptoms.

Similarly, the potential for QDs, semiconductor nanoparticles, to fluoresce under specific circumstances, has been investigated. QDs can target and bind to tau proteins when conjugated with particular ligands, making it possible to identify tauopathies in AD early on [121]. These nanoparticles function as potent biomarkers, providing a cutting-edge method for the early diagnosis and tracking of AD progression.

5.5.2 Theranostics: Combining Therapy and Diagnosis in AD

Theranostics is an area that offers a more effective and individualized approach to managing diseases like AD by integrating pharmacological and diagnostic procedures on a single platform. In the field of theranostics, nanoparticles have two functions:

- Medication delivery systems
- Diagnostic tools

Theranostic nanoparticles have the potential to both detect AD and concurrently deliver therapeutic medicines to the brain regions impacted by the disease. Real-time tracking of the course of the disease and the efficacy of the treatment is made possible by this integrated method [122–124]. Theranostics provides a major benefit in controlling AD, where early intervention and ongoing monitoring are critical, by integrating diagnosis and therapy.

Moreover, preclinical research on AD has demonstrated the promise of polymeric nanoparticles loaded with neuroprotective and imaging medicines. Theranostics-purposed nanoparticles can be functionalized with a variety of substances to carry out both therapeutic and diagnostic tasks. For example, a single nanoparticle can be combined with a therapeutic medication to treat AD and a contrast agent for imaging [125]. This multifunctionality is very helpful for AD patients since the condition progresses and calls for constant care and observation.

Similar to liposomes, lipid-based nanoparticles have been investigated for their capacity to penetrate the BBB, target certain brain regions, and administer therapeutic drugs such as curcumin, a substance with anti-inflammatory and anti-amyloid characteristics [126,127]. Imaging tools can be used to track these nanoparticles, enabling a simultaneous evaluation of medication efficacy and distribution in the brain.

Moreover, preclinical research on AD has demonstrated the promise of polymeric nanoparticles loaded with neuroprotective and imaging medicines. By highlighting pathological abnormalities in the brain, these nanoparticles not only help in the early detection of AD but also offer sustained release of therapeutic medicines, slowing the rate at which neurodegeneration progresses [128]. Theranostics' dual use of nanoparticles is a promising approach to the overall management of AD.

5.6 CLINICAL AND PRECLINICAL STUDIES

The advancements in preclinical and clinical research pertaining to nanomedicine for AD are explored where clinical trials are starting to convert preclinical research utilizing animal models into prospective treatments for human patients.

5.6.1 Preclinical Studies: Overview of Animal Models Used in AD Research with Nanomedicine

To better understand AD and create treatments based on nanomedicine, animal models are essential. Before moving forward with human trials, these models aid in understanding the biology of the illness and in assessing the efficacy and safety of innovative therapeutic approaches. Transgenic mice that overexpress human genes linked to AD, such as tau proteins, presenilin-1 (PS1), and APP, are the most widely used animal models in AD research [129–131].

These models are useful for testing nanomedicine therapies because they mimic important characteristics of AD, such as the build-up of tau tangles, neuroinflammation, and Aβ plaques. For example, the effectiveness of nanoparticle-based therapy in lowering amyloid load and enhancing cognitive function has been widely assessed using the 5xFAD mouse model, which produces Aβ plaques and cognitive impairments quickly [132].

In these models, therapeutic medicines have been delivered using liposomes, dendrimers, and polymeric nanoparticles to target Aβ plaques, modify neuroinflammation, and pass the BBB. Nanoparticles are especially well suited for preclinical research because of their capacity to penetrate the BBB and selectively target brain areas impacted by AD [21].

5.6.1.1 Results and Implications from Key Preclinical Studies

Promising results from preclinical studies employing nanomedicine in animal models of AD indicate the potential of these strategies to improve cognitive function and halt the progression of the illness. Using polylactic glycolic acid (PLGA) nanoparticles loaded with curcumin, a substance recognized for its anti-inflammatory and anti-amyloid qualities, was one noteworthy work. These nanoparticles effectively decreased the burden of Aβ plaque and enhanced cognitive function when given to APP/PS1 transgenic mice [133].

In a significant investigation, 5xFAD mice were given AuNPs functionalized with antibodies against Aβ. The treated mice showed better memory and learning capacities as a result of these nanoparticles' reduction in amyloid load, neuroinflammation, and oxidative stress [120].

5.6.2 Clinical Trials and Human Studies: Status of Current Clinical Trials Involving Nanomedicine for AD

The application of nanomedicine in AD clinical practice is still in its infancy, despite encouraging preclinical research outcomes. Numerous clinical trials are currently being conducted to determine the best dosage, safety, and effectiveness of nanoparticle-based treatments in AD patients. These studies are essential to ascertain whether human benefits may be attributed to the same mechanisms as seen in animal models [134].

Using nanoparticles to deliver siRNA targeting BACE1, an enzyme involved in Aβ generation, was one of the first clinical trials for AD based on nanomedicine. The purpose of this trial was to lower brain levels of Aβ and decrease the rate of cognitive loss in people with mild to moderate AD. While the experiment is still in progress, first findings indicate that the medication is well tolerated, and there may be some indication of decreased levels of Aβ in the CSF.

The use of lipid nanoparticles to deliver a medicinal drug that targets tau protein aggregation is being investigated in another ongoing trial. Preclinical research showing these nanoparticles' capacity to lessen tau pathology and enhance cognitive performance in mice models of AD served as the foundation for this trial [112]. The results of these trials will play a crucial role in dictating the future course of AD nanomedicine.

5.7 CHALLENGES AND FUTURE PERSPECTIVES

AD is a devastating CNS disease, with BBB and BCFB being major pharmaceutical obstacles. BBB-targeted nanomedicine has been developed for treating AD, but clinical translation is challenging due to inadequate understanding of mechanisms, nanocarrier fate, toxicity, biocompatibility, and clearance. Comprehensive toxicological research is needed for brain-targeting nanoformulations. However, polymeric NPs, liposomes, nano-emulsions, and dendrimers have potential toxicity issues [14].

As nanomedicine develops as a potentially effective treatment for AD, several issues and concerns need to be considered to guarantee its safe and efficient application. This chapter addresses the main issues surrounding the toxicity and safety of nanomaterials, the difficulties in translating preclinical research into clinical applications, and the moral and societal ramifications of applying nanotechnology to the treatment of AD.

5.7.1 Safety and Toxicity of Nanomaterials

Although intriguing, the use of nanomaterials in medicine poses serious questions about their safety and potential toxicity. Because of their small size and strong reactivity, nanoparticles can interact with biological systems in unforeseen ways, which can have harmful effects that worsen rather than improve medical conditions. Because of their small size and strong reactivity, nanoparticles can interact with biological systems in unforeseen ways, which can have harmful effects that worsen rather than improve medical conditions. Knowing the toxicological profile of nanomaterials is important in the context of AD, because long-term treatment is frequently necessary [135].

The potential of nanoparticles to get through the BBB is one of the main worries. This characteristic increases the possibility of unintentional interactions with healthy brain tissues, which could result in neuroinflammation, oxidative stress, or even neurodegeneration, even if it is advantageous for drug delivery to the brain [34]. Research has indicated that some nanoparticles, like silver and carbon-based nanomaterials, can cause harmful effects in neural cells, emphasizing the necessity for thorough safety evaluations [136]. Thorough preclinical testing of nanoparticles is necessary to overcome these problems. This entails assessing their potential for both acute and chronic toxicity, as well as their biodistribution, metabolism, and bodily elimination. Furthermore, to forecast the long-term impacts of nanomedicine in AD treatment, more sophisticated in vitro and in vivo models that more closely resemble human physiology should be used.

5.7.2 Regulatory Challenges and Safety Assessments

Because nanoparticles have distinct features that set them apart from their bulk counterparts, regulating nanomedicine poses special issues. It's possible that existing regulatory frameworks—which were mostly created for conventional medications and medical devices—are not entirely appropriate for nanomedicine, calling for the creation of new policies and standards [137].

In an effort to address these issues, regulatory organizations like the European Medicines Agency (EMA) and the Food and Drug Administration (FDA) of the United States have established detailed standards for the assessment of nanoparticles. According to the EFSA Scientific Committee (2018), these guidelines are primarily concerned with characterizing nanomaterials, evaluating their pharmacokinetics and toxicity, and establishing the safety and effectiveness of these materials in clinical trials.

The absence of standardized techniques for assessing the safety of nanomaterials, however, is one of the major regulatory obstacles. This includes differences in the toxicity testing procedures, nanoparticle characterization techniques, and approval standards [138]. International cooperation and harmonization of regulatory standards are crucial to overcoming these obstacles and guaranteeing the safety and efficacy of nanomedicine for AD across diverse populations and healthcare systems.

5.7.3 Translational Challenges

It will be difficult to turn the encouraging findings of preclinical research into efficient treatments for AD. Although nanomedicine has demonstrated considerable promise in lab settings, there are a number of obstacles that must be addressed before it can be applied in clinical practice, including the complexity of human physiology, interindividual variability, and the strict guidelines for clinical trials [139].

The scalability of nanoparticle production is one of the main obstacles. Small batches of nanoparticles are frequently created in carefully monitored laboratory settings for use in preclinical research. One major problem is scaling up manufacturing to satisfy clinical demand without sacrificing the quality, safety, and efficacy of the nanoparticles. Furthermore, maintaining consistent treatment effects depends on the repeatability of nanoparticle manufacturing, especially about size, shape, and surface properties [140].

The incorporation of nanomedicine into current clinical protocols presents another difficulty. This entails teaching medical personnel how to properly use medicines based on nanomedicine in addition to developing novel treatment plans [141]. Furthermore, because of the difficulty in synthesizing and formulating nanoparticles, the cost of nanomedicine may be greater than that of traditional medicines, which could restrict its accessibility and broad acceptance [142].

5.7.4 Issues in Large-Scale Production and Standardization

Production of nanomedicine on a large scale presents several logistical and technical difficulties. For nanoparticles to be safe and effective, the manufacturing process needs to be optimized to generate particles with uniform quality and attributes. This necessitates the creation of reliable, scalable production processes in addition to strict quality assurance procedures [143].

Since there are now no widely recognized guidelines for the characterization and quality assurance of nanoparticles, standardization is another crucial issue. Standardized procedures are therefore required to measure the particle size, surface charge, and other physicochemical characteristics that may affect how nanoparticles behave in biological systems [144]. To obtain regulatory permission for clinical usage and to guarantee the repeatability of results across trials, these standards must be established.

5.7.5 Ethical and Societal Considerations

There are several ethical concerns with using nanomedicine for AD that need to be properly explored. Considering nanomaterials' unique and complicated character, one of the main concerns is the possibility of unexpected effects. Since the long-term consequences of nanomedicine are still being investigated, there is a chance that certain therapies will injure patients or result in unanticipated public health problems [145].

Conscientiousness is yet another crucial ethical concern. Due to their potential cognitive impairment, patients with AD may not be able to give their informed consent to participate in clinical trials employing nanomedicine [146,147]. These requirements are for creating transparent and unambiguous permission procedures that consider the cognitive deficits linked to AD and guarantee that patients and their families are properly educated about the advantages and disadvantages of nanomedicine.

Furthermore, distributing treatments based on nanomedicines fairly is a crucial ethical factor. If these sophisticated therapies are only available to a select few or are too expensive for those who can afford them, there is a chance that they will worsen already existing health inequities. To address these ethical issues, it is imperative to guarantee that nanomedicine is available to all AD patients, irrespective of their financial situation [148].

5.7.6 Public Perception and Acceptance of Nanotechnology

The public's acceptance and perception of nanomedicine as a treatment for AD will be just as important as its scientific and clinical advantages. Despite its promise, nanotechnology is frequently viewed with distrust and anxiety by the general public because of worries about its security and potential for abuse. The general public has little knowledge of nanotechnology, and false beliefs about its advantages and disadvantages may prevent the use of nanomedicine.

To overcome these issues, public participation and effective communication are crucial. Accurate information regarding the advantages and safety of nanomedicine must be given, and any ethical, legal, or societal ramifications must be addressed. Transparency in clinical application, research, and regulation, together with patient and public participation in the decision-making process, are all important ways to promote public trust in nanomedicine [149].

Future research should focus not just on advancing the scientific and technical elements of nanomedicine but also on recognizing and addressing the societal and ethical implications of its use. By doing this, it will be possible to fully realize how nanomedicine can transform AD treatment in a way that is safe, efficient, and considerate of society.

5.8 CONCLUSION

Treatment of AD, nanomedicine offers a novel and promising approach that solves many of the problems with conventional therapeutic and diagnostic techniques. The use of nanotechnology involved possibilities for early diagnosis, targeted medication administration, and potentially the possibility of stopping or even reversing the progression of AD.

Nanoparticles in diagnostic imaging have shown great potential in enhancing MRI and PET scans, enabling early identification of biomarkers associated with AD such as tau proteins and Aβ plaques. Thus, nanomedicine offers new hope for patients and care by representing a holistic and varied approach to AD management.

Numerous possible developments in nanomedicine could completely change the way this debilitating disease is treated in the future. New kinds of nanoparticles with superior properties and developments in nanoparticle design show the effectiveness and safety of nanomedicine in the treatment of AD. The future of nanomedicine in AD treatment is filled with potential advancements that could revolutionize how this devastating disease is managed.

REFERENCES

1. Puranik N, Song M. Insights into the role of microRNAs as clinical tools for diagnosis, prognosis, and as therapeutic targets in Alzheimer's disease. *International Journal of Molecular Sciences* 2024;25:9936. https://doi.org/10.3390/IJMS25189936
2. Kamatham PT, Shukla R, Khatri DK, Vora LK. Pathogenesis, diagnostics, and therapeutics for Alzheimer's disease: Breaking the memory barrier. *Ageing Res Rev* 2024;101:102481. https://doi.org/10.1016/J.ARR.2024.102481
3. Mangialasche F, Kivipelto M, Solomon A, Fratiglioni L. Dementia prevention: Current epidemiological evidence and future perspective. *Alzheimers Res Ther* 2012;4:6. https://doi.org/10.1186/ALZRT104.
4. WHO. A blueprint for dementia research 2022:72.
5. Dementia n.d. https://www.who.int/health-topics/dementia#tab=tab_2 (accessed February 6, 2025).
6. Clinical Trials for Alzheimer's & Dementia | Alzheimer's Association n.d. https://www.alz.org/alzheimers-dementia/research-and-progress/clinical-trials (accessed February 6, 2025).
7. Bloom GS. Amyloid-β and tau: The trigger and bullet in Alzheimer disease pathogenesis. *JAMA Neurol* 2014;71:505–8. https://doi.org/10.1001/JAMANEUROL.2013.5847
8. Rajmohan R, Reddy PH. Amyloid Beta and phosphorylated tau accumulations cause abnormalities at synapses of Alzheimer's disease neurons. *J Alzheimers Dis* 2017;57:975. https://doi.org/10.3233/JAD-160612.
9. Selkoe DJ, Hardy J. The amyloid hypothesis of Alzheimer's disease at 25 years. *EMBO Mol Med* 2016;8:595–608. https://doi.org/10.15252/EMMM.201606210
10. Zhang H, Wei W, Zhao M, Ma L, Jiang X, Pei H et al. Interaction between aβ and tau in the pathogenesis of Alzheimer's disease. *Int J Biol Sci* 2021;17:2181. https://doi.org/10.7150/IJBS.57078
11. Spires-Jones TL, Hyman BT The intersection of amyloid beta and tau at synapses in Alzheimer's disease. *Neuron* 2014;82:756. https://doi.org/10.1016/J.NEURON.2014.05.004.
12. Mir Najib Ullah SN, Afzal O, Altamimi ASA, Ather H, Sultana S, Almalki WH et al. Nanomedicine in the management of Alzheimer's disease: State-of-the-art. *Biomedicines* 2023;11:1752. https://doi.org/10.3390/BIOMEDICINES11061752
13. Khan NH, Mir M, Ngowi EE, Zafar U, Khakwani MMAK, Khattak S et al. Nanomedicine: A promising way to manage Alzheimer's disease. *Front Bioeng Biotechnol* 2021;9:630055. https://doi.org/10.3389/FBIOE.2021.630055
14. Puranik N, Yadav D, Song M. Advancements in the application of nanomedicine in Alzheimer's disease: A therapeutic perspective. *Int J Mol Sci* 2023;24. https://doi.org/10.3390/IJMS241814044
15. Shabani L, Abbasi M, Azarnew Z, Amani AM, Vaez A Neuro-nanotechnology: Diagnostic and therapeutic nano-based strategies in applied neuroscience. *BioMedical Engineering OnLine* 2023 22:1 2023;22:1–41. https://doi.org/10.1186/S12938-022-01062-Y
16. Malik S, Muhammad K, Waheed Y Emerging applications of nanotechnology in healthcare and medicine. *Molecules* 2023;28:6624. https://doi.org/10.3390/MOLECULES28186624
17. Tiwari G, Tiwari R, Bannerjee S, Bhati L, Pandey S, Pandey P et al. Drug delivery systems: An updated review. *Int J Pharm Investig* 2012;2:2. https://doi.org/10.4103/2230-973X.96920
18. Kurul F, Turkmen H, Cetin AE, Topkaya SN Nanomedicine: How nanomaterials are transforming drug delivery, bio-imaging, and diagnosis. *Next Nanotechnology* 2025;7:100129. https://doi.org/10.1016/J.NXNANO.2024.100129
19. Sim S, Wong NK Nanotechnology and its use in imaging and drug delivery (review). *Biomed Rep* 2021;14:42. https://doi.org/10.3892/BR.2021.1418

20. Chakraborty A, Mohapatra SS, Barik S, Roy I, Gupta B, Biswas A Impact of nanoparticles on amyloid β-induced Alzheimer's disease, tuberculosis, leprosy and cancer: A systematic review. *Biosci Rep* 2023;43:BSR20220324. https://doi.org/10.1042/BSR20220324
21. Saraiva C, Praça C, Ferreira R, Santos T, Ferreira L, Bernardino L Nanoparticle-mediated brain drug delivery: Overcoming blood–brain barrier to treat neurodegenerative diseases. *Journal of Controlled Release* 2016;235:34–47. https://doi.org/10.1016/J.JCONREL.2016.05.044
22. Mittal KR, Pharasi N, Sarna B, Singh M, Rachana, Haider S et al. Nanotechnology-based drug delivery for the treatment of CNS disorders. *Transl Neurosci* 2022;13:527. https://doi.org/10.1515/TNSCI-2022-0258.
23. Cacabelos R, Cacabelos P, Torrellas C. Personalized medicine of Alzheimer's disease. *Handbook of Pharmacogenomics and Stratified Medicine* 2014:563. https://doi.org/10.1016/B978-0-12-386882-4.00027-X
24. Puccetti M, Pariano M, Schoubben A, Giovagnoli S, Ricci M Biologics, theranostics, and personalized medicine in drug delivery systems. *Pharmacol Res* 2024;201:107086. https://doi.org/10.1016/J.PHRS.2024.107086
25. Hu L, Tao Y, Jiang Y, Qin F Recent progress of nanomedicine in the treatment of Alzheimer's disease. *Front Cell Dev Biol* 2023;11:1228679. https://doi.org/10.3389/FCELL.2023.1228679
26. Bayda S, Adeel M, Tuccinardi T, Cordani M, Rizzolio F The history of nanoscience and nanotechnology: From Chemical–Physical applications to nanomedicine. *Molecules* 2019;25:112. https://doi.org/10.3390/MOLECULES25010112
27. Khan I, Saeed K, Khan I Nanoparticles: Properties, applications and toxicities. *Arabian Journal of Chemistry* 2019;12:908–31. https://doi.org/10.1016/J.ARABJC.2017.05.011
28. Hsu CY, Rheima AM, Kadhim MM, Ahmed NN, Mohammed SH, Abbas FH et al. An overview of nanoparticles in drug delivery: Properties and applications. *S Afr J Chem Eng* 2023;46:233–70. https://doi.org/10.1016/J.SAJCE.2023.08.009
29. Khan SU, Ullah M, Saeed S, Saleh EAM, Kassem AF, Arbi FM et al. Nanotherapeutic approaches for transdermal drug delivery systems and their biomedical applications. *Eur Polym J* 2024;207:112819. https://doi.org/10.1016/J.EURPOLYMJ.2024.112819
30. Allen TM, Cullis PR Liposomal drug delivery systems: From concept to clinical applications. *Adv Drug Deliv Rev* 2013;65:36–48. https://doi.org/10.1016/J.ADDR.2012.09.037
31. Mura S, Couvreur P Nanotheranostics for personalized medicine. *Adv Drug Deliv Rev* 2012;64:1394–416. https://doi.org/10.1016/J.ADDR.2012.06.006
32. Kadry H, Noorani B, Cucullo L. A blood–brain barrier overview on structure, function, impairment, and biomarkers of integrity. *Fluids and Barriers of the CNS* 2020 17:12020;17():1–24. https://doi.org/10.1186/S12987-020-00230-3
33. Banks WA, Rhea EM, Reed MJ, Erickson MA. The penetration of therapeutics across the blood-brain barrier: Classic case studies and clinical implications. *Cell Rep Med* 2024;5:101760. https://doi.org/10.1016/J.XCRM.2024.101760
34. Oberdörster G, Oberdörster E, Oberdörster J Nanotoxicology: An emerging discipline evolving from studies of ultrafine particles. *Environ Health Perspect* 2005;113:823–39. https://doi.org/10.1289/EHP.7339
35. Jagaran K, Singh M. Nanomedicine for neurodegenerative disorders: Focus on Alzheimer's and Parkinson's diseases. *Int J Mol Sci* 2021;22. https://doi.org/10.3390/IJMS22169082
36. Tapia-Arellano A, Cabrera P, Cortés-Adasme E, Riveros A, Hassan N, Kogan MJ Tau- and α-synuclein-targeted gold nanoparticles: Applications, opportunities, and future outlooks in the diagnosis and therapy of neurodegenerative diseases. *J Nanobiotechnology* 2024;22:248. https://doi.org/10.1186/S12951-024-02526-0
37. Roghani AK, Garcia RI, Roghani A, Reddy A, Khemka S, Reddy RP et al. Treating Alzheimer's disease using nanoparticle-mediated drug delivery strategies/systems. *Ageing Res Rev* 2024;97:102291. https://doi.org/10.1016/J.ARR.2024.102291

38. Abbas M Potential role of nanoparticles in treating the accumulation of amyloid-Beta peptide in Alzheimer's patients. *Polymers* 2021;13:1051 2021;13:1051. https://doi.org/10.3390/POLYM13071051
39. Agraharam G, Saravanan N, Girigoswami A, Girigoswami K Future of Alzheimer's disease: Nanotechnology-based diagnostics and therapeutic approach. *Bionanoscience* 2022;12:1002–17. https://doi.org/10.1007/S12668-022-00998-8/METRICS
40. Jain U, Johari S, Srivastava P Current insights of nanocarrier-mediated Gene therapeutics to treat potential impairment of amyloid Beta protein and tau protein in Alzheimer's disease. *Molecular Neurobiology* 2023 61:4 2023;61:1969–89. https://doi.org/10.1007/S12035-023-03671-7
41. Muolokwu CE, Chaulagain B, Gothwal A, Mahanta AK, Tagoe B, Lamsal B et al. Functionalized nanoparticles to deliver nucleic acids to the brain for the treatment of Alzheimer's disease. *Front Pharmacol* 2024;15:1405423. https://doi.org/10.3389/FPHAR.2024.1405423/BIBTEX
42. Imran Sajid M, Sultan Sheikh F, Anis F, Nasim N, Sumbria RK, Nauli SM et al. siRNA drug delivery across the blood–brain barrier in Alzheimer's disease. *Adv Drug Deliv Rev* 2023;199:114968. https://doi.org/10.1016/J.ADDR.2023.114968
43. Sercombe L, Veerati T, Moheimani F, Wu SY, Sood AK, Hua S. Advances and challenges of liposome assisted drug delivery. *Front Pharmacol* 2015;6. https://doi.org/10.3389/FPHAR.2015.00286
44. Bors LA, Erdö F Overcoming the blood–brain barrier. Challenges and tricks for CNS drug delivery. *Scientia Pharmaceutica* 2019;87:6. https://doi.org/10.3390/SCIPHARM87010006
45. Burgess D, Morris M, Subramanyam M, Juhairiyah F, De Lange ECM Understanding drug delivery to the brain using liposome-based strategies: Studies that provide mechanistic insights are essential. *AAPS J* 2021;23:114. https://doi.org/10.1208/S12248-021-00648-Z
46. Mukherjee S, Ray S, Thakur RS Solid lipid nanoparticles: A modern formulation approach in drug delivery system. *Indian J Pharm Sci* 2009;71:349. https://doi.org/10.4103/0250-474X.57282
47. Müller RH, Mäder K, Gohla S Solid lipid nanoparticles (SLN) for controlled drug delivery – A review of the state of the art. *European Journal of Pharmaceutics and Biopharmaceutics* 2000;50:161–77. https://doi.org/10.1016/S0939-6411(00)00087-4
48. Satapathy MK, Yen TL, Jan JS, Tang RD, Wang JY, Taliyan R et al. Solid lipid nanoparticles (SLNs): An advanced drug delivery system targeting brain through BBB. *Pharmaceutics* 2021;13:1183. https://doi.org/10.3390/PHARMACEUTICS13081183
49. Wei XQ, Zhu JF, Wang XB, Ba K Improving the stability of liposomal curcumin by adjusting the inner aqueous chamber pH of liposomes. *ACS Omega* 2020;5:1120–6. https://doi.org/10.1021/ACSOMEGA.9B03293/ASSET/IMAGES/LARGE/AO9B03293_0006.JPEG
50. Nunes D, Loureiro JA, Pereira MC Drug delivery systems as a strategy to improve the efficacy of FDA-approved Alzheimer's drugs. *Pharmaceutics* 2022;14:2296. https://doi.org/10.3390/PHARMACEUTICS14112296
51. Al Asmari AK, Ullah Z, Tariq M, Fatani A Preparation, characterization, and in vivo evaluation of intranasally administered liposomal formulation of donepezil. *Drug Des Devel Ther* 2016;10:205–15. https://doi.org/10.2147/DDDT.S93937
52. Loureiro JA, Andrade S, Duarte A, Neves AR, Queiroz JF, Nunes C et al. Resveratrol and grape extract-loaded solid lipid nanoparticles for the treatment of Alzheimer's disease. *Molecules* 2017;22. https://doi.org/10.3390/MOLECULES22020277
53. Rahman MH, Akter R, Bhattacharya T, Abdel-Daim MM, Alkahtani S, Arafah MW et al. Resveratrol and neuroprotection: Impact and its therapeutic potential in Alzheimer's disease. *Front Pharmacol* 2020;11:619024. https://doi.org/10.3389/FPHAR.2020.619024
54. Teskač K, Kristl J The evidence for solid lipid nanoparticles mediated cell uptake of resveratrol. *Int J Pharm* 2010;390:61–9. https://doi.org/10.1016/J.IJPHARM.2009.10.011

55. Pinheiro RGR, Granja A, Loureiro JA, Pereira MC, Pinheiro M, Neves AR et al. Quercetin lipid nanoparticles functionalized with transferrin for Alzheimer's disease. *Eur J Pharm Sci* 2020;148. https://doi.org/10.1016/J.EJPS.2020.105314
56. Dhawan S, Kapil R, Singh B Formulation development and systematic optimization of solid lipid nanoparticles of quercetin for improved brain delivery. *J Pharm Pharmacol* 2011;63:342–51. https://doi.org/10.1111/J.2042-7158.2010.01225.X
57. Kesharwani P, Jain K, Jain NK Dendrimer as nanocarrier for drug delivery. *Prog Polym Sci* 2014;39:268–307. https://doi.org/10.1016/J.PROGPOLYMSCI.2013.07.005
58. Palan F, Chatterjee B Dendrimers in the context of targeting central nervous system disorders. *J Drug Deliv Sci Technol* 2022;73:103474. https://doi.org/10.1016/J.JDDST.2022.103474
59. Arbez-Gindre C, Steele BR, Micha-Screttas M Dendrimers in Alzheimer's disease: Recent approaches in multi-targeting strategies. *Pharmaceutics* 2023;15:898. https://doi.org/10.3390/PHARMACEUTICS15030898
60. Adams ML, Lavasanifar A, Kwon GS Amphiphilic block copolymers for drug delivery. *J Pharm Sci* 2003;92:1343–55. https://doi.org/10.1002/JPS.10397
61. Gothwal A, Lamptey RNL, Singh J Multifunctionalized cationic chitosan polymeric micelles polyplexed with pVGF for noninvasive delivery to the mouse brain through the intranasal route for developing therapeutics for Alzheimer's disease. *Mol Pharm* 2023;20:3009–19. https://doi.org/10.1021/ACS.MOLPHARMACEUT.3C00031
62. Kaur J, Gulati M, Kapoor B, Jha NK, Gupta PK, Gupta G et al. Advances in designing of polymeric micelles for biomedical application in brain related diseases. *Chem Biol Interact* 2022;361:109960. https://doi.org/10.1016/J.CBI.2022.109960
63. Begines B, Ortiz T, Pérez-Aranda M, Martínez G, Merinero M, Argüelles-Arias F et al. Polymeric nanoparticles for drug delivery: Recent developments and future prospects. *Nanomaterials* 2020;10:1403. https://doi.org/10.3390/NANO10071403
64. Bhardwaj H, Jangde RK Current updated review on preparation of polymeric nanoparticles for drug delivery and biomedical applications. *Next Nanotechnology* 2023;2:100013. https://doi.org/10.1016/J.NXNANO.2023.100013
65. Adepu S, Ramakrishna S Controlled drug delivery systems: Current status and future directions. *Molecules* 2021;26:5905. https://doi.org/10.3390/MOLECULES26195905
66. Hong Q, Zhou JX, Shao CJ Gold nanoparticles with amyloid-β reduce neurocell cytotoxicity for the treatment and care of Alzheimer's disease therapy. *Gold Bull* 2023;56:135–44. https://doi.org/10.1007/S13404-023-00327-1/METRICS
67. Bruna T, Maldonado-Bravo F, Jara P, Caro N Silver nanoparticles and their antibacterial applications. *Int J Mol Sci* 2021;22:7202. https://doi.org/10.3390/IJMS22137202
68. Carvalho-Silva JM, Reis AC Anti-inflammatory action of silver nanoparticles in vivo: Systematic review and meta-analysis. *Heliyon* 2024;10. https://doi.org/10.1016/j.heliyon.2024.e34564
69. Gonzalez-Carter DA, Leo BF, Ruenraroengsak P, Chen S, Goode AE, Theodorou IG et al. Silver nanoparticles reduce brain inflammation and related neurotoxicity through induction of H2S-synthesizing enzymes. *Sci Rep* 2017;7. https://doi.org/10.1038/SREP42871
70. Qiao R, Fu C, Forgham H, Javed I, Huang X, Zhu J et al. Magnetic iron oxide nanoparticles for brain imaging and drug delivery. *Adv Drug Deliv Rev* 2023;197:114822. https://doi.org/10.1016/J.ADDR.2023.114822
71. Bouché M, Hsu JC, Dong YC, Kim J, Taing K, Cormode DP Recent advances in molecular imaging with gold nanoparticles. *Bioconjug Chem* 2019;31:303. https://doi.org/10.1021/ACS.BIOCONJCHEM.9B00669
72. Kim JH, Ha TL, Im GH, Yang J, Seo SW, Lee IS et al. Magnetic resonance imaging of amyloid plaques using hollow manganese oxide nanoparticles conjugated with antibody aβ1-40 in a transgenic mouse model. *Neuroreport* 2013;24:16–21. https://doi.org/10.1097/WNR.0B013E32835BA850

73. Kowalska A, Adamska E, Grobelna B Medical applications of silver and gold nanoparticles and core-shell nanostructures based on silver or gold core: Recent progress and innovations. *ChemMedChem* 2024;19:e202300672. https://doi.org/10.1002/CMDC.202300672
74. dos Santos Tramontin N, da Silva S, Arruda R, Ugioni KS, Canteiro PB, de Bem Silveira G et al. Gold nanoparticles treatment reverses brain damage in Alzheimer's disease model. *Mol Neurobiol* 2020;57:926–36. https://doi.org/10.1007/S12035-019-01780-W
75. Luo S, Ma C, Zhu MQ, Ju WN, Yang Y, Wang X Application of iron oxide nanoparticles in the diagnosis and treatment of neurodegenerative diseases with emphasis on Alzheimer's disease. *Front Cell Neurosci* 2020;14:21. https://doi.org/10.3389/FNCEL.2020.00021
76. Mohajeri M, Behnam B, Barreto GE, Sahebkar A Carbon nanomaterials and amyloid-beta interactions: Potentials for the detection and treatment of Alzheimer's disease? *Pharmacol Res* 2019;143:186–203. https://doi.org/10.1016/J.PHRS.2019.03.023
77. Jayaprakash N, Elumalai K, Manickam S, Bakthavatchalam G, Tamilselvan P. Carbon nanomaterials: Revolutionizing biomedical applications with promising potential. *Nano Materials Science* 2024. https://doi.org/10.1016/J.NANOMS.2024.11.004
78. Ghosh R, Bag J, Datta A, Pramanick A, Abubakar IH Functionalized carbon nanotubes-a Boon in treating brain diseases. *J Appl Pharm Sci* 2023;13:32–039. https://doi.org/10.7324/JAPS.2023.107158
79. Xiang C, Zhang Y, Guo W, Liang XJ Biomimetic carbon nanotubes for neurological disease therapeutics as inherent medication. *Acta Pharm Sin B* 2019;10:239. https://doi.org/10.1016/J.APSB.2019.11.003
80. Mishra J, Kumar B, Pandey M, Pottoo FH, Fayaz F, Khan FA et al. Carbon nano tubes: Novel drug delivery system in amelioration of Alzheimer's disease. *Comb Chem High Throughput Screen* 2020;24:1528–43. https://doi.org/10.2174/1386207323999200918112538
81. Elsori D, Rashid G, Khan NA, Sachdeva P, Jindal R, Kayenat F et al. Nanotube breakthroughs: Unveiling the potential of carbon nanotubes as a dual therapeutic arsenal for Alzheimer's disease and brain tumors. *Front Oncol* 2023;13. https://doi.org/10.3389/FONC.2023.1265347/BIBTEX
82. Rosenfeld JV, Wong YT. Neurobionics and the brain–computer interface: current applications and future horizons 2017. https://doi.org/10.5694/mja16.01011
83. Wilson DL, Ahlawat J, Narayan M The role of fullerenes in neurodegenerative disorders. *Journal of Nanotheranostics* 2024;5:1–12. https://doi.org/10.3390/JNT5010001
84. Omar Khudhur Z, Maad AH, Ghanimi HA, Abdolmaleki A Fullerene nanoparticle as new therapeutic agent for the nervous system disorders. *Nanomed J* 2024;11:342–59. https://doi.org/10.22038/NMJ.2024.78043.1903
85. Mimona MA, Rimon MIH, Zohura FT, Sony JM, Rim SI, Arup MMR et al. Quantum dot nanomaterials: Empowering advances in optoelectronic devices. *Chemical Engineering Journal Advances* 2025;21:100704. https://doi.org/10.1016/J.CEJA.2025.100704
86. Feng L, Long HY, Liu RK, Sun DN, Liu C, Long LL et al. A quantum dot probe conjugated with aβ antibody for molecular imaging of Alzheimer's disease in a mouse model. *Cell Mol Neurobiol* 2013;33:759–65. https://doi.org/10.1007/S10571-013-9943-6
87. Lin X, Galaqin N, Tainaka R, Shimamori K, Kuragano M, Noguchi TQP et al. Real-time 3D imaging and inhibition analysis of various amyloid aggregations using quantum dots. *Int J Mol Sci* 2020;21:1978. https://doi.org/10.3390/IJMS21061978
88. Soni G, Yadav KS Nanogels as potential nanomedicine carrier for treatment of cancer: A mini review of the state of the art. *Saudi Pharmaceutical Journal* 2016;24:133–9. https://doi.org/10.1016/J.JSPS.2014.04.001
89. Manimaran V, Nivetha RP, Tamilanban T, Narayanan J, Vetriselvan S, Fuloria NK, et al. Nanogels as novel drug nanocarriers for CNS drug delivery. *Front Mol Biosci* 2023;10:1232109. https://doi.org/10.3389/FMOLB.2023.1232109

90. Zhang G, Shen Y, Phipps J, Sun L, Ma S Metal-organic frameworks for the diagnosis and treatment of Alzheimer's disease: Current status and perspectives. *Coord Chem Rev* 2024;518:216059. https://doi.org/10.1016/J.CCR.2024.216059
91. Zhang J, Li M, Liu M, Yu Q, Ge D, Zhang J Metal–Organic framework nanomaterials as a medicine for catalytic tumor therapy: Recent advances. *Nanomaterials* 2024;14:797. https://doi.org/10.3390/NANO14090797
92. Wu D, Chen Q, Chen X, Han F, Chen Z, Wang Y The blood–brain barrier: Structure, regulation and drug delivery. *Signal Transduction and Targeted Therapy* 2023 8:1 2023;8:1–27. https://doi.org/10.1038/s41392-023-01481-w
93. Shilo M, Motiei M, Hana P, Popovtzer R Transport of nanoparticles through the blood–brain barrier for imaging and therapeutic applications. *Nanoscale* 2014;6:2146–52. https://doi.org/10.1039/C3NR04878K
94. van den Broek SL, Shalgunov V, Herth MM Transport of nanomedicines across the blood-brain barrier: Challenges and opportunities for imaging and therapy. *Biomaterials Advances* 2022;141:213125. https://doi.org/10.1016/J.BIOADV.2022.213125
95. Johnsen KB, Bak M, Melander F, Thomsen MS, Burkhart A, Kempen PJ et al. Modulating the antibody density changes the uptake and transport at the blood-brain barrier of both transferrin receptor-targeted gold nanoparticles and liposomal cargo. *Journal of Controlled Release* 2019;295:237–49. https://doi.org/10.1016/J.JCONREL.2019.01.005
96. Lim SH, Yee GT, Khang D Nanoparticle-based combinational strategies for overcoming the blood-brain barrier and blood-tumor barrier. *Int J Nanomedicine* 2024;19:2529. https://doi.org/10.2147/IJN.S450853
97. Hersh AM, Alomari S, Tyler BM Crossing the blood-brain barrier: Advances in nanoparticle technology for drug delivery in neuro-oncology. *Int J Mol Sci* 2022;23:4153. https://doi.org/10.3390/IJMS23084153
98. Torchilin VP Multifunctional, stimuli-sensitive nanoparticulate systems for drug delivery. *Nat Rev Drug Discov* 2014;13:813–27. https://doi.org/10.1038/NRD4333
99. Shrestha B, Wang L, Brey EM, Uribe GR, Tang L Smart nanoparticles for chemo-based combinational therapy. *Pharmaceutics* 2021;13:853. https://doi.org/10.3390/PHARMACEUTICS13060853
100. Mitchell MJ, Billingsley MM, Haley RM, Wechsler ME, Peppas NA, Langer R Engineering precision nanoparticles for drug delivery. *Nature Reviews Drug Discovery* 2020 20:2 2020;20:101–24. https://doi.org/10.1038/s41573-020-0090-8
101. Zhao J, Xu N, Yang X, Ling G, Zhang P The roles of gold nanoparticles in the detection of amyloid-β peptide for Alzheimer's disease. *Colloids and Interface Science Communications* 2022;46. https://doi.org/10.1016/j.colcom.2021.100579
102. Huang Y, Chang Y, Liu L, Wang J Nanomaterials for modulating the aggregation of β-amyloid peptides. *Molecules* 2021;26:4301. https://doi.org/10.3390/MOLECULES26144301
103. Li V, Huang Y. Oligonucleotide therapeutics for neurodegenerative diseases. *NeuroImmune Pharmacology and Therapeutics* 2024;1–11. https://doi.org/10.1515/NIPT-2024-0013
104. Grabowska-Pyrzewicz W, Want A, Leszek J, Wojda U Antisense oligonucleotides for Alzheimer's disease therapy: From the mRNA to miRNA paradigm. *EBioMedicine* 2021;74:103691. https://doi.org/10.1016/J.EBIOM.2021.103691
105. Zhou Y, Zhu F, Liu Y, Zheng M, Wang Y, Zhang D et al. Blood-brain barrier-penetrating siRNA nanomedicine for Alzheimer's disease therapy. *Sci Adv* 2020;6. https://doi.org/10.1126/SCIADV.ABC7031/SUPPL_FILE/ABC7031_SM.PDF
106. Sun ZT, Ma C, Li GJ, Zheng XY, Hao YT, Yang Y et al. Application of antibody fragments against aβ with emphasis on combined application with nanoparticles in Alzheimer's disease. *Front Pharmacol* 2021;12:654611. https://doi.org/10.3389/FPHAR.2021.654611/BIBTEX

107. Maiti P, Paladugu L, Dunbar GL Solid lipid curcumin particles provide greater anti-amyloid, anti-inflammatory and neuroprotective effects than curcumin in the 5xFAD mouse model of Alzheimer's disease. *BMC Neurosci* 2018;19:7. https://doi.org/10.1186/S12868-018-0406-3
108. Sadegh Malvajerd S, Azadi A, Izadi Z, Kurd M, Dara T, Dibaei M et al. Brain delivery of curcumin using solid lipid nanoparticles and nanostructured lipid carriers: Preparation, optimization, and pharmacokinetic evaluation. *ACS Chem Neurosci* 2019;10:728–39. https://doi.org/10.1021/ACSCHEMNEURO.8B00510
109. Gupta J, Fatima MT, Islam Z, Khan RH, Uversky VN, Salahuddin P Nanoparticle formulations in the diagnosis and therapy of Alzheimer's disease. *Int J Biol Macromol* 2019;130:515–26. https://doi.org/10.1016/J.IJBIOMAC.2019.02.156
110. Kuo YC, Chen IY, Rajesh R Use of functionalized liposomes loaded with antioxidants to permeate the blood–brain barrier and inhibit β-amyloid-induced neurodegeneration in the brain. *J Taiwan Inst Chem Eng* 2018;87:1–14. https://doi.org/10.1016/J.JTICE.2018.03.001
111. Kfoury N, Holmes BB, Jiang H, Holtzman DM, Diamond MI Trans-cellular propagation of tau aggregation by fibrillar species. *J Biol Chem* 2012;287:19440–51. https://doi.org/10.1074/JBC.M112.346072
112. Ma R, Mu Q, Xi Y, Liu G, Liu C Nanotechnology for tau pathology in Alzheimer's disease. *Mater Today Bio* 2024;27:101145. https://doi.org/10.1016/J.MTBIO.2024.101145
113. Pawar S, Rauf MA, Abdelhady H, Iyer AK. Tau-targeting nanoparticles for treatment of Alzheimer's disease. *Exploration* 2024;20230137. https://doi.org/10.1002/EXP.20230137
114. Viola KL, Sbarboro J, Sureka R, De M, Bicca MA, Wang J et al. Towards non-invasive diagnostic imaging of early-stage Alzheimer's disease. *Nat Nanotechnol* 2014;10:91. https://doi.org/10.1038/NNANO.2014.254
115. Sillerud LO, Solberg NO, Chamberlain R, Orlando RA, Heidrich JE, Brown DC et al. SPION-enhanced magnetic resonance imaging of Alzheimer's disease plaques in AβPP/PS-1 transgenic mouse brain. *J Alzheimers Dis* 2013;34:349–65. https://doi.org/10.3233/JAD-121171
116. Tafoya MA, Madi S, Sillerud LO Superparamagnetic nanoparticle-enhanced MRI of Alzheimer's disease plaques and activated microglia in 3X transgenic mouse brains: Contrast optimization. *Journal of Magnetic Resonance Imaging* 2017;46:574–88. https://doi.org/10.1002/JMRI.25563
117. Lois C, Gonzalez I, Johnson KA, Price JC PET imaging of tau protein targets: A methodology perspective. *Brain Imaging Behav* 2019;13:333. https://doi.org/10.1007/S11682-018-9847-7
118. Morbelli S, Bauckneht M Amyloid PET imaging: Standardization and integration with other Alzheimer's disease biomarkers. *Methods Mol Biol* 2018;1750:203–12. https://doi.org/10.1007/978-1-4939-7704-8_13
119. Saraiva C, Praça C, Ferreira R, Santos T, Ferreira L, Bernardino L Nanoparticle-mediated brain drug delivery: Overcoming blood-brain barrier to treat neurodegenerative diseases. *J Control Release* 2016;235:34–47. https://doi.org/10.1016/J.JCONREL.2016.05.044
120. Gao G, Zhang M, Gong D, Chen R, Hu X, Sun T The size-effect of gold nanoparticles and nanoclusters in the inhibition of amyloid-β fibrillation. *Nanoscale* 2017;9:4107–13. https://doi.org/10.1039/C7NR00699C
121. Li H, Zhang Y, Ding J, Wu T, Cai S, Zhang W et al. Synthesis of carbon quantum dots for application of alleviating amyloid-β mediated neurotoxicity. *Colloids Surf B Biointerfaces* 2022;212:112373. https://doi.org/10.1016/J.COLSURFB.2022.112373
122. Ahmad J, Akhter S, Rizwanullah M, Khan MA, Pigeon L, Addo RT et al. Nanotechnology based theranostic approaches in Alzheimer's disease management: Current status and future perspective. *Curr Alzheimer Res* 2017;14:1164. https://doi.org/10.2174/1567205014666170508121031

123. Tripathi P, Shukla P, Bieberich E Theranostic applications of nanomaterials in Alzheimer's disease: A multifunctional approach. *Curr Pharm Des* 2022;28:116–32. https://doi.org/10.2174/1381612827666211122153946
124. Toader C, Dumitru AV, Eva L, Serban M, Covache-Busuioc RA, Ciurea AV Nanoparticle strategies for treating CNS disorders: A comprehensive review of drug delivery and theranostic applications. *International Journal of Molecular Sciences* 2024;25:13302. https://doi.org/10.3390/IJMS252413302
125. Liu L, He H, Du B, He Y Nanoscale drug formulations for the treatment of Alzheimer's disease progression. *RSC Adv* 2025;15:4031–78. https://doi.org/10.1039/D4RA08128E
126. Fernandes F, Dias-Teixeira M, Delerue-Matos C, Grosso C Critical review of lipid-based nanoparticles as carriers of neuroprotective drugs and extracts. *Nanomaterials* 2021;11:563. https://doi.org/10.3390/NANO11030563
127. Teixeira MI, Lopes CM, Amaral MH, Costa PC Surface-modified lipid nanocarriers for crossing the blood-brain barrier (BBB): A current overview of active targeting in brain diseases. *Colloids Surf B Biointerfaces* 2023;221:112999. https://doi.org/10.1016/J.COLSURFB.2022.112999
128. Zhang W, Mehta A, Tong Z, Esser L, Voelcker NH Development of polymeric nanoparticles for blood–brain barrier transfer—Strategies and challenges. *Advanced Science* 2021;8:2003937. https://doi.org/10.1002/ADVS.202003937
129. Xu QQ, Yang W, Zhong M, Lin ZX, Gray NE, Xian YF Animal models of Alzheimer's disease: Preclinical insights and challenges. *Acta Materia Medica* 2023;2:192–215. https://doi.org/10.15212/AMM-2023-0001
130. Van Dam D, De Deyn PP Animal models in the drug discovery pipeline for Alzheimer's disease. *Br J Pharmacol* 2011;164:1285. https://doi.org/10.1111/J.1476-5381.2011.01299.X
131. Drummond E, Wisniewski T Alzheimer's disease: Experimental models and reality. *Acta Neuropathol* 2016;133:155. https://doi.org/10.1007/S00401-016-1662-X
132. Oakley H, Cole SL, Logan S, Maus E, Shao P, Craft J et al. Intraneuronal β-amyloid aggregates, neurodegeneration, and neuron loss in transgenic mice with five familial Alzheimer's disease mutations: Potential factors in amyloid plaque formation. *Journal of Neuroscience* 2006;26:10129–40. https://doi.org/10.1523/JNEUROSCI.1202-06.2006
133. Anand B, Wu Q, Nakhaei-Nejad M, Karthivashan G, Dorosh L, Amidian S et al. Significance of native PLGA nanoparticles in the treatment of Alzheimer's disease pathology. *Bioact Mater* 2022;17:506–25. https://doi.org/10.1016/J.BIOACTMAT.2022.05.030
134. Boyton I, Valenzuela SM, Collins-Praino LE, Care A Neuronanomedicine for Alzheimer's and Parkinson's disease: Current progress and a guide to improve clinical translation. *Brain Behav Immun* 2024;115:631–51. https://doi.org/10.1016/J.BBI.2023.11.004
135. Fadeel B, Garcia-Bennett AE Better safe than sorry: Understanding the toxicological properties of inorganic nanoparticles manufactured for biomedical applications. *Adv Drug Deliv Rev* 2010;62:362–74. https://doi.org/10.1016/J.ADDR.2009.11.008
136. Borm PJA, Robbins D, Haubold S, Kuhlbusch T, Fissan H, Donaldson K et al. The potential risks of nanomaterials: A review carried out for ECETOC. *Part Fibre Toxicol* 2006;3. https://doi.org/10.1186/1743-8977-3-11
137. Etheridge ML, Campbell SA, Erdman AG, Haynes CL, Wolf SM, McCullough J. The big picture on nanomedicine: The state of investigational and approved nanomedicine products. *Nanomedicine* 2013;9:1–14. https://doi.org/10.1016/J.NANO.2012.05.013
138. Ramos TI, Villacis-Aguirre CA, López-Aguilar KV, Padilla LS, Altamirano C, Toledo JR et al. The Hitchhiker's guide to human therapeutic nanoparticle development. *Pharmaceutics* 2022;14:247. https://doi.org/10.3390/PHARMACEUTICS14020247

139. Mak IWY, Evaniew N, Ghert M. Lost in translation: Animal models and clinical trials in cancer treatment. *Am J Transl Res* 2014;6:114.
140. Dobrovolskaia MA, Mcneil SE. Strategy for selecting nanotechnology carriers to overcome immunological and hematological toxicities challenging clinical translation of nucleic acid-based therapeutics. *Expert Opin Drug Deliv* 2015;12:1163–75. https://doi.org/10.1517/17425247.2015.1042857
141. Huertas JD, Fuentes YV, Garcia JC, Bustos RH. The role of education in nanomedicine as a current need for academic programs related to the healthcare field: A scoping review. *Adv Med Educ Pract* 2024;15:65–74. https://doi.org/10.2147/AMEP.S431359
142. Farjadian F, Ghasemi A, Gohari O, Roointan A, Karimi M, Hamblin MR. Nanopharmaceuticals and nanomedicines currently on the market: Challenges and opportunities. *Nanomedicine* 2018;14:93. https://doi.org/10.2217/NNM-2018-0120
143. Paliwal R, Babu RJ, Palakurthi S. Nanomedicine scale-up technologies: Feasibilities and challenges. *AAPS PharmSciTech* 2014;15:1527. https://doi.org/10.1208/S12249-014-0177-9
144. Gao X, Lowry GV. Progress towards standardized and validated characterizations for measuring physicochemical properties of manufactured nanomaterials relevant to nano health and safety risks. *NanoImpact* 2018;9:14–30. https://doi.org/10.1016/J.IMPACT.2017.09.002
145. Ma X, Tian Y, Yang R, Wang H, Allahou LW, Chang J et al. Nanotechnology in healthcare, and its safety and environmental risks. *Journal of Nanobiotechnology* 2024 22:12024;22():1–81. https://doi.org/10.1186/S12951-024-02901-X
146. Kim SYH. The ethics of informed consent in Alzheimer disease research. *Nat Rev Neurol* 2011;7:410. https://doi.org/10.1038/NRNEUROL.2011.76
147. Prusaczyk B, Cherney SM, Carpenter CR, DuBois JM. Informed consent to research with cognitively impaired adults: Transdisciplinary challenges and opportunities. *Clin Gerontol* 2016;40:63. https://doi.org/10.1080/07317115.2016.1201714
148. Uskoković V. Nanomedicine for the poor: A lost cause or an idea whose time has yet to come? *Nanomedicine* 2021;16:10.2217/nnm-2021–0024. https://doi.org/10.2217/NNM-2021-0024
149. Wasti S, Lee IH, Kim S, Lee JH, Kim H. Ethical and legal challenges in nanomedical innovations: A scoping review. *Front Genet* 2023;14:1163392. https://doi.org/10.3389/FGENE.2023.1163392/FULL

6 Gold Nanoparticles-Based Drug Delivery for Treatment and Management of Alzheimer's Disease

Pooja Singh and Rohit Kumar Singh

6.1 INTRODUCTION

Alzheimer's disease (AD) is a progressive neurodegenerative disorder that poses an escalating global healthcare crisis. Currently affecting over 50 million people worldwide, the prevalence of AD continues to rise dramatically due to increasing life expectancy and aging populations (Cummings et al., 2021). In the United States alone, AD ranks as the sixth-leading cause of death, with 121,499 deaths recorded in 2019 (Poudel and Park, 2022). Based on revised calculation, it was estimated that by 2050, approximately 12.7 million Americans over the age of 65 will be living with Alzheimer's dementia (Alzheimer's Association, 2012). AD leads to devastating cognitive functions including memory, reasoning, and executive abilities while inducing significant behavioral changes in older adults. The disease's pathological cascade begins with the accumulation of amyloid-beta (Aβ) proteins, triggering the formation of neurofibrillary tangles (NFTs) and ultimately leading to progressive neuronal degeneration. Neuropathologically, AD is characterized by two hallmark features: the extracellular deposition of Aβ plaques and the intracellular accumulation of hyperphosphorylated tau proteins (Jack et al., 2013; Nguyen et al., 2021). Aβ formation occurs through the proteolytic processing of amyloid precursor protein (APP), with elevated levels detectable in both cerebrospinal fluid and plasma of AD patients. While dual-target therapeutic strategies aim to both reduce Aβ plaque deposition and inhibit tau fibril formation (Murman and Colenda, 2005). While extensive research has investigated the crosstalk between Aβ and tau pathways, the precise molecular mechanisms by which Aβ drives AD pathogenesis remain incompletely understood, despite numerous studies exploring their interaction through various molecular signaling cascades (Vossel et al., 2010; Congdon and Sigurdsson, 2018; Nguyen et al., 2021).

Current therapeutic approaches for AD face significant limitations. While existing medications targeting cognitive decline primarily focus on modulating neurotransmitters and enzymes through intranasal delivery routes, their clinical efficacy remains

DOI: 10.1201/9781003543381-6

suboptimal (Sood et al., 2014; Khan et al., 2021). Treatment failures are frequently reported due to multiple challenges, including poor neuronal membrane penetration, limited drug stability, potential neurotoxicity, and unfavorable pharmacokinetic and pharmacodynamic profiles. Despite these therapeutic interventions, treatment failures occur frequently due to multiple pharmacological challenges, including poor neuronal membrane permeability, molecular instability, neurotoxicity, and suboptimal pharmacokinetic and pharmacodynamic properties (Khan et al., 2021).

Nanomaterials have become transformative tools for the diagnosis and treatment of neurological disorders, with their commercial and industrial applications expanding dramatically (Siddiqi et al., 2018; Asil et al., 2020). As an innovative field, nanomedicine leverages engineered nanomaterials (NMs) to overcome traditional therapeutic limitations, particularly in targeting complex organs like the brain. These advanced delivery systems enhance drug bioavailability and pharmacokinetic profiles while providing crucial protection for therapeutic compounds to damaged tissues (Singh and Singh, 2024). The field encompasses various nanostructures including metal nanoparticles, nanocarriers, nanotubes, microparticles, and polymeric nanomaterials (Figure 6.1). Each nanostructure engineered to facilitate

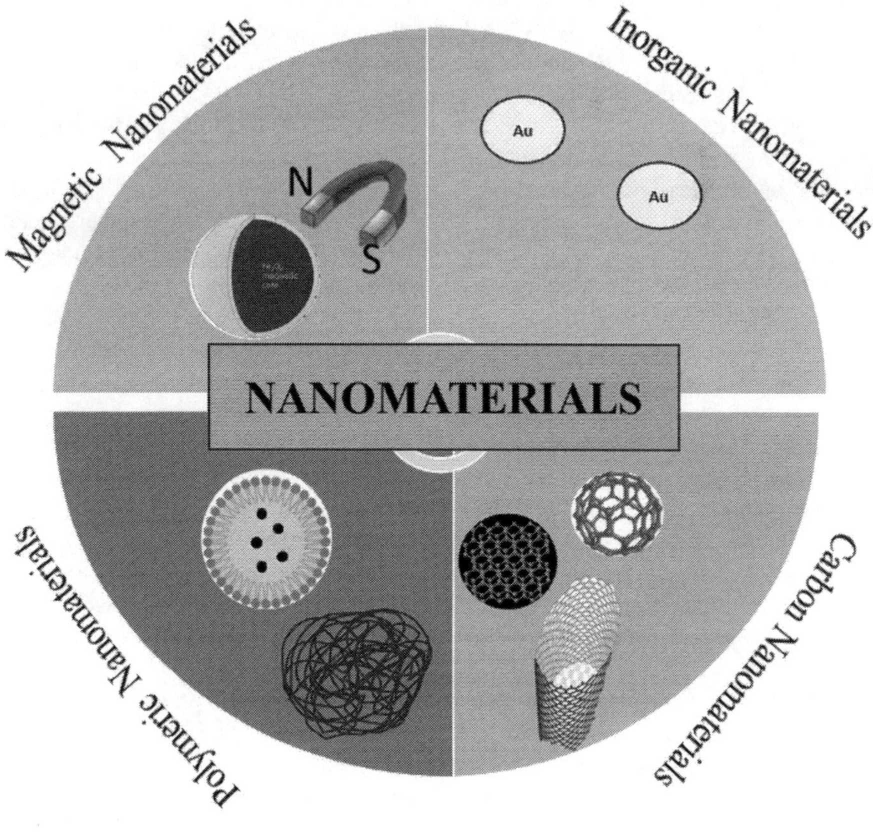

FIGURE 6.1 Carbon nanomaterials for Alzheimer's disease therapy.

accurate drug delivery to certain molecular targets (Saraiva et al., 2016). A key advantage of nano-based delivery systems lies in their ability to achieve controlled, sustained drug release, optimizing therapeutic efficacy while minimizing dosing frequency and potential side effects (Asil et al., 2020). These nanostructures can be precisely designed with specific size, surface charge, and functionalization to enhance brain penetration through the highly selective blood–brain barrier (BBB), a critical obstacle drug delivery. Their versatility allows for multiple therapeutic advantages: they can be engineered to carry higher drug payloads, provide controlled release kinetics, offer targeted delivery to specific brain regions, and potentially reduce systemic side effects. Furthermore, these nanocarriers can be modified with specific ligands to facilitate receptor-mediated transcytosis across the BBB, while simultaneously protecting their therapeutic cargo from premature degradation in the bloodstream. This multifunctional capability positions engineered NPs as particularly promising vehicles for addressing the complex pathophysiology of AD, where traditional therapeutic approaches have shown limited success (Mukherjee et al., 2020; Khan et al., 2021).

Gold nanoparticles (AuNPs) exhibit exceptional physicochemical properties that make them unique for diverse biomedical applications (Bansal et al., 2020; Nguyen and Falagan-Lotsch, 2023). These distinctive characteristics arise from their precise nanoscale dimensions, highly tunable surface chemistry, and unique optical and electronic properties, which collectively enable their versatile functionality in biological systems (Liu et al., 2021; Sarfraz and Khan, 2021). The fundamental properties of AuNPs can be attributed to their nanoscale architecture, which typically ranges from 1 to 100 nm in diameter, positioning them ideally for interactions with cellular and molecular components (Liu et al., 2021). The dimensional characteristics of AuNPs play a crucial function in their biological interactions and therapeutic efficacy. Their nanoscale size facilitates remarkable cellular permeability, enabling them to cross various biological barriers, including cell membranes and, under specific conditions, the BBB (Dreaden et al., 2012). This cellular internalization occurs primarily through endocytic pathways, making AuNPs excellent carriers for targeted therapeutic and diagnostic agents.

A particularly significant attribute of AuNPs is their exceptional surface-area-to-volume ratio, which provides an extensive platform for functionalization and molecular interactions. This high surface area enables efficient loading of various therapeutic molecules, including drugs, proteins, and nucleic acids, while maintaining the stability and bioactivity of the attached compounds (Liu and Peng, 2017). The surface chemistry of AuNPs can be precisely engineered through various modification strategies, including the attachment of targeting ligands, therapeutic agents, and protective coatings, which collectively enhance their therapeutic efficacy and biocompatibility. The ability to fine-tune these parameters allows for the optimization of AuNPs for specific biomedical applications, ranging from targeted drug delivery to molecular imaging and biosensing (Hammami and Alabdallah, 2021; Nguyen and Falagan-Lotsch, 2023). Moreover, their distinct optical characteristics, such as localized surface plasmon resonance (LSPR), allow them to be used in variety of diagnostic and therapeutic applications, including molecular imaging and photothermal treatment.

6.2 ALZHEIMER'S DISEASE

AD is a severe, often lethal, progressive neurological disorder that diminishes cognitive functions (Wilson and Geetha, 2020; Puranik et al., 2023). The predominant hypotheses regarding the etiology of AD involve the overproduction and plaque-forming aggregation of Aβ peptides and aberrant hyperphosphorylation of microtubule-associated tau protein, which results in the development of NFTs in the brains of AD patients. Furthermore, disrupted calcium signaling, impaired autophagy, glial cell activation, and neuronal demyelination are recognized as significant contributors to the pathophysiology of AD. Recent studies have indicated that persistent oxidative stress (OS), dysregulation of hormonal levels, impairment of mitochondrial function, inflammatory processes, genetic predispositions, and disruption of the BBB may significantly impact the etiology of AD (Nation et al., 2019). At present, the therapeutic interventions sanctioned by the Food and Drug Administration (FDA) primarily focus on two distinct biochemical pathways in AD, namely the aggregation of Aβ peptides and the formation of NFTs constituted by hyperphosphorylated tau protein. Nevertheless, these treatments exhibit limited efficacy in managing AD, emphasizing the urgent need for alternative therapeutic approaches. Development of new therapies for AD may be facilitated by the identification of additional molecular targets through the discovery of novel biomarkers (Cano et al., 2021; Puranik et al., 2023).

6.3 CURRENT CHALLENGES IN TREATMENT OF AD

The brain is the most well-protected organ in the body, which is protected by several defensive mechanisms. The brain maintains multiple protective layers – the skull, cerebrospinal fluid, meninges, and BBB. While these structures protect against harmful agents, they also impede therapeutic drug delivery to neural tissue. In diseased conditions, these protective structures impair the brain's ability to receive therapeutic medications (Hanif et al., 2020). The key barriers, involving the BBB, multidrug resistance proteins (MDRPs), and the blood–cerebrospinal fluid barrier (BCFB), are concisely discussed.

6.3.1 Blood–Brain Barrier Issues in Drug Delivery

The BBB is the main obstacle preventing nanomedicines from accessing the brain, limiting their capability to detect and cure AD. In order to enhance their ability to accumulate in the brain, nanomedicines should be carefully developed. The primary barrier to treating neurological disorders is the BBB, which keeps various drugs from reaching the brain in sufficient amounts (Tian et al., 2021). The BBB consist of pericytes, astrocytes, endothelial cells, and basal membranes with tight junctions providing it special properties. As a result, the BBB prevents medications that are helpful in treating a range of neurological disorders from entering the body. Brain capillaries have nearly no intercellular or interstitial gaps, making cellular transit necessary for most substances. The BBB may be easily crossed by Lipid-soluble substances since they can flow freely through endothelial membranes

(Mittal et al., 2022). Recent studies have explored a variety of approaches including as direct injection, the nose-to-brain route, BBB opening, efflux transporter inhibition, and nanocarrier systems to improve drug delivery across the BBB. Among these, nanocarriers have emerged as the most promising and effective approach (Puranik et al., 2023).

The utilization of advanced therapeutic nano-delivery systems has the potential to address the challenge of traversing the BBB (Jagaran and Singh, 2021; Yadav et al., 2022; Puranik et al., 2023). Due to their unique physicochemical characteristics and ability to cross the BBB, engineered nanoparticles measuring less than 100 nm possess several purposes in mitigating these pharmacological and biological challenges (Ghalamfarsa et al., 2016). The capacity of nanoparticles to penetrate the BBB enhances the prospects for initial diagnosis and effective treatment of neurological disorders. Six potential mechanisms for BBB penetration include paracellular diffusion (for hydrophilic molecules), transcellular diffusion, carrier-mediated transport, receptor-mediated transport, adsorptive-mediated transport, and cell-mediated transport (Sánchez-Dengra et al., 2023). Paracellular transport represents a passive mechanism by which substances are transported across epithelial tissue. The main rate-limiting barrier in the paracellular passage of bigger molecules across the epithelium is tight junctions. Adsorption-mediated transcytosis has garnered significant attention due to its potential for efficiently delivering large-molecule drugs to the brain (Puranik et al., 2023).

6.3.2 The Blood–Cerebrospinal Fluid Barrier

The BCFB, formed by choroid plexus epithelial cells, represents a critical checkpoint for drug transport into the central nervous system (CNS) beyond the BBB. The choroid plexus epithelium (CPE) is highly specialized, featuring sophisticated secretory systems that regulate cellular transport. Like the BBB, this epithelial barrier maintains strict separation between blood and cerebrospinal fluid (CSF). The CPE's tight junctions facing the CSF create a robust barrier, while its array of detoxifying enzymes and efflux transporters actively prevent potentially harmful substances from entering the CNS (Hersh et al., 2016; Pawar et al., 2022). While numerous drug delivery strategies have been developed for the BBB's microvascular endothelium, successful CNS drug delivery requires targeting both barriers, with particular attention to the BCFB's unique properties (Guo et al., 2023). The BCFB, though less studied than the BBB, presents an important therapeutic opportunity for enhancing CNS drug delivery and neuroprotection. Developing reliable in vitro BCFB models enables researchers to efficiently predict drug behavior at this barrier, reducing unnecessary experimentation. Future CNS drug delivery strategies could leverage the natural transport capabilities of choroid plexus epithelial cells. Although the choroid plexus has been historically overlooked as a drug delivery route to the brain, current in vitro BCFB models allow for preliminary assessment of transport mechanisms and efficiency. Three primary transport systems could potentially be targeted for drug delivery across the BCFB: solute carriers, protein receptors, and amino acid transporters (Dabbagh et al., 2022; Puranik et al., 2023).

6.3.3 Multidrug Resistance Proteins

The BBB is comprised with specialized endothelial cells in brain capillaries, which are endowed with several defense mechanisms. These cells have energy-dependent efflux transport proteins and a variety of metabolic enzymes, such as glutathione transferases, alkaline phosphatases, and cytochrome P450 enzymes. Among these transporters, P-glycoprotein (P-gp), MDRPs, and breast cancer resistance protein (BCRP; ABCG2) are crucial because of their asymmetrical arrangement, which effectively forms a barrier against foreign chemicals (Meyer et al., 1990). These transporters, which are members of the ATP-binding cassette (ABC) superfamily and specifically P-gp and BCRP, protect the brain by restricting the entry of a wide range of molecules (Aryal et al., 2017). While this protective function is crucial, it can also impede therapeutic success by preventing drugs from reaching their aimed targets and limiting drug accumulation in brain tissue (Yalamarty et al., 2023).

MDRP plays a particularly significant role in constraining the distribution of pharmaceuticals to the brain through its powerful efflux activity. Variations in the expression levels of MDRP can markedly influence the concentrations of drugs within both cerebral and spinal cord tissues. One potential strategy for improving drug delivery involves inhibiting P-gp function and expression. A key challenge in current pharmaceutical research is developing methods to effectively deliver medications across the MDRP system into the CNS. To effectively predict drug behavior in the CNS, this effort must be coupled with a deeper understanding of ABC transporter activity at both the BBB and BCFB (Puranik et al., 2023).

6.4 GOLD NANOPARTICLES AS THERAPEUTIC AGENTS

The complex pathophysiology of AD highlights the potential advantages of combination therapies over monotherapy in slowing cognitive decline and alleviating associated behavioral and social challenges. Currently, the FDA has authorized two principal pharmacological categories for AD management: acetylcholinesterase (AChE) inhibitors, comprising galantamine, donepezil, and rivastigmine; and N-methyl-D-aspartate (NMDA) receptor antagonists, represented by memantine. Clinical efficacy evaluation of these therapeutic agents typically employs standardized assessment instruments, including the Alzheimer's Disease Assessment Scale-Cognitive Subscale and the Disability Assessment in Dementia (DAD) scale (Singh and Singh, 2024). Despite the current therapeutic drugs, significant clinical challenges persist due to relapse frequently occurs as aging progresses, and the limited capacity of these pharmacological agents to effectively traverse the BBB that substantially restricts their therapeutic efficacy. To overcome these limitations, researchers have developed advanced drug delivery systems including metallic nanocarriers such as AuNPs, lipid and polymer-based nanostructures, hydrogel formulations, and drug-conjugate systems (Singh et al., 2024). These advanced delivery vehicles offer substantial advantages over conventional approaches by enhancing critical pharmacokinetic parameters including absorption, distribution, metabolism, and elimination profiles of therapeutic agents. Furthermore, these innovative systems can significantly improve drug solubility and facilitate enhanced permeation across biological barriers, particularly the restrictive BBB, thereby potentially increasing therapeutic concentrations at target sites within the CNS (Singh and Singh, 2024).

AuNPs have emerged as promising candidates in nanomedicine due to their exceptional physicochemical properties, comprising their tunable size, shape, surface chemistry, and optical characteristics. These unique properties enable their diverse applications across multiple medical conditions, particularly in neurological disorders. In the context of AD, AuNPs demonstrate remarkable potential through their ability to interact with Aβ peptides. This interaction occurs through multiple mechanisms, including directly attaching to Aβ monomers and oligomers, which stops them from clumping together to form neurotoxic plaques, which are the main pathogenic features of AD. The neuroprotective capabilities of AuNPs extend beyond their anti-aggregation properties, as they effectively function as antioxidant agents by scavenging reactive oxygen species (ROS) and attenuating OS-induced neuronal damage (Puranik et al., 2023; Chiang et al., 2024).

In the field of stroke therapy, AuNPs exhibit multifaceted therapeutic potential. They contribute to neuroprotection and regeneration through several pathways: modulating inflammatory responses by reducing pro-inflammatory cytokine production, mitigating OS through their intrinsic antioxidant properties, and promoting neuronal survival and regeneration in the ischemic brain environment. The distinctive properties of AuNPs, including their ability to penetrate the BBB, their low toxicity when properly functionalized, and their capacity for targeted drug delivery, make them particularly suitable for therapeutic interventions in neurological conditions. However, AuNP-based therapies face several critical challenges that require careful consideration. These include establishing standardized manufacturing procedures, maintaining uniform biodistribution and clearance, and maximizing therapeutic efficacy while avoiding possible toxicity by optimizing their size and surface chemistry (Chiang et al., 2024).

6.4.1 Biocompatibility and Safety Profiles of Gold Nanoparticles

AuNPs possess several additional characteristics that make them exceptionally valuable for biomedical applications. A primary advantage is their remarkable biocompatibility – gold's inherent chemical inertness and stability in biological systems minimize the risk of adverse immune responses and cytotoxicity. This intrinsic biocompatibility, combined with their controllable synthesis and stability, makes AuNPs particularly suitable for in vivo applications and long-term therapeutic interventions (Zhang et al., 2020).

The surface chemistry of AuNPs offers unprecedented versatility through facile functionalization processes. Their surface can be readily modified with a diverse array of molecules, including targeting ligands, antibodies, therapeutic agents, and imaging probes (Zhang et al., 2020). This exceptional flexibility in surface modification enables the creation of multifunctional platforms where different molecular entities can be integrated onto a single nanoparticle surface. Such customization allows for the development of precisely engineered nanoparticles that can simultaneously perform multiple functions, such as targeting specific cell types while delivering therapeutic payloads and enabling real-time imaging (Huang et al., 2023). AuNPs serve as sophisticated carriers that can significantly enhance therapeutic efficacy. They provide a protective environment for sensitive therapeutic compounds, shielding them from premature degradation in biological environments and maintaining their structural integrity until reaching the target site. The surface chemistry of AuNPs can be engineered to achieve controlled and sustained drug release profiles, optimizing the pharmacokinetics and bioavailability of the therapeutic agents. Stimulus-responsive components that initiate drug release in response to particular biological or environmental stimuli can be added to further improve this controlled release capacity.

The capacity of AuNPs to pass across biological barriers, especially the BBB, is one of their greatest benefits. Through careful surface engineering and functionalization strategies, AuNPs can be designed to efficiently cross this highly selective barrier, opening new avenues for treating neurological disorders (Khongkow et al., 2019). The surface modification can include specific targeting moieties that recognize BBB transporters or receptors, facilitating receptor-mediated transcytosis across the barrier. This capability, combined with their ability to carry therapeutic payloads, makes AuNPs particularly promising for treating various neurological conditions that have traditionally been challenging to address due to limited drug delivery across the BBB.

The toxicity and safety profile of AuNPs constitutes a critical area requiring comprehensive investigation, particularly for long-term neurological applications. Despite their promising therapeutic potential, the assessment of potential adverse effects demands careful consideration across multiple dimensions of safety and biocompatibility. In AuNP toxicity profiles, size emerges as a primary determinant. Smaller nanoparticles frequently demonstrate heightened toxicity attributable to their intensified surface reactivity and increased propensity to elicit cellular stress responses. This size-dependent relationship significantly influences the design parameters for safe and effective AuNP formulations (Kumar and Lim, 2021). The pharmacokinetic behavior of AuNPs, including their biodistribution patterns and clearance mechanisms, directly impacts their safety profile. Notably, smaller nanoparticles may experience rapid renal elimination, which affects both their systemic circulation time and potential accumulation in critical organs such as brain. Comprehending these complex pharmacokinetic relationships proves essential for evaluating long-term safety implications (Koushki et al., 2021; Chiang et al., 2024).

Surface modification strategies play a crucial role in enhancing AuNP safety profiles. The application of biocompatible coatings, such as specialized polymers or surfactants, significantly improves their biological compatibility while minimizing potential toxic effects associated with exposed nanoparticle surfaces. The evaluation of neurotoxicity requires particular attention to direct cellular impacts. This involves a thorough evaluation of any possible impairments to synapse activity, cellular survival, and neuronal function. Predicting the safety of AuNPs in neurological applications requires an understanding of their long-term impact on neural network integrity. Another important factor to consider is the possibility that AuNPs can trigger immunological reactions, which could result in inflammation or immune system stimulation. This issue becomes more important when considering neurological disorders, since long-term inflammation may make pre-existing pathological problems worse.

6.4.2 Potential Use of AuNPs in Alzheimer's Disease Therapy

AuNPs are currently being explored as a potentially effective therapeutic strategy for the management of AD owing to their distinctive characteristics (Aili et al., 2023). This section elucidates various applications of AuNPs. Neuroprotection: AuNPs may reduce inflammation and promote neuronal survival to have neuroprotective effects (Song et al., 2021). This mechanism could contribute to the preservation of cognitive abilities and the deceleration of disease advancement (Figure 6.2).

Promotion of neurogenesis: According to research studies, AuNPs have been demonstrated to facilitate neurogenesis, which may assist in the regeneration of injured neurons.

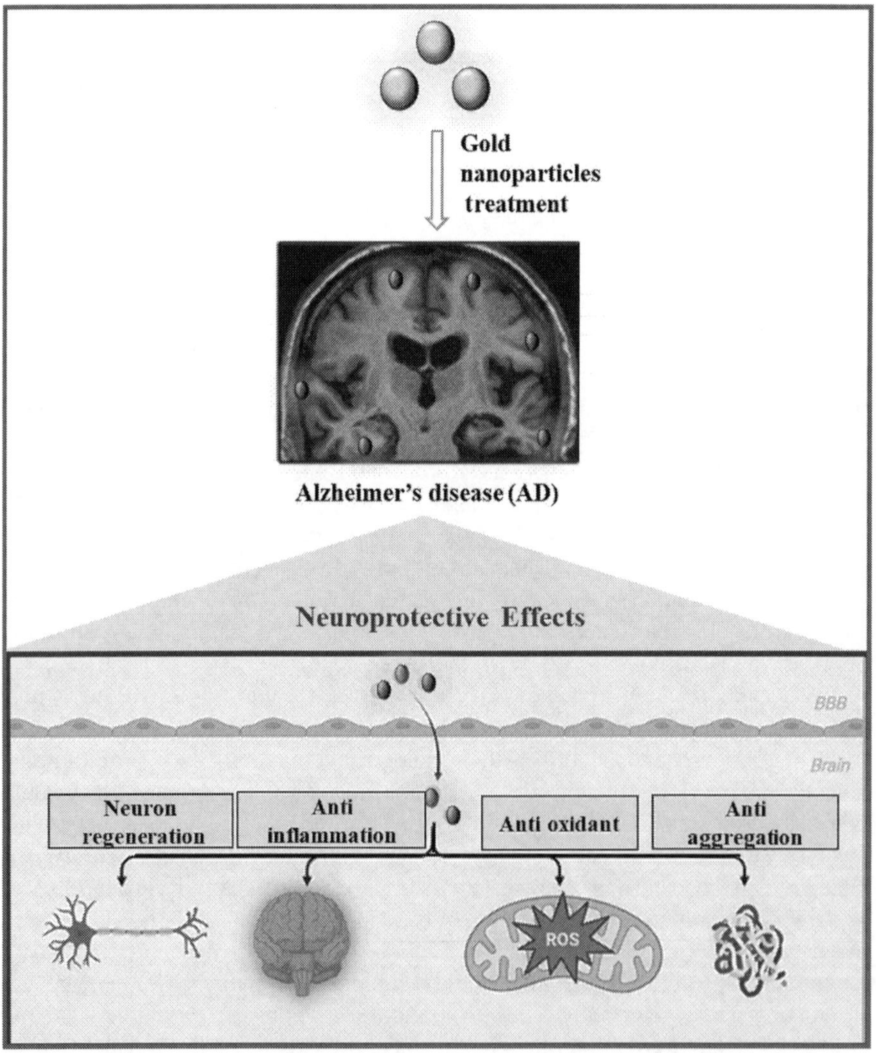

FIGURE 6.2 Neuroprotective effects of gold nanoparticles in Alzheimer's disease.

Immunological response modulation: AuNPs possess the capability to alter immunological responses, thereby potentially diminishing neuroinflammation, a prevalent characteristic of AD.

Effects of antioxidants: Certain AuNPs display antioxidant characteristics, which can be instrumental in alleviating OS. AD progression is linked to OS, which results in neuronal damage.

Anti-aggregation: Aβ protein aggregation may be inhibited by AuNPs, hence avoiding the production of harmful lesions that lead to neuronal injury and cognitive impairment (Table 6.1).

TABLE 6.1
Gold Nanoparticles-Based Drug Delivery for Alzheimer's Disease Treatment

Drug-loaded Gold Nanoparticle Type	Surface Functionalization	Therapeutic Findings	References
Gold nanoparticles	Glutathione	GSH-AuNPs showed the Aβ-induced reduction in the expression of nuclear factor erythroid 2-related factor 2 (Nrf2) and Nrf2 downstream antioxidant target genes (SOD-1, SOD-2, Gpx, Catalase, and HO-1)	(Chiang and Nicol, 2022)
Gold nanoparticles	L- and D-glutathione	chiral nanoparticles effectively cross the blood–brain barrier and prevent Aβ42 aggregation following intravenous administration without inducing systemic toxicity.	(Hou et al., 2020)
Anthocyanin-loaded gold nanoparticles	Polyethylene glycol	Anthocyanin-conjugated gold nanoparticles demonstrate neuroprotective effects in both in vitro and in vivo Alzheimer's disease models by attenuating $A\beta_{1-42}$-induced inflammation and apoptosis through suppression of the p-JNK/NF-κB/p-GSK3β signaling cascade.	(Kim et al., 2017)
Gold nanoparticles	Mimosine, plant-based amino acid	Mimo-AuNPs were able to suppress the spontaneous and seed-induced $A\beta_{1-42}$ aggregation.	(Anand et al., 2021)
Chondroitin sulphate-gold nanoparticle	TAT peptide	TAT-CS@Au effectively inhibited the accumulation of Aβ1–40, and significantly reduced Aβ1–40-induced apoptosis in SH-SY5Y cells. Additionally, the particles also decrease the levels of inflammatory factors, specifically TNF-α, IL-6, and IL-1β, by inhibiting NF-κB nuclear translocation by activating MAPK signaling pathways.	(Feng et al., 2023)

Drug delivery: AuNPs have the potential to be designed to target certain AD-affected parts of the brain and carry pharmaceutical substances over the BBB. They might provide therapeutic substances that prevent the development of tau tangles or Aβ plaques, which are the disease's clinical hallmarks.

Metal chelation: By attaching to metals that promote amyloid aggregation, such as copper and zinc, AuNPs may act as metal chelators. This interaction may prevent amyloid plaques from accumulating. In conclusion, AuNPs have shown a lot of promise in Alzheimer's research due to their neuroprotective and anti-inflammatory properties. The therapeutic efficacy of AuNPs in neurodegenerative disorders such as AD has been evaluated in a number of studies. This neuroprotective capability is vital for obstructing disease progression and maintaining cognitive function. Because of their anti-inflammatory properties, AuNPs may be able to reduce nerve inflammation. In individuals with AD, AuNPs might contribute to the protection of neuronal cells and the enhancement of overall cerebral function by modulating the inflammatory response (Chiang et al., 2024).

6.5 IN VITRO AND IN VIVO STUDIES ON AD MODEL

Preclinical and in vitro studies have indicated the interaction of AuNPs with Aβ within the framework of AD. Based on their engagement with Aβ, these investigations assess the feasibility of employing AuNPs as a targeted therapeutic intervention for AD. Numerous in vitro examinations have affirmed the capacity of AuNPs to associate with Aβ aggregates. It has been shown that AuNPs functionalized with specific ligands or peptides exhibiting an affinity for Aβ interact and adhere to Aβ plaques in an efficient manner. Some research suggests that AuNPs may hinder the aggregation of Aβ peptides, a pivotal process in the formation of the amyloid plaques that demonstrate AD. Preclinical in vivo experiments, frequently executed in transgenic murine models of AD, have scrutinized the targeting potential of AuNPs. For diagnostic imaging applications, the interaction between AuNPs and Aβ has been studied. Aβ plaques may be seen and detected in vivo more easily when AuNPs are functionalized with imaging agents like fluorophores or contrast materials. AuNPs can be functionalized with ligands or peptides that have a strong affinity for Aβ, allowing for selective administration. This selectivity is essential for reducing off-target effects and increasing the effectiveness of treatment for Aβ disease. Through their interaction with Aβ, AuNPs have the potential to mitigate the neurotoxic effects of Aβ aggregates. This might potentially reduce AD-related pathology and have a neuroprotective impact. The foundation for targeted therapeutic approaches resides in the surface modifications of AuNPs. Such functionalization empowers AuNPs to selectively target Aβ aggregates. Lv et al. (2024) have explained an innovative electrochemical detection methodology in their study to enhance sensitivity in detecting Aβ1–42 oligomers by employing a dual amplification strategy that utilizes AuNPs as the electrode substrate alongside a covalent organic framework (COF)-based probe. This biosensing technology has an ultralow detection limit of 4.27 fg mL^{-1} and a linear range of 0.01 pg mL^{-1} to 180 pg mL^{-1}. Yang et al. (2023) have designed a novel gold nanomaterial, AuNPs@PEG@MIL-101, worked as Aβ inhibitor. This hybrid nanomaterial may effectively break the produced Aβ fibers and reduce extracellular Aβ monomer fibrillation and exhibit promising attributes for prospective therapeutic applications in AD. In cellular studies utilizing PC12 cells, AuNPs@PEG@MIL-101 displayed protective effects toward Aβ40-induced microtubular defects and cellular membrane damage. In their comprehensive review of the field, Warerkar et al. (2024) highlight the potential of coated nanoparticles in preventing the production of amyloid fibrils while addressing the difficulties in developing medications for neurodegenerative diseases.

Chang et al. (2024) have explained a novel methodology for the synthesis of stable and biocompatible AuNPs with the conjugation of cysteine-Aβ peptides aimed at detecting subfemtomolar concentrations of Aβ peptides in human plasma. Cys-Aβ@AuNP offers advantages over traditional thioflavin-T fluorescence methods by enabling early-stage detection of Aβ oligomerization. When combined with centrifugation, this system not only detects but also redirects Aβ aggregation pathways, potentially preventing the formation of toxic oligomers and fibrils. This dual capability for early detection and inhibition of Aβ aggregation represents a promising advance in both diagnostics and therapeutic development for AD. Chiang et al. (2022) have explained the anti-inflammatory properties of AuNPs by synthesizing glutathione-conjugated gold nanoparticles (GSH-AuNPs) to protect human neural stem cells (hNSCs) from Aβ-induced damage through multiple mechanisms. GSH-AuNPs enhance cell survival by reducing caspase activity, maintaining antioxidant gene expression through Nrf2 signaling, normalizing ER stress markers and calcium levels, and preserving mitochondrial function and energy metabolism. These comprehensive protective effects suggest GSH-AuNPs could serve as a promising therapeutic approach for AD (Table 6.2).

TABLE 6.2
Neuroprotective and Anti-inflammatory Properties of Gold Nanoparticles for Alzheimer's Disease

Nanomaterial Utilized	Biological Model	Neuroprotective/ Anti-Inflammatory Findings	References
Gold nanoparticles	Male Wistar rats were induced with okadaic acid and treated with 20-nm AuNP.	AuNPs prevented oxidative stress in brain structures and long-term AuNP treatment prevented the neuroinflammation, modulation of mitochondrial function, and impaired cognition.	(Dos Santos Tramontin et al., 2020)
Gold nanoparticles	Rat animal models were injected with gold nanoparticles intrahippocampal (IH) and intraperitoneal (IP).	AuNPs could improve the acquisition and retention of spatial learning and memory in Aβ treated rats. Additionally, cAMP response element binding protein, CREB, expression of brain-derived neurotrophic factor (BDNF), and stromal interaction molecules were also increased.	(Sanati et al., 2019)

(Continued)

TABLE 6.2 *(Continued)*
Neuroprotective and Anti-inflammatory Properties of Gold Nanoparticles for Alzheimer's Disease

Nanomaterial Utilized	Biological Model	Neuroprotective/ Anti-Inflammatory Findings	References
Polypeptide-functionalized gold nanoparticles	Human neuroblastoma SH-SY5Y cells	Polypeptide gold nanoparticles protected neurons by inhibiting beta-amyloid aggregation and binding copper ions.	(Zhou et al., 2022)
Peptide-chondroitin sulphate-gold nanoparticles	Apoptosis induced in SH-SY5Y cells	Gold nanoparticles reduced neurodegeneration by controlling tau phosphorylation, inflammation, and oxidative damage through modulation of GSK3β and NF-κB pathways and regulation of MDA and GSH-Px levels.	(Feng et al., 2023)
Gold nanoparticles	Aβ-induced toxicity in human neural stem cells	Gold nanoparticles restored normal levels of inflammatory proteins (TNF-α, IL-1β), NF-κB (p65), and Nrf2, while reducing beta-amyloid aggregation in human neural stem cells.	(Chiang et al., 2022)

6.6 CONCLUSION

AD is one of the most challenging CNS disorders to treat, mainly because of the brain's protective barriers: the BCFB and the BBB. While BBB-targeted nanomedicine has become a viable strategy, with various nanoformulations showing encouraging results in laboratory and clinical studies, the translation to effective clinical treatments faces significant challenges. This chapter explores the distinguishing features of AuNPs as promising therapeutic agents for neurological disorders, with particular focus on their role in targeting neuroinflammation. The distinctive physicochemical properties of AuNPs incorporating their controllable surface chemistry, tunable size, and biocompatibility that make it enable for multiple neuroprotective mechanisms. These include OS reduction, pro-inflammatory cytokine suppression, signaling pathway regulation, and the enhancement of anti-inflammatory factors. The synthesis and functionalization of AuNPs critically influence their therapeutic potential through effects on stability, biocompatibility, and neural cell interactions. Their neuroprotective effects operate through multiple pathways: antioxidant activity, mitochondrial protection, antiapoptotic properties, neurotrophic support, enhanced neuronal connectivity, and possible reduction in protein aggregation.

While AuNPs show promising biocompatibility at appropriate concentrations, their clinical translation requires careful consideration of safety through size optimization, dosage control, surface modification, and targeted delivery strategies. Their ability to improve drug delivery through the BBB positions them as valuable tools for improving therapeutic efficacy in neurological disorders, though long-term effects and patient variability require further investigation.

REFERENCES

Aili, M., Zhou, K., Zhan, J., Zheng, H. and Luo, F., 2023. Anti-inflammatory role of gold nanoparticles in the prevention and treatment of Alzheimer's disease. *Journal of Materials Chemistry B*, *11*(36), pp.8605–8621.

Alzheimer's Association, 2012. Alzheimer's disease facts and figures. *Alzheimer's & Dementia*, *8*(2), pp.131–168.

Anand, B.G., Wu, Q., Karthivashan, G., Shejale, K.P., Amidian, S., Wille, H. and Kar, S., 2021. Mimosine functionalized gold nanoparticles (mimo-AuNPs) suppress β-amyloid aggregation and neuronal toxicity. *Bioactive Materials*, *6*(12), pp.4491–4505.

Aryal, M., Fischer, K., Gentile, C., Gitto, S., Zhang, Y.Z. and McDannold, N., 2017. Effects on p-glycoprotein expression after blood-brain barrier disruption using focused ultrasound and microbubbles. *PLoS One*, *12*(1), p.e0166061.

Asil, S.M., Ahlawat, J., Barroso, G.G. and Narayan, M., 2020. Nanomaterial based drug delivery systems for the treatment of neurodegenerative diseases. *Biomaterials Science*, *8*(15), pp.4109–4128.

Bansal, S.A., Kumar, V., Karimi, J., Singh, A.P. and Kumar, S., 2020. Role of gold nanoparticles in advanced biomedical applications. *Nanoscale Advances*, *2*(9), pp.3764–3787.

Cano, A., Turowski, P., Ettcheto, M., Duskey, J.T., Tosi, G., Sánchez-López, E., García, M.L., Camins, A., Souto, E.B., Ruiz, A. and Marquié, M., 2021. Nanomedicine-based technologies and novel biomarkers for the diagnosis and treatment of Alzheimer's disease: From current to future challenges. *Journal of Nanobiotechnology*, *19*(1), p.122.

Chang, Y.J., Chien, Y.H., Chang, C.C., Wang, P.N., Chen, Y.R. and Chang, Y.C., 2024. Detection of femtomolar amyloid-β peptides for early-stage identification of Alzheimer's amyloid-β aggregation with functionalized gold nanoparticles. *ACS Applied Materials & Interfaces*, *16*(3), pp.3819–3828.

Chiang, M.C. and Nicol, C.J., 2022. GSH-AuNP anti-oxidative stress, ER stress and mitochondrial dysfunction in amyloid-beta peptide-treated human neural stem cells. *Free Radical Biology and Medicine*, *187*, pp.185–201.

Chiang, M.C., Yang, Y.P., Nicol, C.J. and Wang, C.J., 2024. Gold nanoparticles in neurological diseases: A review of neuroprotection. *International Journal of Molecular Sciences*, *25*(4), p.2360.

Congdon, E.E. and Sigurdsson, E.M., 2018. Tau-targeting therapies for Alzheimer disease. *Nature Reviews Neurology*, *14*(7), pp.399–415.

Cummings, J., Lee, G., Zhong, K., Fonseca, J. and Taghva, K., 2021. Alzheimer's disease drug development pipeline: 2021. *Alzheimer's & Dementia: Translational Research & Clinical Interventions*, *7*(1), p.e12179.

Dabbagh, F., Schroten, H. and Schwerk, C., 2022. In vitro models of the blood–cerebrospinal fluid barrier and their applications in the development and research of (neuro) pharmaceuticals. *Pharmaceutics*, *14*(8), p.1729.

Dos Santos Tramontin, N., da Silva, S., Arruda, R., Ugioni, K.S., Canteiro, P.B., de Bem Silveira, G., Mendes, C., Silveira, P.C.L. and Muller, A.P., 2020. Gold nanoparticles treatment reverses brain damage in Alzheimer's disease model. *Molecular Neurobiology*, *57*, pp.926–936.

Dreaden, E.C., Austin, L.A., Mackey, M.A. and El-Sayed, M.A., 2012. Size matters: Gold nanoparticles in targeted cancer drug delivery. *Therapeutic Delivery*, *3*(4), pp.457–478.

Feng, Y., Li, X., Ji, D., Tian, J., Peng, Q., Shen, Y. and Xiao, Y., 2023. Functionalised penetrating peptide-chondroitin sulphate-gold nanoparticles: Synthesis, characterization, and applications as an anti-Alzheimer's disease drug. *International Journal of Biological Macromolecules*, *230*, p.123125.

Ghalamfarsa, G., Hojjat-Farsangi, M., Mohammadnia-Afrouzi, M., Anvari, E., Farhadi, S., Yousefi, M. and Jadidi-Niaragh, F., 2016. Application of nanomedicine for crossing the blood–brain barrier: Theranostic opportunities in multiple sclerosis. *Journal of Immunotoxicology*, *13*(5), pp.603–619.

Guo, Z.H., Khattak, S., Rauf, M.A., Ansari, M.A., Alomary, M.N., Razak, S., Yang, C.Y., Wu, D.D. and Ji, X.Y., 2023. Role of nanomedicine-based therapeutics in the treatment of CNS disorders. *Molecules*, *28*(3), p.1283.

Hammami, I. and Alabdallah, N.M., 2021. Gold nanoparticles: Synthesis properties and applications. *Journal of King Saud University-Science*, *33*(7), p.101560.

Hanif, S., Muhammad, P., Chesworth, R., Rehman, F.U., Qian, R.J., Zheng, M. and Shi, B.Y., 2020. Nanomedicine-based immunotherapy for central nervous system disorders. *Acta Pharmacologica Sinica*, *41*(7), pp.936–953.

Hersh, D., Wadajkar, A., Roberts, N., Perez, J., Connolly, N., Frenkel, V., Winkles, J., Woodworth, G. and Kim, A., 2016. Evolving drug delivery strategies to overcome the blood brain barrier. *Current Pharmaceutical Design*, *22*(9), pp.1177–1193.

Hou, K., Zhao, J., Wang, H., Li, B., Li, K., Shi, X., Wan, K., Ai, J., Lv, J., Wang, D. and Huang, Q., 2020. Chiral gold nanoparticles enantioselectively rescue memory deficits in a mouse model of Alzheimer's disease. *Nature Communications*, *11*(1), p.4790.

Huang, H., Liu, R., Yang, J., Dai, J., Fan, S., Pi, J., Wei, Y. and Guo, X., 2023. Gold nanoparticles: Construction for drug delivery and application in cancer immunotherapy. *Pharmaceutics*, *15*(7), p.1868.

Jack, C.R., Knopman, D.S., Jagust, W.J., Petersen, R.C., Weiner, M.W., Aisen, P.S., Shaw, L.M., Vemuri, P., Wiste, H.J., Weigand, S.D. and Lesnick, T.G., 2013. Tracking pathophysiological processes in Alzheimer's disease: An updated hypothetical model of dynamic biomarkers. *The Lancet Neurology*, *12*(2), pp.207–216.

Jagaran, K. and Singh, M., 2021. Nanomedicine for neurodegenerative disorders: Focus on Alzheimer's and Parkinson's diseases. *International Journal of Molecular Sciences*, *22*(16), p.9082.

Khan, N.H., Mir, M., Ngowi, E.E., Zafar, U., Khakwani, M.M.A.K., Khattak, S., Zhai, Y.K., Jiang, E.S., Zheng, M., Duan, S.F. and Wei, J.S., 2021. Nanomedicine: A promising way to manage Alzheimer's disease. *Frontiers in Bioengineering and Biotechnology*, *9*, p.630055.

Khongkow, M., Yata, T., Boonrungsiman, S., Ruktanonchai, U.R., Graham, D. and Namdee, K., 2019. Surface modification of gold nanoparticles with neuron-targeted exosome for enhanced blood–brain barrier penetration. *Scientific Reports*, *9*(1), p.8278.

Kim, M.J., Rehman, S.U., Amin, F.U. and Kim, M.O., 2017. Enhanced neuroprotection of anthocyanin-loaded PEG-gold nanoparticles against Aβ1-42-induced neuroinflammation and neurodegeneration via the NF-KB/JNK/GSK3β signaling pathway. *Nanomedicine: Nanotechnology, Biology and Medicine*, *13*(8), pp.2533–2544.

Koushki, K., Keshavarz Shahbaz, S., Keshavarz, M., Bezsonov, E.E., Sathyapalan, T. and Sahebkar, A., 2021. Gold nanoparticles: Multifaceted roles in the management of autoimmune disorders. *Biomolecules*, *11*(9), p.1289.

Kumar, P.P.P. and Lim, D.K., 2021. Gold-polymer nanocomposites for future therapeutic and tissue engineering applications. *Pharmaceutics*, *14*(1), p.70.

Liu, J. and Peng, Q., 2017. Protein-gold nanoparticle interactions and their possible impact on biomedical applications. *Acta Biomaterialia*, *55*, pp.13–27.

Liu, X.Y., Wang, J.Q., Ashby, C.R. Jr, Zeng, L., Fan, Y.F. and Chen, Z.S., 2021. Gold nanoparticles: Synthesis, physiochemical properties and therapeutic applications in cancer. *Drug Discovery Today*, *26*(5), pp.1284–1292.

Lv, Y., Zhou, Y., Dong, H., Xu, M., Zhang, J. and Yan, M., 2024. Ultrasensitive electrochemical detection of amyloid-beta oligomers using double amplification strategy by MXene substrate and covalent organic framework-based probe. *Talanta*, *266*, p.125134.

Meyer, J., Mischeck, U., Veyhl, M., Henzel, K. and Galla, H.J., 1990. Blood-brain barrier characteristic enzymatic properties in cultured brain capillary endothelial cells. *Brain Research*, *514*(2), pp.305–309.

Mittal, K.R., Pharasi, N., Sarna, B., Singh, M., Rachana, Haider, S., Singh, S.K., Dua, K., Jha, S.K., Dey, A. and Ojha, S., 2022. Nanotechnology-based drug delivery for the treatment of CNS disorders. *Translational Neuroscience*, *13*(1), pp.527–546.

Mukherjee, S., Madamsetty, V.S., Bhattacharya, D., Roy Chowdhury, S., Paul, M.K. and Mukherjee, A., 2020. Recent advancements of nanomedicine in neurodegenerative disorders theranostics. *Advanced Functional Materials*, *30*(35), p.2003054.

Murman, D.L. and Colenda, C.C., 2005. The economic impact of neuropsychiatric symptoms in Alzheimer's disease: Can drugs ease the burden? *Pharmacoeconomics*, *23*, pp.227–242.

Nation, D.A., Sweeney, M.D., Montagne, A., Sagare, A.P., D'Orazio, L.M., Pachicano, M., Sepehrband, F., Nelson, A.R., Buennagel, D.P., Harrington, M.G. and Benzinger, T.L., 2019. Blood–brain barrier breakdown is an early biomarker of human cognitive dysfunction. *Nature Medicine*, *25*(2), pp.270–276.

Nguyen, N.H. and Falagan-Lotsch, P., 2023. Mechanistic insights into the biological effects of engineered nanomaterials: A focus on gold nanoparticles. *International Journal of Molecular Sciences*, *24*(4), p.4109.

Nguyen, T.T., Nguyen, T.T.D., Nguyen, T.K.O. and Vo, T.K., 2021. Advances in developing therapeutic strategies for Alzheimer's disease. *Biomedicine & Pharmacotherapy*, *139*, p.111623.

Pawar, B., Vasdev, N., Gupta, T., Mhatre, M., More, A., Anup, N. and Tekade, R.K., 2022. Current update on transcellular brain drug delivery. *Pharmaceutics*, *14*(12), p.2719.

Poudel, P. and Park, S., 2022. Recent advances in the treatment of Alzheimer's disease using nanoparticle-based drug delivery systems. *Pharmaceutics*, *14*(4), p.835.

Puranik, N., Yadav, D. and Song, M., 2023. Advancements in the application of nanomedicine in Alzheimer's disease: A therapeutic perspective. *International Journal of Molecular Sciences*, *24*(18), p.14044.

Sanati, M., Khodagholi, F., Aminyavari, S., Ghasemi, F., Gholami, M., Kebriaeezadeh, A., Sabzevari, O., Hajipour, M.J., Imani, M., Mahmoudi, M. and Sharifzadeh, M., 2019. Impact of gold nanoparticles on amyloid β-induced Alzheimer's disease in a rat animal model: Involvement of STIM proteins. *ACS Chemical Neuroscience*, *10*(5), pp.2299–2309.

Sánchez-Dengra, B., González-Álvarez, I., Bermejo, M. and González-Álvarez, M., 2023. Access to the CNS: Strategies to overcome the BBB. *International Journal of Pharmaceutics*, *636*, p.122759.

Saraiva, C., Praça, C., Ferreira, R., Santos, T., Ferreira, L. and Bernardino, L., 2016. Nanoparticle-mediated brain drug delivery: Overcoming blood–brain barrier to treat neurodegenerative diseases. *Journal of Controlled Release*, *235*, pp.34–47.

Sarfraz, N. and Khan, I., 2021. Plasmonic gold nanoparticles (AuNPs): Properties, synthesis and their advanced energy, environmental and biomedical applications. *Chemistry–An Asian Journal*, *16*(7), pp.720–742.

Siddiqi, K.S., Husen, A., Sohrab, S.S. and Yassin, M.O., 2018. Recent status of nanomaterial fabrication and their potential applications in neurological disease management. *Nanoscale Research Letters*, *13*(1), p.17.

Singh, B., Day, C.M., Abdella, S. and Garg, S., 2024. Alzheimer's disease current therapies, novel drug delivery systems and future directions for better disease management. *Journal of Controlled Release*, *367*, pp.402–424.

Singh, P. and Singh, L.K., 2024. Myeloperoxidase enzyme-catalyzed breakdown of zero-dimension carbon quantum dots. *Frontiers in Medical Technology*, *6*, p.1493288.

Song, G., Zhao, M., Chen, H., Lenahan, C., Zhou, X., Ou, Y. and He, Y., 2021. The role of nanomaterials in stroke treatment: Targeting oxidative stress. *Oxidative Medicine and Cellular Longevity*, *2021*(1), p.8857486.

Sood, S., Jain, K. and Gowthamarajan, K., 2014. Intranasal therapeutic strategies for management of Alzheimer's disease. *Journal of Drug Targeting*, *22*(4), pp.279–294.

Tian, X., Fan, T., Zhao, W., Abbas, G., Han, B., Zhang, K., Li, N., Liu, N., Liang, W., Huang, H. and Chen, W., 2021. Recent advances in the development of nanomedicines for the treatment of ischemic stroke. *Bioactive Materials*, *6*(9), pp.2854–2869.

Vossel, K.A., Zhang, K., Brodbeck, J., Daub, A.C., Sharma, P., Finkbeiner, S., Cui, B. and Mucke, L., 2010. Tau reduction prevents aβ-induced defects in axonal transport. *Science*, *330*(6001), pp.198–198.

Warerkar, O., Mudliar, N. and Momin, M. and Singh, P., Targeting Amyloids with coated Nanoparticles: A review on lucrative combinations of nanoparticles and its bio-compatible coating. *Critical Reviews in Therapeutic Drug Carrier Systems*, *41*, pp.85–119.

Wilson, B. and Geetha, K.M., 2020. Neurotherapeutic applications of nanomedicine for treating Alzheimer's disease. *Journal of Controlled Release*, *325*, pp.25–37.

Yadav, D., Kwak, M., Chauhan, P.S., Puranik, N., Lee, P.C. and Jin, J.O., 2022, November. Cancer immunotherapy by immune checkpoint blockade and its advanced application using bio-nanomaterials. In *Seminars in Cancer Biology* (Vol. 86, pp. 909–922). Academic Press.

Yalamarty, S.S.K., Filipczak, N., Li, X., Subhan, M.A., Parveen, F., Ataide, J.A., Rajmalani, B.A. and Torchilin, V.P., 2023. Mechanisms of resistance and current treatment options for glioblastoma multiforme (GBM). *Cancers*, *15*(7), p.2116.

Yang, L., Chen, Y., Jia, Z., Yuan, X. and Liu, J., 2023. Electrostatic assembly of gold nanoparticle and metal–organic framework nanoparticles attenuates amyloid β aggregate-mediated neurotoxicity. *Journal of Materials Chemistry B*, *11*(20), pp.4453–4463.

Zhang, J., Mou, L. and Jiang, X., 2020. Surface chemistry of gold nanoparticles for health-related applications. *Chemical Science*, *11*(4), pp.923–936.

Zhou, B., Sheng, X., Xie, H., Zhou, S., Zhong, M. and Liu, A., 2022. Inhibition of Alzheimer's Aβ1-42 fibrillogenesis and removal of copper ions by polypeptides modified gold nanoparticles. *Chemistry & Biodiversity*, *19*(11), p.e202200342.

7 Lipid-Based Nanocarrier in the Management of Alzheimer's Disease

Ragini Singh and Neha Sharma

7.1 INTRODUCTION

Alzheimer's disease (AD) is a persistent neurodegenerative sickness. Because of AD, patients suffer from quick-time period memory loss, vocal memory loss, temper swings, loss of enthusiasm and intellectual coordination abilities. The disease is characterized by cholinergic insufficiency, dysfunction of mitochondria, oxidative stress, hormonal imbalances, synthesis of abnormal proteins, particularly amyloid plaques and tau tangles, which damage and disrupt brain cells (Figure 7.1). In AD, therapies target multiple mechanisms, including amyloid-beta aggregation, tau hyperphosphorylation, and neuroinflammation. Strategies aim to reduce amyloid plaque buildup, prevent tau tangles, and modulate inflammatory responses. Additionally, oxidative stress reduction and neuroprotection through antioxidant or neurotrophic factors help preserve neuronal function and slow disease progression (Garbuz et al., 2021).

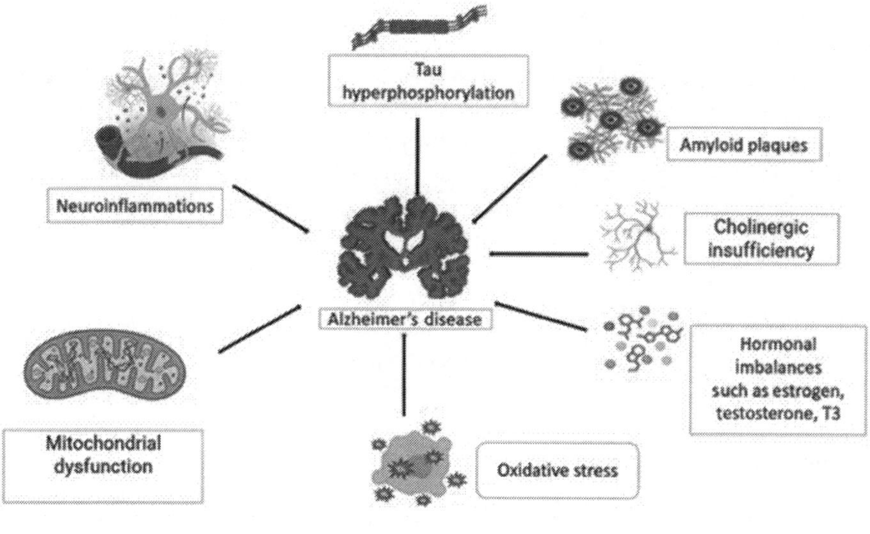

FIGURE 7.1 Causes of Alzheimer disease.

DOI: 10.1201/9781003543381-7

Lipid-based nanocarriers are new drug delivery approaches that enhance therapeutic efficacy and precision. They are composed of biocompatible and biodegradable lipid materials, making them suitable for application in medical facilities. These nanocarriers are versatile and include various types such as liposomes, solid lipid nanoparticles (SLNs), and nanostructured lipid carriers (NLCs), each offering unique advantages in drug encapsulation, stability, and release profiles (Arduino et al., 2020). Their ability to encapsulate both hydrophilic and hydrophobic drugs enables them to deliver a wide range of therapeutic agents. Moreover, lipid-based nanocarriers are particularly advantageous in overcoming biological barriers, such as the blood–brain barrier (BBB), resulting in treating neurodegenerative illnesses like AD highly challenging (Taliyan et al., 2022). Their tenable surface properties and potential for functionalization allow for targeted delivery, reduced side effects, and improved therapeutic approach. These characteristics position lipid-based nanocarriers as a promising platform in advancing drug delivery strategies for complex diseases (Peng et al., 2020).

Advanced platforms known lipid-based delivery systems are generated to enhance the pharmacokinetics and therapeutic efficacy of medications. These systems utilize lipids, such as phospholipids, cholesterol, and triglycerides, as core components to create carriers like liposomes, SLNs, and NLCs (Barba et al., 2019). They are capable of encapsulating both hydrophilic and lipophilic drugs, offering versatility in drug delivery applications. Enhancing the solubility, stability, and bioavailability of medications—especially those with low water solubility—is one of their most important benefits (Preeti et al., 2023). Also, lipid-based systems can enable controlled and extended release of therapeutic medications, lowering dose frequency and decreasing side effects. Their biocompatibility and biodegradability further enhance their safety profile. Moreover, these can be engineered for targeted delivery through surface modification, enabling specific interaction with diseased cells or tissues, such as crossing the BBB in neurological disorders (Preeti et al., 2023). These features make lipid-based delivery systems a vital resource in modern drug delivery technologies, especially for complex and chronic illnesses. To overcome these issues, drug delivery systems (DDSs) such as hydrogels, nanoparticles (NPs), NP-loaded hydrogel (NLH) systems, and micro formulations (microneedles, microparticles, microspheres, and microemulsions) have been employed extensively. Because NPs and microparticles shield drugs from deterioration, boost their bioavailability, and enable more focused and prolonged release, they can increase the therapeutic efficacy of pharmaceuticals (Nunes et al., 2022).

7.2 TYPES OF LIPID-BASED NANOCARRIERS

Lipid-based nanocarriers are a wide range of DDSs which employ lipids to improve the therapeutic potential of the pharmaceutical drugs. Liposomes, SLNs, and NLCs are three of the most widely investigated varieties, all of which have their own set of advantages and applications.

Liposomes are spherical vesicles made up of one or more phospholipid bilayers around an aqueous core. They are highly flexible and can encapsulate both hydrophilic and hydrophobic drugs, making them suitable for a number of therapeutic

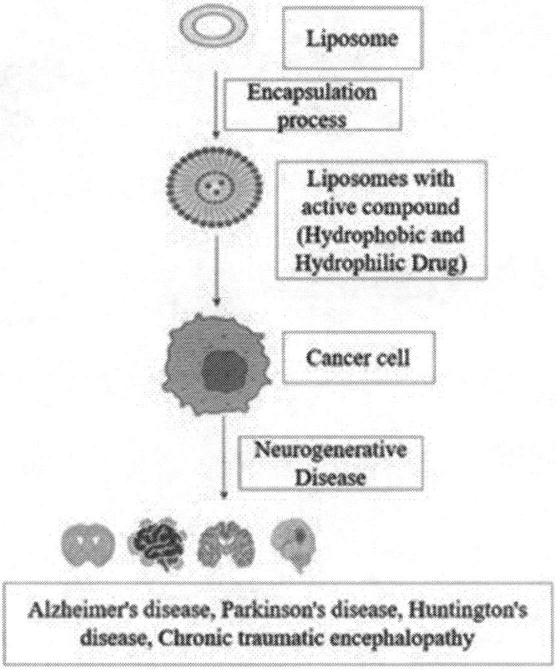

FIGURE 7.2 Liposome-based drug delivery in neurodegenerative diseases.

applications (Figure 7.2). Liposomes can be functionalized with targeting ligands on their surface to improve specificity, which is extremely effective in cancer and neurological disorders. Liposomes have been widely used in therapeutic settings because of their biocompatibility and low toxicity. Multiple FDA-approved formulations are available (Yi et al., 2016).

SLNs are solid lipid-based carriers that are submicron in size and stable at body and room temperatures. Monoglycerides, diglycerides, or triglycerides such as tristearin, glyceryl behenate, and glycerol monostearate can comprise the lipid core. Additionally, it contains surfactants that can be stabilized with emulsifiers to stop particle agglomeration, which include fatty acids, steroids, or waxes (Mehnert and Mäder, 2012). SLNs offer great stability, inhibit encapsulated medicines from degradation, and have controlled release qualities. Their manufacture is scalable and cost-effective, making them ideal for pharmaceutical applications. However, the crystalline lipid matrix may limit drug loading capacity (Patidar et al., 2010; Figure 7.3).

NLCs, which feature a disordered inner lipid matrix made up of solid and liquid lipids, are another possible method for targeted drug delivery. NLCs can handle large loads and are more stable. NLCs are employed for carrying medications from the nose to the brain and in Alzheimer's treatment connected with microglial activation (Gobbi et al., 2010; Costa et al., 2021). Examples of SLNs and NLCs with their targets and functions are described in Table 7.1.

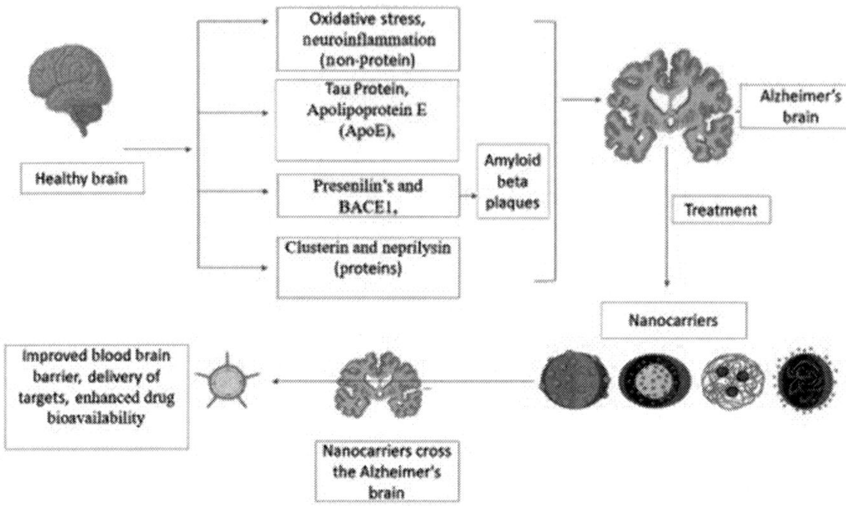

FIGURE 7.3 Cause of Alzheimer's brain and its treatment with nanocarriers.

NLCs were developed to solve the limitations of SLNs through the combination of solid and liquid lipids. This results in an amorphous lipid matrix with improved drug-loading capacity and stability. NLCs exhibit enhanced entrapment efficiency and provide more controlled and prolonged drug release, making them suitable for the delivery of a wide range of therapeutics, including poorly water-soluble drugs. Other lipid-based nanocarriers include nanoemulsions, micelles, and lipid-drug conjugates, each tailored for specific therapeutic needs. Collectively, these systems represent a promising frontier in drug delivery, offering improved efficacy, safety, and targeted therapeutic outcomes (Patidar et al., 2010).

Lipid nanoemulsions consisting of lipid droplets dispersed in water, are being explored for Alzheimer's treatment. They can encapsulate neuroprotective agents or anti-inflammatory compounds, enhancing their delivery to the brain. By improving drug solubility and stability, lipid emulsions may help reduce amyloid-beta plaque buildup and slow cognitive decline in Alzheimer's patients (Yi et al., 2015).

Niosome increase therapeutic efficacy to target brain regions, sorbitan esters and cholesterol are used in the film hydration approach to create niosomes (Estabragh et al., 2018). AD pathologies are significantly impacted when a niosome–lipid nanocarrier system loaded with artemisia-absinthium is administered to prevent amyloid accumulation (Khan et al., 2021). To improve drug exposure and address the blockage of folic acid transport across the BBB in AD therapy, different formulations such as pentamide-loaded chitosan glutamate-coated niosomes and different doses of folic acid-niosomes have been created (Ravouru et al. 2013; Rinaldi et al. 2018). In addition to the foregoing, rivastigmine can be used in AD therapy to improve brain function (Estabragh et al., 2018).

Nanoemulsions are produced using homogenization and ultrasonication procedures (Table 7.2). It is used to load memantine for intranasal delivery in AD therapy,

TABLE 7.1
Types of SLNs, Targets and Their Functions

S. No.	Types	Targets and Functions	References
1	Transferrin-functionalized nanostructured lipid carriers	Induce the expression of p-glycoprotein and breast cancer resistance protein transporters in brain endothelial cells via targeting the MC11 ligands.	(Arduino et al., 2020)
2	Solid lipid NPs loaded with donepezil	Provides non-targeted drugs delivery. There is potential for enhancing the delivery of drugs to the brain via the intranasal route.	(Al Asmari et al, 2016; Yasir et al., 2018a; Yasir et al., 2018b)
3	Curcumin-loaded lipid-core nanocapsules	Neuroprotective advantages against Aβ1-42-induced behavioral and neurochemical changes in an AD mouse model.	(Sadegh Malvajerd et al., 2018; Sadegh Malvajerd et al., 2019; Yavarpour-Bali et al., 2019)
4	Pomegranate extract-loaded lipidic nanoparticles	Decreased neurofibrillary tangles and Aβ deposition.	(Almuhayawi et al, 2020)
5	α-Bisabolol-loaded cholesterol lipidic nanoparticles	Prevent neuro-2α cells from Aβ-induced neurotoxicity and minimize Aβ aggregation.	(Sathya et al, 2018)
6	EPO-encapsulated lipidic nanoparticles	Decrease oxidative stress, Aβ deposition, and enhance spatial memory.	(Dara et al, 2019)
7	Lipid nanocapsules (LNCs) with a lipid core and loaded with indomethacin (Ind)	Potential to prevent neuroinflammation and cell damage induced by Aβ1-42.	(Bernardi et al, 2012)

hence resolving the BBB obstacle. Naringerin nanoemulsion is a possible strategy to combat Aβ neurotoxicity and amyloidogenesis, resulting in improved clinical efficiency (Md et al., 2018; Kaur et al., 2020; Nirale et al., 2020).

Cubosomes have the potential application for drug delivery to the brain like donepezil-HCL delivery through cubosomal mucoadhesive in situ nasal gel show that formulated gel could be considered as a promising carrier for drug delivery to target the affected parts of the brain (Patil et al., 2019; Gaballa et al., 2020).

Amylolipid Nanovesicles, the research of the self-assembled lipid-modified starch hybrid system demonstrates that intranasal delivery of curcumin loaded into amylolipid nanovesicles significantly affects AD pathology and has a higher capacity to cross the BBB. Accordingly, the data show that this carrier system is a potential way to transport drugs to the brain tissues of people with Alzheimer's (Sintov et al., 2020).

TABLE 7.2
Types of Nanocarriers and Their Impact on AD

S. No.	Types of Nanocarriers	Impact of Nanocarriers on AD	References
1	Liposomes	Spherical vesicles composed of phospholipid bilayers are used to deliver hydrophilic and hydrophobic drugs.	(Yi et al., 2015)
2	Solid Lipid Nanoparticles (SLNs)	Solid lipid particles that provide controlled release of encapsulated drugs.	(Patidar et al., 2010)
3	Nanostructured Lipid Carriers (NLCs)	Similar to SLNs, but with a mixture of solid and liquid lipids, that enhances drug loading and stability.	(Patidar et al., 2010)
4	Lipid Emulsions	Colloidal systems that contain lipid droplets dispersed in water, often used for intravenous drug delivery.	(Yi et al., 2015)
5	Niosomes	Niosomes improve drug stability, speed up circulation, reduce adverse effects, and increase target site absorption. The present work aims to determine the efficacy and neuroprotective. Amygdaline and its niosome formulation perform an essential role in Alzheimer's disease prevention.	(El-Banna et al., 2024)
6	Nano emulsion	It is used to load memantine for intranasal delivery for AD therapy and overcome the problem of blood–brain barrier.	(Nirale et al., 2020)
7	Cubosomes	Cubosomes have the capability to deliver drugs to the brain.	(Gaballa et al., 2020)
8	Amylolipid Nanovesicles	Amylolipid nanovesicles have an enhanced capacity to pass the blood–brain barrier and exhibit a considerable effect on Alzheimer's disease pathology.	(Sintov et al., 2020)

7.3 FORMULATION AND DESIGN OF LIPID-BASED NANOCARRIERS

The formulation and design of lipid-based nanocarriers involve selecting appropriate lipids, surfactants, and stabilizers to encapsulate drugs effectively. Key considerations include optimizing particle size, surface charge, and stability, as well as functionalizing carriers for targeted delivery. Techniques like extrusion, solvent evaporation, and high-pressure homogenization are used for production (Musacchio et al., 2011).

1. **Composition of lipid-based carriers (phospholipids, surfactants, cholesterol)**: Lipid-based carriers are composed of a variety of lipids that contribute to their stability, drug-loading capacity, and biocompatibility. Phospholipids are the primary structural components, forming bilayers that encapsulate drugs, mimicking natural cell membranes (Musacchio et al., 2011). They can be derived from sources like soy lecithin or egg yolk phosphatidylcholine. Surfactants, such as polyethoxylated surfactants, are used to stabilize the lipid matrix, reduce surface tension, and improve dispersion in aqueous environments (Musacchio et al., 2011). Cholesterol is often included to enhance the rigidity and stability of the carrier, preventing premature drug release and maintaining structural integrity. These components are carefully selected to optimize the carrier's performance in drug delivery (Musacchio et al., 2011).
2. **Surface functionalization for targeted delivery**: Surface functionalization of lipid-based nanocarriers increases their ability to selectively target certain cells or tissues, resulting in better therapeutic outcomes and fewer adverse effects. This is done by binding targeted ligands, including as antibodies, peptides, or small molecules, to the nanocarrier's surface. These ligands bind to specific receptors or biomarkers that are overexpressed on target cells, including cancer cells or neurons in AD (Del Amo et al., 2021). Functionalization may also involve modifications such as polyethylene glycol (PEG) coating, which increases circulation time and reduces immune recognition. By changing the surface features, lipid-based nanocarriers may deliver drugs precisely to the targeted site of action, enhancing efficacy and safety (Del Amo et al., 2021).

7.4 MECHANISMS OF LIPID-BASED NANOCARRIER IN THE MANAGEMENT OF ALZHEIMER'S DISEASE

Lipid-based nanocarriers play an essential role in improving drug delivery and therapeutic efficacy in the management of AD. Their mechanisms of action include:

1. **Enhanced BBB Penetration**: Compared to traditional medications, lipid-based nanocarriers like liposomes and SLNs are made to pass the BBB more effectively. Their lipophilic nature allows them to penetrate the tightly packed endothelial cells of the BBB, enabling the delivery of therapeutic agents directly to the brain (Pottoo et al., 2020).
2. **Targeted Delivery**: Functionalization of nanocarriers with targeting ligands, such as antibodies, peptides, or small molecules, enables selective delivery to specific regions of the brain. In AD, targeting amyloid-beta plaques or tau tangles can enhance therapeutic efficacy by focusing treatment on disease-related proteins (Gopalan et al., 2020).

3. **Controlled and Sustained Drug Release**: Lipid-based nanocarriers offer controlled and sustained release profiles, reducing the need for frequent dosing and minimizing side effects. This allows therapeutic agents to be released gradually over time, ensuring consistent drug concentrations and prolonged therapeutic effects (Witika et al., 2022).
4. **Combination Therapies**: Nanocarriers can encapsulate multiple drugs simultaneously, enabling combination therapies. In Alzheimer's, they can deliver anti-amyloid drugs, antioxidants, neuroprotective agents, and anti-inflammatory agents in a single formulation, addressing the multifactorial nature of the disease (Guo et al., 2023).
5. **Neuroprotective and Antioxidant Effects**: Lipid-based nanocarriers can encapsulate antioxidants or neuroprotective agents that help reduce oxidative stress and inflammation in the brain, protecting neurons from damage and preserving cognitive function (Daraban et al., 2024).
6. **Pathophysiology of AD**: AD is a neurological disorder defined by the accumulation of amyloid-beta plaques and tau neurofibrillary tangles, which cause neuronal malfunction and death. This leads to synapse loss, persistent neuroinflammation, and brain shrinkage, especially in the hippocampus and cortex, which causes progressive memory loss, cognitive decline, and behavior deficits (Li et al., 2022).
7. **Use of Nanocarriers for Combination Therapies**: Nanocarriers enable combination therapies by simultaneously delivering multiple therapeutic agents to target complex diseases like Alzheimer's (Sahoo et al., 2018). These systems can co-encapsulate drugs with complementary mechanisms, such as anti-amyloid agents, antioxidants, and anti-inflammatory drugs, enhancing therapeutic efficacy. Functionalized nanocarriers improve targeting, directing the payload to specific cells or tissues, such as amyloid-beta plaques in the brain. By overcoming biological barriers like the BBB and minimizing systemic side effects, nanocarriers enhance the effectiveness of combination therapies, offering a promising approach to tackle multifactorial diseases with improved patient outcomes (Sahoo et al., 2018).

7.5 MOLECULAR TARGETS IN ALZHEIMER'S DISEASE

AD is triggered by complex molecular mechanisms, and addressing these processes is critical for effective treatment. The main targets are amyloid-beta (Aβ) peptides, which combine to form plaques that damage synaptic function and cause neuroinflammation. Drug development aims to reduce Aβ synthesis, aggregation, and clearance (Bhute et al., 2020). Table 7.3 shows the different types of proteins and their impact on brain with molecular targets.

Neurodegeneration is made worse through the association of tau tangles with amyloid-beta plaques. It has been established that tau hyperphosphorylation is caused by amyloid-beta buildup, which connects the two disorders in a vicious cycle. This combination of actions speeds up neuroinflammation, synapse loss, and brain atrophy, especially in areas like the cortex and hippocampus that are important for memory and learning. In an attempt to slow or stop the progression of AD,

TABLE 7.3
Different Types of Proteins and Their Impact on Brain with Molecular Targets

S. No.	Types of Proteins	Impact on Brain	References
1	Amyloid-beta (Aβ)	The primary targets are amyloid-beta (Aβ) peptides, which combine to form plaques that damage synaptic function and cause neuroinflammation. Drug development aims to reduce Aβ manufacturing, aggregation, and enhance clearance.	(Ehtiati et al., 2023)
2	Tau Tangle	Tau tangles, or intracellular clumps, develop when tau protein is hyperphosphorylated. Tau is a microtubule-associated protein required for intracellular transport and microtubule stability. When tau is hyperphosphorylated, it loses its normal function and forms irreversible tangles within neurons. These tangles cause neuronal dysfunction and death by disrupting microtubule dynamics, impeding axonal transport, and causing cytoskeletal collapse.	(Boutajangout et al., 2011)
3	Apolipoprotein E (ApoE)	ApoE plays a part in Alzheimer's disease because it impacts lipid metabolism and amyloid-beta plaque clearance. ApoE appears in several isoforms, with ApoE4 being a major inherited risk factor for Alzheimer's. ApoE4 is thought to hinder the brain's ability to remove amyloid-beta, resulting in plaque formation and neurodegeneration. In contrast, ApoE2 may give some protective effects against the development of Alzheimer's.	(Kim et al., 2009)
4	Clusterin	Clusterin is a multipurpose protein which participates in cell survival, protein folding, and elimination. Clusterin facilitates the clearance of amyloid-beta plaques, which are a distinctive characteristic of Alzheimer's disease. It may assist to eliminate amyloid-beta from the brain by attaching to it. However, its ability to eliminate amyloid-beta may be hampered by changes in clusterin expression or dysfunction, which could result in plaque formation, neuroinflammation, and cognitive decline.	(Breijyeh & Karaman, 2020)

(Continued)

TABLE 7.3 *(Continued)*
Different Types of Proteins and Their Impact on Brain with Molecular Targets

S. No.	Types of Proteins	Impact on Brain	References
5	Presenilin's (PS1 and PS2)	The gamma-secretase complex, which cleaves amyloid precursor protein (APP) to produce amyloid-beta, is primarily made up of Presenilins (PS1 and PS2). Familial Alzheimer's disease is linked to mutations in the presenilin genes, which result in an excess of amyloid-beta peptide production. These peptides then accumulate in the brain as plaques. These mutations disrupt APP's normal processing, resulting in synaptic dysfunction, neurodegeneration, and cognitive decline. Thus, presenilins play an important part in the pathophysiology of Alzheimer's disease.	(De Strooper et al., 2007)
6	Ephexin 5	Ephexin 5 is a protein that regulates the dynamics of the actin cytoskeleton and synaptic signaling. Cognitive failure in Alzheimer's disease has been linked to abnormal Ephexin 5 activity, which can alter synaptic plasticity and neuronal transfer. According to studies, Ephexin 5 may interact with tau and amyloid-beta, two proteins critical to the etiology of Alzheimer's disease. It may have the potential to improve synapse function and decrease disease development via modulating Ephexin 5 activity.	(Cook et al., 2019)
7	Glutamate Receptors	Glutamate receptors, particularly NMDA receptors, are targeted to reduce excitotoxicity caused by excessive glutamate signaling, which contributes to neuronal death. Other emerging targets include neuroinflammation mediated by overactive microglia and astrocytes, as well as pathways involved in oxidative stress and mitochondrial dysfunction, which exacerbate neuronal damage. Furthermore, dysregulated lipid metabolism and the role of ApoE in amyloid deposition present novel areas for intervention.	(Puranik and Song, 2024)

tau tangles and amyloid-beta plaques work together as important therapeutic targets (Bejanin et al., 2017).

Advantages of Lipid-based Nanocarriers in AD Management—Lipid-based nanocarriers offer advantages in AD management by enhancing drug bioavailability and enabling efficient delivery across the BBB. They provide controlled and sustained drug release, minimize systemic side effects, and can be functionalized for targeted therapy (Agosti et al., 2024). These properties improve therapeutic efficacy and patient outcomes in Alzheimer's treatment such as:

1. **Enhanced drug bioavailability**: Enhanced drug bioavailability refers to the improved absorption and systemic availability of therapeutic agents, particularly those with poor solubility or stability. Lipid-based nanocarriers play a crucial role in achieving this by encapsulating hydrophobic drugs within their lipid matrix, protecting them from enzymatic degradation, and enhancing solubility (Agosti et al., 2024).

   These nanocarriers also improve drug transport across biological barriers, such as the BBB, ensuring efficient delivery to target sites. Additionally, their nanoscale size increases cellular uptake through endocytosis, while their sustained release properties maintain therapeutic drug levels over extended periods. Collectively, these features significantly enhance the effectiveness of drugs in treating diseases like Alzheimer's (Agosti et al., 2024).
2. **Improved BBB**: Improved BBB penetration is a significant advantage of lipid-based nanocarriers in the treatment of neurological conditions such as Alzheimer's. The BBB is a highly selective barrier that stops many drugs from penetrating the brain (Al-Azzawi et al., 2018). Lipid-based nanocarriers, such as liposomes and NLCs, improve drug delivery by imitating the BBB's lipophilic nature, permitting passive diffusion or receptor-mediated transport. Surface changes, such as coating with targeted ligands or polyethylene glycol (PEG), enhance nanocarrier interactions with BBB transport pathways. These technologies enable the efficient delivery of therapeutic medicines to the brain, solving a significant obstacle in neurodegenerative disease management (Al-Azzawi et al., 2018).
3. **Controlled and sustained drug release**: Controlled and sustained drug release ensures a steady therapeutic drug concentration over an extended period, minimizing dosing frequency and reducing side effects. Lipid-based nanocarriers achieve this by encapsulating drugs within their lipid matrix, allowing gradual release. This improves treatment efficacy and patient compliance, particularly in managing chronic conditions like AD (Di Stefano et al., 2011).

7.6 THERAPEUTIC AGENTS DELIVERED VIA LIPID-BASED NANOCARRIERS

Lipid-based nanocarriers can deliver a wide range of therapeutic agents, including anti-amyloid drugs, neuroprotective agents like antioxidants, gene therapies, and RNA-based treatments. These nanocarriers are especially useful for targeting difficult-to-reach areas, such as the brain, by enhancing drug solubility, stability, and penetration across the BBB (Yi et al., 2015). Some therapeutic agents are:

1. **Anti-amyloid drugs**: The main purpose of anti-amyloid medications is to target and reduce the generation of amyloid-beta plaques, which are a key component of AD. These medications help to prevent amyloid-beta peptides from developing, aggregating, or removing them from the brain. aducanumab and lecanemab are monoclonal antibodies that bind to and help remove amyloid-beta clumps. Beta-secretase and gamma-secretase inhibitors aim to halt the enzymes that generate amyloid-beta (Panza et al., 2019).
2. **Antioxidants and neuroprotective agents**: In AD, antioxidants and neuroprotective agents play a role to minimize oxidative stress and neuronal damage. Free radicals get neutralized by antioxidants including vitamin E, vitamin C, and flavonoids, which reduce oxidative damage to neurons and maintain cellular integrity (Jiang et al., 2016). Neuroprotective agents that promote cellular repair and protect neurons against apoptosis include curcumin, resveratrol, and N-acetylcysteine (NAC). Additionally, compounds like omega-3 fatty acids and neurotrophic factors promote the survival, growth, and function of neurons (Jiang et al., 2016).
3. **Gene therapy and RNA-based therapies**: Targeting the genetic and molecular origins of neurodegeneration, gene therapy, and RNA therapy give fascinating strategies to treating AD. Delivering therapeutic genes to the brain to replace or repair defective genes that cause tau phosphorylation, amyloid growth, or other disease-related processes is referred to as gene therapy (Pena et al., 2020). RNA-based therapies, such as antisense oligonucleotides and small interfering RNA (siRNA), target the RNA transcripts that produce harmful proteins like tau or amyloid-beta. These therapies function by chemically altering or suppressing gene expression (Pena et al., 2020).

7.7 CHALLENGES IN LIPID-BASED NANOCARRIER DEVELOPMENT

Challenges in lipid-based nanocarrier development include achieving optimal drug loading capacity and maintaining stability under physiological conditions. Ensuring controlled and sustained release without premature drug leakage is difficult, especially for hydrophobic drugs. Additionally, scalability of production, biocompatibility, and the potential for immune response are concerns. Overcoming these obstacles requires refining formulation strategies, improving targeting capabilities, and ensuring efficacy and safety for clinical applications (Mishra et al., 2018).

1. **Stability and scalability of nanocarriers**: The stability of nanocarriers involves maintaining their structure, drug entrapment, and functionality over time under physiological conditions. Scalability refers to the ability to produce nanocarriers efficiently in large quantities. Both factors are crucial for ensuring consistent quality, reproducibility, and cost-effectiveness in clinical applications, particularly for widespread use in drug delivery (Alshawwa et al., 2022).

2. **Potential toxicity and biocompatibility issues**: Potential toxicity and biocompatibility issues in lipid-based nanocarriers arise from the materials used, their degradation products, and unintended interactions with biological systems. Cytotoxicity can occur if the nanocarriers cause cell membrane disruption or inflammation. Immunogenicity may lead to immune responses, while prolonged circulation or accumulation in tissues could cause toxicity. Ensuring biocompatibility and non-toxicity requires thorough evaluation of lipid materials, surface modifications, and the overall safety profile for clinical use (Lim et al., 2012).
3. **Regulatory and clinical translation barriers**: Regulatory and clinical translation barriers for lipid-based nanocarriers include navigating complex approval processes, ensuring compliance with safety and efficacy standards, and meeting Good Manufacturing Practice (GMP) requirements. Demonstrating consistent batch-to-batch quality and scalability is crucial. Additionally, long-term safety and immune responses must be rigorously evaluated. Overcoming these challenges requires thorough preclinical studies, clinical trials, and collaboration with regulatory agencies to achieve successful product development and market approval (Souto et al., 2024).

7.8 LIMITATIONS OF CURRENT STUDIES

Current research on lipid-based nanocarriers has major limitations. Many preclinical research use animal models, which do not properly represent the intricacy of human diseases such as Alzheimer's. The process of selecting an animal model for biomedical research is quite complex, as not all models are suitable due to numerous restrictions. Many criteria should be considered when choosing an appropriate animal model for biomedical experiments (Mukherjee et al., 2022). The most significant factor is accurate model selection based on the physiological and/or pathophysiological similarities between animal species and humans. The long-term safety and toxicity of these nanocarriers have not been thoroughly investigated, particularly in terms of breakdown products and immunological responses. Also, issues in achieving consistency (Mukherjee et al., 2022).

7.9 FUTURE ASPECTS AND EMERGING TRENDS

Future directions in lipid-based nanocarriers focus on enhancing targeted delivery, stability, and clinical applicability. Emerging trends include the development of multifunctional nanocarriers that combine diagnostic and therapeutic capabilities for real-time monitoring of treatment efficacy. Advances in surface functionalization, such as ligand conjugation for precise targeting, are being explored to improve delivery across the BBB (Giordano et al., 2024). Emerging fields like gene therapy and RNA-based therapies can also benefit from lipid-based nanocarriers for efficient delivery to the brain. Addressing these limitations through interdisciplinary research, robust clinical trials, and standardized evaluation protocols is essential. Stimuli-responsive nanocarriers, triggered by pH, temperature, or enzymes, offer controlled drug release at specific sites. Future studies should concentrate on developing more sophisticated nanoparticle systems, improving the precision of targeting, and guaranteeing secure and economical production procedures. Moving this technology from the lab to the clinic will require interdisciplinary cooperation between chemists, biologists, engineers, and medical specialists. To guarantee a successful clinical translation in the near future, researchers will need to close the gap between in vitro findings and reality (Giordano et al., 2024).

7.10 CONCLUSION

This book chapter presents an overview of lipid-based nanocarriers, which have emerged as promising methods for solving AD treatment problems, including crossing the BBB and improving targeted medication delivery. A variety of proteins, including Aβ, Tau Tangle, ApoE, Clusterin, Presenilins (PS1 and PS2), Ephexin, and Glutamate Receptors, have a role in AD. Lipid-based nanocarriers, such as liposomes, SLNs, NLCs, lipid nanoemulsion, niosomes, nanoemulsion, cubosomes, and amylolipid nanovesicles, have emerged as promising DDSs for AD treatment. These carriers increase the bioavailability and stability of medicinal substances while allowing for controlled and prolonged release. Future prospects include the creation of multifunctional nanocarriers that combine therapeutic delivery with diagnostic capabilities, allowing for real-time monitoring of treatment.

REFERENCES

Agosti, E., Zeppieri, M., Antonietti, S., Battaglia, L., Ius, T., Gagliano, C., Fontanella, M. M., & Panciani, P. P. (2024). Navigating the nose-to-brain route: A systematic review on lipid-based nanocarriers for Central nervous system disorders. *Pharmaceutics*, *16*(3), 329. https://doi.org/10.3390/pharmaceutics16030329

Al Asmari, A. K., Ullah, Z., Tariq, M., & Fatani, A. (2016). Preparation, characterization, and in vivo evaluation of intranasally administered liposomal formulation of donepezil. *Drug Design, Development and Therapy*, 205–215.

Al-Azzawi, S., Masheta, D., Guildford, A. L., Phillips, G., & Santin, M. (2018). Dendrimeric poly (epsilon-lysine) delivery systems for the enhanced permeability of flurbiprofen across the blood-brain barrier in Alzheimer's disease. *International Journal of Molecular Sciences*, *19*(10), 3224.

Almuhayawi, M. S., Ramadan, W. S., Harakeh, S., Al Jaouni, S. K., Bharali, D. J., Mousa, S. A., & Almuhayawi, S. M. (2020). The potential role of pomegranate and its nanoformulations on cerebral neurons in aluminum chloride induced Alzheimer rat model. *Saudi Journal of Biological Sciences*, *27*(7), 1710–1716.

Alshawwa, S. Z., Kassem, A. A., Farid, R. M., Mostafa, S. K., & Labib, G. S. (2022). Nanocarrier drug delivery systems: Characterization, limitations, future perspectives and implementation of artificial intelligence. *Pharmaceutics*, *14*(4), 883.

Ansari, M., & Eslami, H. (2020). Preparation and study of the inhibitory effect of nanoniosomes containing essential oil from *Artemisia absinthium* on amyloid fibril formation. *Nanomed. J*, *7*(3), 243–50.

Arduino, I., Iacobazzi, R. M., Riganti, C., Lopedota, A. A., Perrone, M. G., Lopalco, A., Cutrignelli, A., Cantore, M., Laquintana, V., Franco, M., Colabufo, N. A., Luurtsema, G., Contino, M., & Denora, N. (2020). Induced expression of P-gp and BCRP transporters on brain endothelial cells using transferrin functionalized nanostructured lipid carriers: A first step of a potential strategy for the treatment of Alzheimer's disease. *International Journal of Pharmaceutics*, *591*, 120011.

Arpicco, S., Battaglia, L., Brusa, P., Cavalli, R., Chirio, D., Dosio, F., & Ceruti, M. (2016). Recent studies on the delivery of hydrophilic drugs in nanoparticulate systems. *Journal of Drug Delivery Science and Technology*, *32*, 298–312.

Barba, A. A., Bochicchio, S., Dalmoro, A., & Lamberti, G. (2019). Lipid delivery systems for nucleic-acid-based-drugs: From production to clinical applications. *Pharmaceutics*, *11*(8), 360.

Bejanin, A., Schonhaut, D. R., La Joie, R., Kramer, J. H., Baker, S. L., Sosa, N., & Rabinovici, G. D. (2017). Tau pathology and neurodegeneration contribute to cognitive impairment in Alzheimer's disease. *Brain*, *140*(12), 3286–3300.

Bernardi, A., Frozza, R. L., Meneghetti, A., Hoppe, J. B., Battastini, A. M. O., Pohlmann, A. R., & Salbego, C. G. (2012). Indomethacin-loaded lipid-core nanocapsules reduce the damage triggered by Aβ1-42 in Alzheimer's disease models. *International Journal of Nanomedicine*, 4927–4942.

Bhute, S., Sarmah, D., Datta, A., Rane, P., Shard, A., Goswami, A., & Bhattacharya, P. (2020). Molecular pathogenesis and interventional strategies for Alzheimer's disease: Promises and pitfalls. *ACS Pharmacology & Translational Science*, *3*(3), 472–488.

Boutajangout, A., Sigurdsson, E. M., & Krishnamurthy, P. K. (2011). Tau as a therapeutic target for Alzheimer's disease. *Current Alzheimer Research*, *8*(6), 666–677. https://doi.org/10.2174/156720511796717195.

Breijyeh, Z., & Karaman, R. (2020). Comprehensive review on Alzheimer's disease: Causes and treatment. *Molecules*, *25*(24), 5789.

Cook, E. K., Sell, G. L., Schaffer, T. B., & Margolis, S. S. (2019). The emergence of Ephexin5 as a therapeutic target in Alzheimer's disease. *Expert Opinion on Therapeutic Targets*, *23*(4), 263–265. https://doi.org/10.1080/14728222.2019.1586884

Costa, C. P., Moreira, J. N., Lobo, J. M. S., & Silva, A. C. (2021). Intranasal delivery of nanostructured lipid carriers, solid lipid nanoparticles and nanoemulsions: A current overview of in vivo studies. *Acta Pharmaceutica Sinica B*, *11*(4), 925–940.

Dara, T., Vatanara, A., Sharifzadeh, M., Khani, S., Vakilinezhad, M. A., Vakhshiteh, F., Meybodi, M. N., Malvajerd, S. S., Hassani, S., & Mosaddegh, M. H. (2019). Improvement of memory deficits in the rat model of Alzheimer's disease by erythropoietin-loaded solid lipid nanoparticles. *Neurobiol. Learn. Mem*, *166*, 107082. doi: 10.1016/j.nlm.2019.107082.

Daraban, B. S., Popa, A. S., & Stan, M. S. (2024). Latest perspectives on Alzheimer's disease treatment: The role of blood-brain barrier and antioxidant-based drug delivery systems. *Molecules*, *29*(17), 4056.

Del Amo, L., Cano, A., Ettcheto, M., Souto, E. B., Espina, M., Camins, A., & Sánchez-López, E. (2021). Surface functionalization of PLGA nanoparticles to increase transport across the BBB for Alzheimer's disease. *Applied Sciences*, *11*(9), 4305.

De Strooper, B. (2007). Loss-of-function presenilin mutations in Alzheimer disease. Talking point on the role of presenilin mutations in Alzheimer disease. *EMBO Reports*, *8*(2), 141–146. https://doi.org/10.1038/sj.embor.7400897.

Di Stefano, A., Iannitelli, A., Laserra, S., & Sozio, P. (2011). Drug delivery strategies for Alzheimer's disease treatment. *Expert Opinion on Drug Delivery*, *8*(5), 581–603.

Ehtiati, S., Alizadeh, M., Farhadi, F., Khalatbari, K., Ajiboye, B. O., Rahimi, V. B., & Askari, V. R. (2023). Promising influences of caffeic acid and caffeic acid phenethyl ester against natural and chemical toxins: A comprehensive and mechanistic review. *Journal of Functional Foods*, *107*, 105637.

El-Banna, A. H., Abo El-Ela, F. I., Abdel-Wahab, A., Gamal, A., Abdel-Razik, A. R. H., El-Banna, H. A., & Abdelghany, A. K. (2024). Therapeutic efficacy of amygdaline and amygdaline-loaded niosomes in a rat model of Alzheimer's disease via oxidative stress, brain neurotransmitters, and apoptotic pathway. *Beni-Suef University Journal of Basic and Applied Sciences*, *13*(1), 117.

Estabragh, M. A. R., Hamidifar, Z., & Pardakhty, A. (2018). Formulation of rivastigmine niosomes for Alzheimer disease. *International Pharmacy Acta*, *1*(1), 104–104.

Gaballa, S. A., El Garhy, O. H., & Abdelkader, H. (2020). Cubosomes: Composition, preparation, and drug delivery applications. *Journal of Advanced Biomedical and Pharmaceutical Sciences*, *3*(1), 1–9.

Garbuz, D. G., Zatsepina, O. G., & Evgen'ev, M. B. (2021). Beta amyloid, tau protein, And neuroinflammation: An attempt to integrate different hypotheses of Alzheimer's disease pathogenesis. *Molecular Biology*, *55*, 670–682.

Giordano, A., Provenza, A. C., Reverchon, G., Baldino, L., & Reverchon, E. (2024). Lipid-based nanocarriers: Bridging diagnosis and cancer therapy. *Pharmaceutics*, *16*(9), 1158.

Gobbi, M., Re, F., Canovi, M., Beeg, M., Gregori, M., Sesana, S., & Masserini, M. E. (2010). Lipid-based nanoparticles with high binding affinity for amyloid-β1–42 peptide. *Biomaterials*, *31*(25), 6519–6529.

Gopalan, D., Pandey, A., Udupa, N., & Mutalik, S. (2020). Receptor specific, stimuli responsive and subcellular targeted approaches for effective therapy of Alzheimer: Role of surface engineered nanocarriers. *Journal of Controlled Release*, *319*, 183–200.

Guo, Q., Li, Y., Xu, S., Wang, P., Qian, K., Yang, P., & Zhang, Q. (2023). Brain-neuron targeted nanoparticles for peptide synergy therapy at dual-target of Alzheimer's disease. *Journal of Controlled Release*, *355*, 604–621.

Jiang, T., Sun, Q., & Chen, S. (2016). Oxidative stress: A major pathogenesis and potential therapeutic target of antioxidative agents in Parkinson's disease and Alzheimer's disease. *Progress in Neurobiology*, *147*, 1–19.

Kaur, H., Pancham, P., Kaur, R., Agarwal, S., & Singh, M. (2020). Synthesis and characterization of *Citrus limonum* essential oil based nanoemulsion and its enhanced antioxidant activity with stability for transdermal application. *Journal of Biomaterials and Nanobiotechnology*, *11*(4), 215–236.

Kelkar, S. S., & Reineke, T. M. (2011). Theranostics: Combining imaging and therapy. *Bioconjugate Chemistry*, *22*(10), 1879–1903.

Khan, N. H., Mir, M., Ngowi, E. E., Zafar, U., Khakwani, M. M. A. K., Khattak, S., & Ji, X. Y. (2021). Nanomedicine: A promising way to manage Alzheimer's disease. *Frontiers in Bioengineering and Biotechnology*, *9*, 630055.

Kim, J., Basak, J. M., & Holtzman, D. M. (2009). The role of apolipoprotein e in Alzheimer's disease. *Neuron*, *63*(3), 287–303.

Li, T., Lu, L., Pember, E., Li, X., Zhang, B., & Zhu, Z. (2022). New insights into neuroinflammation involved in pathogenic mechanism of Alzheimer's disease and its potential for therapeutic intervention. *Cells*, *11*(12), 1925.

Lim, S. B., Banerjee, A., & Önyüksel, H. (2012). Improvement of drug safety by the use of lipid-based nanocarriers. *Journal of Controlled Release*, *163*(1), 34–45.

Md, S., Gan, S. Y., Haw, Y. H., Ho, C. L., Wong, S., & Choudhury, H. (2018). In vitro neuroprotective effects of naringenin nanoemulsion against β-amyloid toxicity through the regulation of amyloidogenesis and tau phosphorylation. *International Journal of Biological Macromolecules*, *118*, 1211–1219.

Mehnert, W., & Mäder, K. (2012). Solid lipid nanoparticles: Production, characterization and applications. *Advanced Drug Delivery Reviews*, *64*, 83–101.

Mishra, D. K., Shandilya, R., & Mishra, P. K. (2018). Lipid based nanocarriers: A translational perspective. *Nanomedicine: Nanotechnology, Biology and Medicine*, *14*(7), 2023–2050.

Mukherjee, P., Roy, S., Ghosh, D., & Nandi, S. K. (2022). Role of animal models in biomedical research: A review. *Laboratory Animal Research*, *38*(1), 18. https://doi.org/10.1186/s42826-022-00128-1.

Musacchio, T., & Torchilin, V. P. (2011). Recent developments in lipid-based pharmaceutical nanocarriers. *Front Biosci*, *16*(1388), 412.

Nirale, P., Paul, A., & Yadav, K. S. (2020). Nanoemulsions for targeting the neurodegenerative diseases: Alzheimer's, Parkinson's and Prion's. *Life Sciences*, *245*, 117394.

Nunes, D., Loureiro, J. A., & Pereira, M. C. (2022). Drug delivery systems as a strategy to improve the efficacy of FDA-approved Alzheimer's drugs. *Pharmaceutics*, *14*(11), 2296. https://doi.org/10.3390/pharmaceutics14112296

Panza, F., Lozupone, M., Logroscino, G., & Imbimbo, B. P. (2019). A critical appraisal of amyloid-β-targeting therapies for Alzheimer disease. *Nature Reviews Neurology*, *15*(2), 73–88.

Patidar, A., Thakur, D. S., Kumar, P., & Verma, J. (2010). A review on novel lipid based nanocarriers. *Int J Pharm Pharm Sci*, *2*(4), 30–35.

Patil, S. P., Ayappa, I. A., Caples, S. M., Kimoff, R. J., Patel, S. R., & Harrod, C. G. (2019). Treatment of adult obstructive sleep apnea with positive airway pressure: An American Academy of Sleep Medicine Clinical Practice Guideline. *Journal of Clinical Sleep Medicine*, *15*(2), 335–343.

Pena, S. A., Iyengar, R., Eshraghi, R. S., Bencie, N., Mittal, J., Aljohani, A., & Eshraghi, A. A. (2020). Gene Therapy for neurological disorders: Challenges and recent advancements. *Journal of Drug Targeting*, *28*(2), 111–128.

Peng, C., Huang, Y., & Zheng, J. (2020). Renal clearable nanocarriers: Overcoming the physiological barriers for precise drug delivery and clearance. *Journal of Controlled Release: Official Journal of the Controlled Release Society*, *322*, 64–80. https://doi.org/10.1016/j.jconrel.2020.03.020

Pottoo, F. H., Sharma, S., Javed, M. N., Barkat, M. A., Harshita, Alam, M. S., & Ashraf, G. M. (2020). Lipid-based nanoformulations in the treatment of neurological disorders. *Drug Metabolism Reviews*, *52*(1), 185–204.

Preeti, Sambhakar, S., Saharan, R., Narwal, S., Malik, R., Gahlot, V., Khalid, A., Najmi, A., Zoghebi, K., Halawi, M. A., Albratty, M., & Mohan, S. (2023). Exploring LIPIDs for their potential to improves bioavailability of lipophilic drugs candidates: A review. *Saudi Pharmaceutical Journal: SPJ: the Official Publication of the Saudi Pharmaceutical Society*, *31*(12), 101870. https://doi.org/10.1016/j.jsps.2023.101870

Puranik, N., & Song, M. (2024). Glutamate: Molecular mechanisms and signaling pathway in Alzheimer's disease, a potential therapeutic target. *Molecules*, *29*(23), 5744.

Ravouru, N., Kondreddy, P., & Korakanchi, D. (2013). Formulation and evaluation of niosomal nasal drug delivery system of folic acid for brain targeting. *Current Drug Discovery Technologies*, *10*(4), 270–282.

Rinaldi, C., & Wood, M. J. (2018). Antisense oligonucleotides: The next frontier for treatment of neurological disorders. *Nature Reviews Neurology*, *14*(1), 9–21.

Roda, A. R., Serra-Mir, G., Montoliu-Gaya, L., Tiessler, L., & Villegas, S. (2022). Amyloid-beta peptide and tau protein crosstalk in Alzheimer's disease. *Neural Regeneration Research*, *17*(8), 1666–1674.

Sadegh Malvajerd, S., Azadi, A., Izadi, Z., Kurd, M., Dara, T., Dibaei, M., & Hamidi, M. (2018). Brain delivery of curcumin using solid lipid nanoparticles and nanostructured lipid carriers: Preparation, optimization, and pharmacokinetic evaluation. *ACS Chemical Neuroscience*, *10*(1), 728–739.

Sadegh Malvajerd, S., Izadi, Z., Azadi, A., Kurd, M., Derakhshankhah, H., Sharifzadeh, M., & Hamidi, M. (2019). Neuroprotective potential of curcumin-loaded nanostructured lipid carrier in an animal model of Alzheimer's disease: Behavioral and biochemical evidence. *Journal of Alzheimer's Disease*, *69*(3), 671–686.

Sahoo, A. K., Dandapat, J., Dash, U. C., & Kanhar, S. (2018). Features and outcomes of drugs for combination therapy as multi-targets strategy to combat Alzheimer's disease. *Journal of Ethnopharmacology*, *215*, 42–73.

Sathya, S., Shanmuganathan, B., Manirathinam, G., Ruckmani, K., & Devi, K. P. (2018). α-Bisabolol loaded solid lipid nanoparticles attenuates Aβ aggregation and protects neuro-2a cells from Aβ-induced neurotoxicity. *Journal of Molecular Liquids*, *264*, 431–441.

Singh, B., Day, C. M., Abdella, S., & Garg, S. (2024). Alzheimer's disease current therapies, novel drug delivery systems and future directions for better disease management. *Journal of Controlled Release*, *367*, 402–424.

Sintov, A. C. (2020). Amylolipid nanovesicles: A self-assembled lipid-modified starch hybrid system constructed for direct nose-to-brain delivery of curcumin. *Int J Pharm*, Oct 15;*588*, 119725. doi: 10.1016/j.ijpharm.2020.119725. Epub 2020 Aug 5. PMID: 32763387.

Souto, E. B., Blanco-Llamero, C., Krambeck, K., Kiran, N. S., Yashaswini, C., Postwala, H., & Maheshwari, R. (2024). regulatory insights into nanomedicine and Gene vaccine innovation: Safety assessment, challenges, and regulatory perspectives. *Acta Biomaterialia*, *180*, 1–17.

Taliyan, R., Kakoty, V., Sarathlal, K. C., Kharavtekar, S. S., Karennanavar, C. R., Choudhary, Y. K., & Kesharwani, P. (2022). Nanocarrier mediated drug delivery as an impeccable therapeutic approach against Alzheimer's disease. *Journal of Controlled Release*, *343*, 528–550.

Witika, B. A., Poka, M. S., Demana, P. H., Matafwali, S. K., Melamane, S., Malungelo Khamanga, S. M., & Makoni, P. A. (2022). Lipid-based nanocarriers for neurological disorders: A review of the state-of-the-art and therapeutic success to Date. *Pharmaceutics*, *14*(4), 836.

Yasir, M., Willcox, M. D. P., & Dutta, D. (2018). Action of antimicrobial peptides against bacterial biofilms. *Materials*, *11*(12), 2468.

Yavarpour-Bali, H., Ghasemi-Kasman, M., & Pirzadeh, M. (2019). Curcumin-loaded nanoparticles: A novel therapeutic strategy in treatment of central nervous system disorders. *International Journal of Nanomedicine*, 4449–4460.

Yi, X., & Gao, H. (2016). Incorporation of soft particles into lipid vesicles: Effects of particle size and elasticity. *Langmuir*, *32*(49), 13252–13260.

Yi Xue, H., Guo, P., Wen, W. C., & Lun Wong, H. (2015). Lipid-based nanocarriers for RNA delivery. *Current Pharmaceutical Design*, *21*(22), 3140–3147.

8 Chitosan-Based Nanoparticles in the Treatment of Alzheimer's Disease

Dibyananda Majhi, Priyanka Yadav, Pravat Kumar Sahu, Jayachandran Venkatesan, and Ch. Subrahmanyam

8.1 INTRODUCTIONS

Alzheimer's disease (AD) is becoming the most fatal and dangerous affecting people worldwide. According to reports, there are more than 55 million patients with still a steep increase in cases over the years [1]. This progressive and neurodegenerative disease is effecting both young as well as old age people. AD is a specific type dementia (Figure 8.1a). Although it is most commonly seen in case of old people over the age of 65, nowadays, early-onset AD risks are also increasing, which may be due to an unhealthy lifestyle and poor mental state management. While the exact cause remains unknown, overall a combination of genetic, lifestyle, and environmental

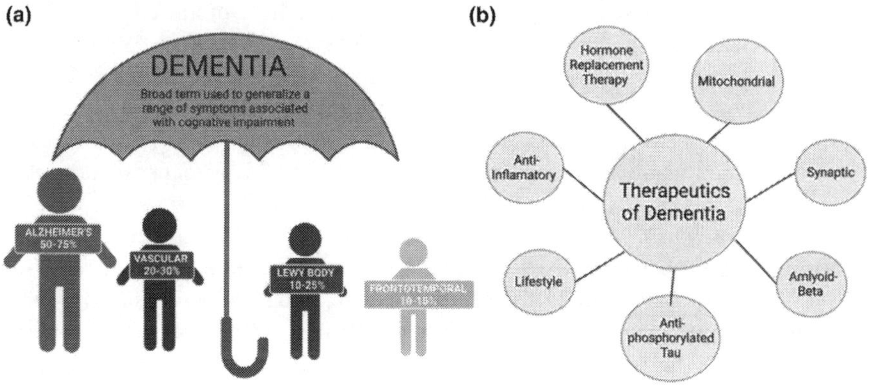

FIGURE 8.1 (a) The significant types of dementia are Alzheimer's disease, Lewy body dementia, vascular dementia, and frontotemporal dementia and (b) management of Alzheimer's disease. (Reproduced with permission from [5].)

DOI: 10.1201/9781003543381-8

factors is believed to contribute to the development of this fatal disease [2]. Most cases of AD are sporadic, with an increased risk in old age, while less than 2.5% are attributed to genetic predisposition. It is becoming an alarming health issue as it involves in damaging both personal and professional life. Currently, there are no available treatments for a complete cure of AD. However, current treatments with changing life style can help in decreasing the severity and progression (Figure 8.1b). Many treatment procedures have been employed including immunotherapy, gene therapy, and contemporary therapeutic approaches depending on the condition of AD. Different Food and Drug Administration (FDA) approved neurologic drugs including donepezil, rivastigmine, and galantamine are also used for slowing down the harsh effect of AD [3]. Still tremendous efforts have been put forwarded by the research community in search of an efficient treatment. Among various methods, nanotechnology-assisted drug delivery has been an effective approach for AD therapy. Nanocarriers in combination with different drugs play an important role in increasing the concentration of drugs, optimal drug release and exceptional bioavailability. Metal nanoparticles and polymeric nanoparticle-assisted AD treatments can cross the so-called blood–brain barrier (BBB) problem and deliver the drugs to the brain [4]. Nanoparticles can be designed for target-specific binding to the cell surface, which can help in improved AD eradication.

8.2 ALZHEIMER'S DISEASE

Alzheimer's disease is the most common cause of dementia characterized by a loss of memory and cognitive abilities. Accumulation of hyperphosphorylated tau-containing intracellular neurofibrillary tangles (NFTs) and amyloid-β (Aβ) containing extracellular neuritic plaques (NPs) are the central pathological events in AD [6–8]. In AD, before neurodegeneration or fibril formation, synaptic dysfunction occurs, which leads to memory loss and personality changes [9]. Hence, AD is a neurodegenerative disorder marked by extracellular Aβ plaques and intracellular NFTs, which are aggregates of hyperphosphorylated tau, a microtubule-associated protein (MAP), within neurons (Frisoni et al. 2021). Aβ protein is produced through the sequential cleavage of amyloid precursor protein (APP) by β- and γ-secretases.

In AD, mutation in genes involved in Aβ formation, APP generation, PSEN1 and PSEN2 (encoding presenilin 1 and presenilin 2, respectively), and tau encoding MAPT gene causes familial AD [10]. In 1984, Aβ was first isolated from the cerebrovascular amyloid of AD patients and identified as the primary component of senile plaques [11]. Aβ spontaneously aggregates into β-sheet structures, forming higher-order oligomers, protofibrils, and fibrils. Aβ pathology is thought to unfold in distinct and reproducible spatial patterns over the course of the disease. However, recent studies have uncovered that specific FAD mutations influence the spatiotemporal dynamics of Aβ aggregation. In 1986, MAP tau was first described as a major component of NFTs [12,13]. Tau pathology disseminates throughout the Alzheimer's brain in a fixed, orderly sequence across neural circuits [14]. The progress of tau pathology is closely linked to the loss of neurons [15]. NFTs are chiefly composed of intracellular paired helical filaments (PHF), with tau protein as the predominant structural constituent. The amyloid hypothesis is a recent perception that contributes to understanding AD. The disease results in brain atrophy caused by neuronal loss and synapse degeneration. Synaptic loss strongly correlates with cognitive decline in both human and animal models of AD. Evidence suggests that soluble forms of Aβ and tau can cause synaptotoxicity and spread through neural circuits. AD is a genetic and sporadic neurodegenerative disease that causes an amnestic cognitive impairment in its prototypical presentation and non-amnestic cognitive impairment in its less common variants. Short-term memory loss is the most frequent symptom, though impairments in expressive speech, visuospatial skills, and executive functions are also observed. Most cases of AD are not inherited in a dominant pattern, and the genetic factors involved often display complex interactions. For the diagnosis of AD, three biomarkers have been well-established and validated in cerebrospinal fluid (CSF): Aβ, total tau, and phospho-tau (P-tau) at 181th position.

8.3 TREATMENT FOR ALZHEIMER'S DISEASE

AD has been a serious threat over the years due to its escalating cases globally and even leading cause of deaths in a few countries. The data revealed that billions of dollars per year used for the treatment, which is an economic burden to any country. It is posing significant challenges to the society as well as healthcare systems. Although there is no treatment procedure for a complete cure of this disease, several treatment procedures have been adopted over the years to slow down the worsening effect and progress of the disease.

In managing the progress of AD, the FDA has approved drugs which are further categorized into two types: (i) cholinesterase inhibitors (ChEIs) and (ii) N-methyl-D-aspartate (NMDA) receptor blockers. ChEIs drugs can be used in the early stages, and the latter category drugs can be used for moderate to severe conditions of AD. A few FDA-approved drugs e.g., Tacrine, donepezil, rivastigmine, galantamine, and memantine, are the first four ChEIs, and the fifth is an NMDA receptor [16]. AD drugs and their evolution over the years are presented in Figure 8.2. These conventional drugs are provided in tablet and capsule form. Various clinical and non-clinical data revealed that these drugs are helpful in slowing down the disease progression to a great extent, and cognitive improvements are also seen after medications.

Physiological factors such as the BBB, drug efflux mediated by p-glycoprotein, and the blood-cerebrospinal fluid barrier (B-CSF) limit the ability of conventional AD drugs to effectively reach the central nervous system (CNS). To address the challenge of drugs crossing the BBB, innovative approaches in drug development have become essential. These challenges can be addressed by integrating therapeutics with nanotechnology, which enhances the therapeutic potential and allows for better regulation of drug molecule properties [18,19]. Liposomes, discovered in the 1960s, have evolved into well-established and clinically validated nanocarriers that have been thoroughly studied for many years [20]. These nanocarriers are valued for their unique properties, including non-immunogenicity, biodegradability, low toxicity, antimicrobial properties, neuroprotective, and biocompatibility [21–23]. Liposomes, with their lipophilic properties, elegantly enable the transport of drugs across the brain's endothelial membrane, offering remarkable efficiency in brain uptake. The release of drugs from liposomes primarily occurs through two key mechanisms:

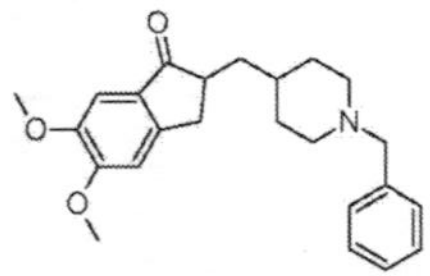	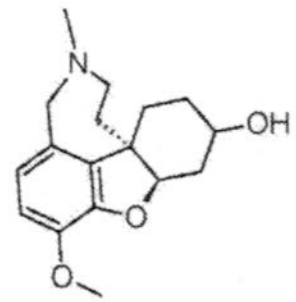	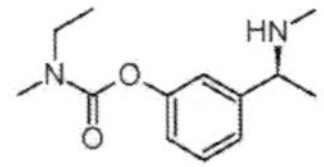	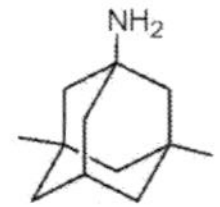
Donepezil, AChE inhibitor, approved in 1997	Galantamine, AChE inhibitor, approved in 1995	Rivastigmine, AChE inhibitor, approved in 1997	Memantine, NMDA receptor, antagonist approved in 2003
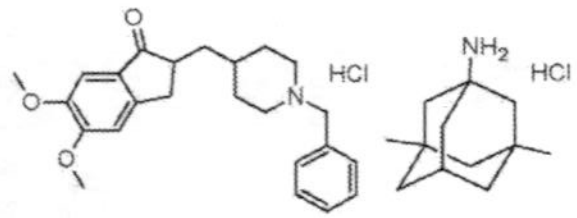	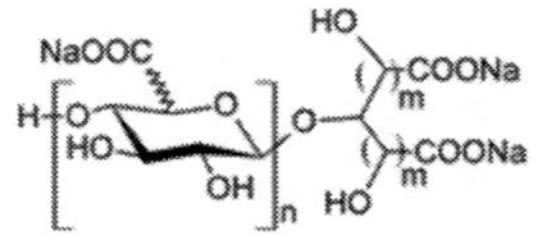		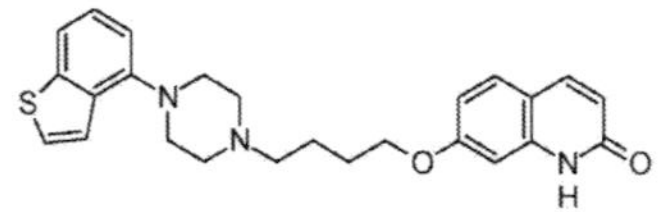
NAMZARIC® (memantine HCl and donepezil HCl), approved in 2014	Sodium oligomannate (development code GV-971)-mixture of oligosaccharides isolated from *Ecklonia kurome* used in China, approved in 2019	Aducanumab, approved in 2021	Brexpiprazole, for the treatment of major depressive disorder, approved in 2023 Lecanemab, approved in 2023 Donanemab, approved in 2024

FIGURE 8.2 Few current anti-AD drugs approved by FDA/China. (Reproduced with permission from [17].)

drug diffusion and liposome endocytosis [24]. Vesicle size and lipid composition significantly impact both their transmission through systemic circulation and their efficiency in cellular uptake within brain cells. In 1994, curcumin-loaded liposomes were developed that reduced amyloid plaque deposition and protected brain cells by binding to amyloid proteins and creating an aggregation-free environment [25]. In 2008, a stable retro-inverso peptide was developed that crosses the BBB and reaches to CNS and inhibits Aβ aggregation and brain toxins [26]. In 2008, it was demonstrated that intranasal administration of rivastigmine-loaded liposomes enhanced drug release, improved patient compliance, and increased both the levels and half-life of rivastigmine in brain cells [27]. Donepezil's challenges in crossing the BBB were mitigated by loading it into liposomes for intranasal administration, which improved bioavailability and reduced side effects. This method significantly enhanced drug absorption and uptake in the brain, with no observed morphological changes in tissues [28].

Inorganic nanoparticles (INPs) are highly valued in biomedical applications due to their large surface area, nontoxic nature, and exceptional stability under physiological conditions, which can be finely controlled by manipulating parameters such as size, morphology, surface chemistry, and interfacial interactions. Gold nanoparticles (AuNPs), silica (SiO_2), and silicon quantum dots are particularly noteworthy for their intrinsic biocompatibility, profound cellular uptake efficiency, and ability to traverse the BBB without requiring surface modifications, making them ideal candidates for both therapeutic and diagnostic applications in nanomedicine (as AuNPs, AgNPs, size range 2–100 nm) [29]. AuNPs inhibit Aβ aggregation and fibril formation, impacting memory cells within 72 hours post-injection [30–32]. To improve the BBB permeation, iron oxide nanoparticles were coated with polyethylene glycol (PEG) [33]. Magnetic iron oxide nanoparticles (MIONs), approved by the FDA as MRI contrast agents, have been functionalized to target Aβ plaques in transgenic mice, though concerns remain about the feasibility of BBB manipulation for human use [34]. Magnetic γ-Fe_2O_3 nanoparticles selectively label Aβ1-40 fibrils and can remove fibrils from solubilized Aβ samples via an external magnetic field [35,36].

Polymeric nanoparticles are preferred over other types of nanoparticles due to their biodegradability, biocompatibility, stability during storage, and extended shelf-life. They also offer effective control and sustained release of their payload. These nanoparticles are designed to protect hydrophobic drugs from degradation and environmental deactivation, while also enhancing the drug's bioavailability and controlling the release of the drug [37]. In pharmaceutical applications, lactic-co-glycolic acid (LGA) is the most used polysaccharide NP among [38]. Biodegradable polysaccharide PLGA NPs are used in treating AD by neuroprotective effect. Biodegradable polysaccharide nanoparticles made from poly(lactic-co-glycolic acid) (PLGA) are used in the treatment of AD due to their neuroprotective effects [39]. Rescued the memory in an AD mouse model and to reduce the cytotoxicity of Aβ coenzyme Q10 (CoQ10)-loaded PLGA NPs are used [40,41]. Among many polymeric nanoparticles, chitosan nanoparticles (ChNPs) possesses extreme potential for AD treatments mainly due to its effective penetration of the BBB. Other properties, particularly for such applications include biocompatibility, biodegradability, multifunctionality, and environmental impact of the nanoparticles.

8.4 CHITOSAN NANOPARTICLES

Among various nature-derived polymeric nanoparticles, chitosan, and chitosan-based nanoparticles have diverse applications in health-life formulations. Chitosan is basically derived from naturally occurring chitin mostly by deacetylation. Particularly, chitosan derived by N-deacetylation is a valuable biopolymer which can form nanoparticles bearing a unique polycationic character [42]. In detail, this natural polysaccharide exhibits free amine moiety, which facilitates the formation of NPs through crosslinking or spontaneous self-assembly (Figure 8.3).

ChNPs acquired special attention than other nature-derived polymeric materials due to its inherent antimicrobial properties. Including its non-toxicity and biocompatibility, it showcases both adsorption-enhancing properties and mucoadhesive nature with minimal immune reaction [42]. Owing to its above-mentioned important properties, these ChNPs are widely used in drug delivery systems (DDS) with improved sensitivity, specificity, and biodistribution. In particular, for AD disease treatment it is a wonder material due to the presence of D-glucosamine group resembling to sugar which are often used as cryoprotectants. This characteristic feature helps in the course of lyophilization of anti-Alzheimer therapeutics. Multifunctional properties coupled with biocompatibility of ChNPs, motivates the potential use of this material as nanocarriers of several potential AD drugs. For example, ChNPs have been coupled with many acetylcholinesterase inhibitors for effective treatment of AD. In addition, various herbal active materials (e.g., curcumin, piperine, etc.) are also loaded over ChNPs, which served as a complementary approach for AD therapy [43]

8.4.1 CHITOSAN NANOPARTICLES PREPARATION AND CHARACTERIZATION

ChNPs are prepared in various methods depending on the need and applications. Properties of the NPs depend on the synthesis method adopted. Following are a few broad class of synthesis methodologies used in fabricating ChNPs and insight into their characterization.

Ionotropic Gelation Method: The ionotropic gelation method implies using an ionic cross-linker to synthesize nanoparticles. Typically, tripolyphosphate (TPP) serves as the ionic cross-linker, facilitating the formation of chitosan (CS) nanoparticles through electrostatic interactions [44]. These interactions occur between the polyanionic TPP and the positively charged amino groups of CS molecules,

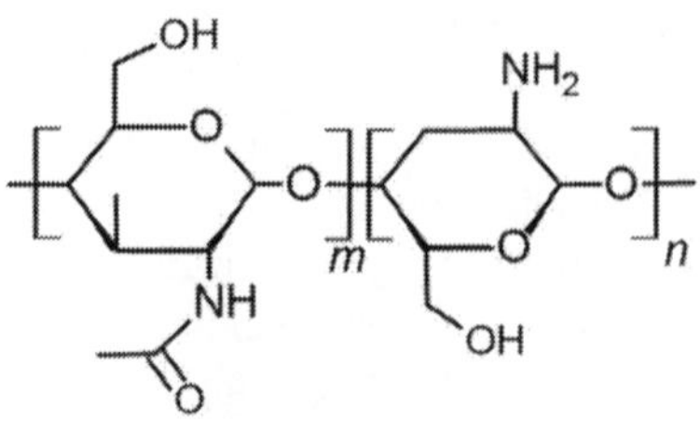

FIGURE 8.3 Structure of chitosan. (Figure reproduced with permission from [42].)

resulting in the formation of CS nanoparticles [45]. The advantage of this technique is the ability to easily control the size of the nanoparticles by adjusting the concentration of the precursor materials [46]. By employing this method, Zameer et al. prepared spherical-shaped alendronate (ALN)-loaded chitosan nanoparticles (CS-ALN-NPs) having an average size range of 200 nm by optimizing the concentration of sodium TPP (cross-linker) in ALN loaded CS solution for the treatment of AD [47].

Microemulsion method: The microemulsion is formed using the reverse micellization method, which involves adding an appropriate surfactant to an organic solvent, followed by the addition of an aqueous acidic solution of chitosan. Commonly used surfactants in this process include sodium bis(2-ethylhexyl) sulfosuccinate or cetyltrimethylammonium bromide (CTAB), typically in an organic solvent such as n-hexane [48]. The polymerization reaction occurs within the micelle core, where monomers and other hydrophilic compounds are cross-linked to form CS nanoparticles in the aqueous solution, encapsulated by a layer of surfactant molecules dispersed in the organic solvent [49]. The key advantage of this process is that the reverse micelle's core, being of nanometric dimensions, ensures that all growth processes result in nanoparticles of consistent size.

Cross-linking method: The nanoparticles of CS are formed by the stable chemical covalent interaction between the primary amino groups of the chitosan and the functional cross-linker. Generally, in the form of crosslinkers like glutaraldehyde, dicarboxylic acid, polyethene glycol (PEG), p-phthaldehyde, ascorbyl palmitate, and dehydroascorbyl palmitate to form a stable covalently bonded complex. In this method, chitosan micro-/nanoparticles are formed through a chemical interaction between a cross-linking agent and the primary amino groups of chitosan. Common cross-linkers are glutaraldehyde, p-phthaldehyde, ascorbyl palmitate, and dehydroascorbyl palmitate. Chitosan microparticles prepared using ascorbyl and dehydroascorbyl palmitate have lower toxicity and high insulin-loading efficiency, and release insulin in a controlled-release manner, for approximately 80 hours, when compared to that produced using di-aldehydes, glutaraldehyde, and p-phthaldehyde as chemical cross-linkers. Chemical cross-linking may take place either through one or two steps. The procedure involves formation of a water/oil (w/o) emulsion in which chitosan and the therapeutic agent are in the aqueous phase that is emulsified into external immiscible solvent. The cross-linking agent is gradually added and, finally, the prepared particles are separated and washed with appropriate solvent to yield the desired particle [50].

Self-assembly method: The self-assembly method, also known as the polyelectrolyte complex method for nanoparticle preparation, involves the ionic interaction between chitosan (CS) and an oppositely charged counterion or polymer, resulting in the formation of a charge-neutralized hydrophobic complex. This process allows for precise control over nanoparticle size by adjusting factors such as the molecular weight, concentration, and pH of the chitosan solution, leading to particles with a size range of 50 to 700 nm. Nanoparticles produced via self-assembly are particularly well-suited for encapsulating both hydrophilic and lipophilic drugs, providing a stable environment for active ingredients within a customizable, biocompatible matrix [51].

8.4.2 Chitosan Nanoparticles as Drug Delivery System

A comprehensive idea about the importance, unique properties, and effectiveness of ChNPs for AD therapy is already discussed in the prior texts of this chapter. Various AD drugs, herbal ingredients, and protein conjugate along with acetylcholinesterase inhibitors have been trialed for AD therapy where ChNPs were used as one complementary counterpart. A few of them are discussed below.

8.4.3 Chitosan-Curcumin Nanoparticles

Curcumin ((1E,6E)-1,7-bis(4-hydroxy-3-methoxyphenyl)-1,6-heptadiene-3,5-dione) is a highly studied natural compound due to its extensive bioactivity, including its potential anti-AD effects. Curcumin (CUR) has additionally been identified as an MRI contrast agent for the detection of Aβ plaques [51]. Curcumin has neuroprotective potential due to its anti-amyloidogenic, metal-chelating, and anti-oxidative properties. It also modulates macrophage polarization by obstructing the toll-like receptor. In contrast, curcumin shows very low aqueous solubility, poor absorption in the intestines, and great clearance rate, which potentially limits the therapeutic power [52]. The applicability of this important biologically active ingredient is further hindered by its low permeability via the BBB. In order to address these problems as well to improve the phagocytosis of the Aβ-peptide, curcumin wrapped with chitosan nanocapsule or nanocarrier is developed which improves delivery and stability and enables the crossing of the BBB. Cellular uptake of Chitosan-CUR NPs is also higher as compared to bare CUR. This resulted in good AD therapy and decrease of cognitive dysfunction [53].

8.4.4 Chitosan-Piperine Nanoparticles

Piperine (PIP, (2E,4E)-5-(1,3-benzodioxol-5-yl)-1-(piperidin-1-ylpenta)-2,4-dien-1-one) is naturally occurring pungent alkaloid from the plant *Piper nigrum* [53]. It has been used from centuries as an anticancer, antidepressant, antioxidant, and so many other applications in healthcare. Piperine containing a tertiary nitrogen like ACh, can also decrease the cognitive dysfunction in AD by AChE inhibition or by helping brain's cholinergic system. However, to overcome the pre-systemic metabolism and hydrophobicity issues of delivering in the brain intranasal ChNPs were coupled. These nanoparticles improved cognitive function like donepezil, offered AChE inhibition and antioxidant effects, reduced nasal irritation, and were brain-safe, enabling a 20-fold reduction in the oral dose for AD treatment [53].

8.4.5 Chitosan-AChE Inhibitors

Rivastigmine (RT) ([3-[(1S)-1-(dimethylamino)ethyl]phenyl] N-ethyl-N-methylcarbamate) is widely used for mild as well as moderate case of AD [53,54]. But the utilization of ChNPs for delivering rivastigmine in the context of AD is an important strategy for the treatment process [55]. Like other drugs, Rivastigmine also faces difficulties in crossing the BBB because of its hydrophobic properties, necessitating repeated dosing. To enhance the bioavailability, and uptake of rivastigminc, intranasal delivery with ionic gelation of rivastigmine-loaded chitosan NPs were prepared. This method significantly enhances drug delivery efficiency compared to both rivastigmine in solution and intravenously administered NPs. Notably, intranasal delivery of these NPs demonstrated a remarkable 355% increase in drug targeting efficiency (DTF) and achieved a drug targeting potential (DTP) of 71.8% [56].

8.4.6 Chitosan-Therapeutic Agents

Various therapeutic agents are also loaded onto ChNPs for efficient treatment of AD. 17-α-Estradiol (E_2) is a well-known female sex hormone also helps in brain development and useful in improvement and prevention of AD [57]. However, like most of the drugs, delivery efficiency after intranasal administration is limited by poor permeability of the nasal mucosa and mucociliary clearance. Chitosan NPs is probed to be an excellent material improving the delivery of E_2 to targeted brain tissue. A convincing delivery of E2 is noted in CSF after compositing with ChNPs [53,58]. Some specific Aβ-peptide sub-fragments are also exhibiting therapeutic efficacy on AD by reducing the amyloid deposition. Aβ sub-fragment with ChNPs can surpass the BBB and enhance the targeted brain cell uptake which is a great step towards AD treatment. Many other therapeutic agents including Memantine and different immunotherapy drugs are also studied in conjugation with ChNPs for improved AD therapy [53].

8.4.7 Chitosan-Protein Conjugates

In addition to the above-mentioned methods, ChNPs have shown promising results for AD therapy in conjugation with different useful protein delivery. Brain-derived neurotrophic factor (BDNF) is one of the most explored and well-known neurotrophic factors in the CNS [59]. It operates many controls of different cellular processes related to the maintenance and development of normal brain function. BDNF also plays a significant role in synaptic plasticity that helps in memory function of normal adult brain. A noted decrease of BDNF proteins occurs in AD brains which may cause cognitive dysfunction leading to the said disease [58]. So with the urgent need for a carrier to deliver BDNF to the target disease tissue, chitosan-based composite materials proven to be an effective material for the same. It can also co-deliver different drug molecules like cannabidiol (CBD) along with BDNF delivery for AD therapy.

8.5 POTENTIAL CHALLENGES AND FUTURE PERSPECTIVE

Limited BBB Penetration, short drug half-life, risk of off-target effects, and clinical translation difficulties are potential challenges in the treatment of AD. Till date, many approaches are being employed to solve the issues. Advanced surface modifications and receptor-specific targeting, stimuli-responsive, incorporating sustained-release formulations, optimized manufacturing systems, site-specific drug release, and robust safety testing protocols are significant future directions for getting an effective solution for improved treatment of this fatal and life-threatening disease. In contrast to traditional AD treatments, future approaches to chitosan-based nanomaterials for

AD focus on enhancing targeted drug delivery, integrating diagnostics, and enabling personalized and regenerative therapies. With continued advancements in nanotechnology, precision medicine, and bioengineering chitosan nanomaterials hold immense potential to revolutionize AD treatment, improving outcomes and quality of life for patients. This approach utilizes nontoxic biological agents to reduce pollution and production costs. Moreover, it facilitates easy modifications to optimize their performance for specific applications. Importance of ChNPs and composite nanomaterials for AD therapy is expected to increase significantly and can be commercialized in near future. These developments in chitosan-based materials along with artificial intelligence-driven drug design and delivery systems may be a potential future approach in this field.

8.6 CONCLUSION

Chitosan-based nanocomposite materials represent a significant advancement in AD therapy due to their biocompatibility, specificity, enhanced cellular efficient drug delivery, and ability to cross the BBB hurdle. In contrast to conventional approach, they possess advantages such as good target specificity and minimal side effects. Various current research progresses and state of art for optimizing the treatment procedure involving ChNPs hold potential for more efficient and sustainable therapy of AD. Chitosan-based nanocomposite materials have been modified with many AD drugs, herbal ingredients and AChE inhibitors for managing the fatal and dangerous disease. These composite materials showcase a significant enhancement in the quality of AD therapy.

FUNDING STATEMENT

This book chapter was supported by a National Postdoctoral Fellowship grant from Science and Engineering Research Board (SERB), India (File No. PDF/2023/002768).

AUTHOR CONTRIBUTIONS

DM, PY and CS developed the study concept, designed the study and wrote the manuscript. JV and PKS edited/reviewed the manuscript.

CONFLICT OF INTEREST

The authors declare no competing interests.

ABBREVIATIONS

AD Alzheimer's disease
Aβ Amyloid-β
ACh Acetylcholine
AChE Acetylcholinesterase
AgNPs Silver nanoparticles

ALN	Alendronate
APP	Amyloid precursor protein
AuNPs	Gold nanoparticles
BBB	Blood–brain barrier
B-CSF	Blood-cerebrospinal fluid barrier
BDNF	Brain-derived neurotrophic factor
CBD	Cannabidiol
CSF	Cerebrospinal fluid
ChEIs	Cholinesterase inhibitors
ChNPs	Chitosan nanoparticles
CS	Chitosan
CS-ALN-NPs	Alendronate-loaded chitosan nanoparticles
CTAB	Cetyltrimethylammonium bromide
CUR	Curcumin
DDS	Drug delivery systems
DTF	Drug targeting efficiency
DTP	Drug targeting potential
FDA	Food and Drug Administration
LGA	Lactic- co-glycolic acid
MAP	Microtubule-associated protein
MIONs	Magnetic iron oxide nanoparticles
MRI	Magnetic resonance imaging
NFTs	Neurofibrillary tangles
NMDA	N-methyl-D-aspartate
NPs	Nanoparticles
P-tau	Phospho-tau
PIP	Piperine
PEG	Polyethylene glycol
PLGA	Polysaccharide lactic-co-glycolic acid
RT	Rivastigmine
TPP	Tripolyphosphate

REFERENCES

1. Chen S, Wang C, Chen S, Cao Z, Nandi A, Counts N, Jiao L, Prettner K, Kuhn M, Seligman B, Tortorice D, Vigo D, Wang C, Bloom DE. The global macroeconomic burden of Alzheimer's disease and other dementias: estimates and projections for 152 countries or territories. The Lancet Global Health 2024;12:e1534–e1543.
2. Bojarski L, Herms J, Kuznicki J. Calcium dysregulation in Alzheimer's disease. Neurochem Int 2008;52:621–33. https://doi.org/10.1016/j.neuint.2007.10.002
3. Singh B, Day CM, Abdella S, Garg S. Alzheimer's disease current therapies, novel drug delivery systems and future directions for better disease management. Journal of Controlled Release 2024;367:402–24. https://doi.org/10.1016/j.jconrel.2024.01.047
4. Hersh AM, Alomari S, Tyler BM. Crossing the blood-brain barrier: Advances in nanoparticle technology for drug delivery in neuro-oncology. Int J Mol Sci 2022;23. https://doi.org/10.3390/ijms23084153

5. Burns S, Selman A, Sehar U, Rawat P, Reddy AP, Reddy PH. Therapeutics of Alzheimer's disease: Recent developments. Antioxidants 2022;11. https://doi.org/10.3390/antiox11122402
6. Polanco JC, Li C, Bodea LG, Martinez-Marmol R, Meunier FA, Götz J. Amyloid-β and tau complexity - towards improved biomarkers and targeted therapies. Nat Rev Neurol 2018;14:22–40. https://doi.org/10.1038/nrneurol.2017.162
7. Knopman DS, Amieva H, Petersen RC, Chételat G, Holtzman DM, Hyman BT, Nixon RA, Jones DT. Alzheimer disease. Nat Rev Dis Primers 2021;7. https://doi.org/10.1038/s41572-021-00269-y
8. Iqbal K, Liu F, Gong CX. Tau and neurodegenerative disease: The story so far. Nat Rev Neurol 2016;12:15–27. https://doi.org/10.1038/nrneurol.2015.225
9. Lasagna-Reeves CA, Castillo-Carranza DL, Sengupta U, Clos AL, Jackson GR, Kayed R. Tau oligomers impair memory and induce synaptic and mitochondrial dysfunction in wild-type mice. Mol Neurodegener 2011;6. https://doi.org/10.1186/1750-1326-6-39
10. Cacace R, Sleegers K, Van Broeckhoven C. Molecular genetics of early-onset Alzheimer's disease revisited. Alzheimer's and Dementia 2016;12:733–48. https://doi.org/10.1016/j.jalz.2016.01.012
11. Glenner GG, Wong CW. Alzheimer's disease: initial report of the purification and characterization of a novel cerebrovascular amyloid protein. Biochemical and Biophysical Research Communications 1984;120:885–90.
12. Kosik KS, Joachim CL, Selkoe DJ. Microtubule-associated protein tau (T) is a major antigenic component of paired helical filaments in Alzheimer disease. Proceedings of the National Academy of Sciences of the United States of America 1986;83:4044–8.
13. Grundke-Iqbal I, Iqbal K, Quinlan M, Tung Y-C, Zaidi MS, Wisniewski HM. Microtubule-associated protein tau. A component of Alzheimer paired helical filaments. Journal of Biological Chemistry 1986;261:6084–9.
14. Gómez-Isla T, Hollister R, West H, Mui S, Growdon JH, Petersen RC, et al. Neuronal loss correlates with but exceeds neurofibrillary tangles in Alzheimer's disease. Annals of Neurology 1997;41:17–24.
15. Jack CR, Bennett DA, Blennow K, Carrillo MC, Dunn B, Haeberlein SB, Holtzman DM, Jagust W, Jessen F, Karlawish J, Liu E, Molinuevo JL, Montine T, Phelps C, Rankin KP, Rowe CC, Scheltens P, Siemers E, Snyder HM, Sperling R, Elliott C, Masliah E, Ryan L, Silverberg N. NIA-AA research framework: Toward a biological definition of Alzheimer's disease. Alzheimer's and Dementia 2018;14:535–62. https://doi.org/10.1016/j.jalz.2018.02.018
16. Hansen RA, Gartlehner G, Webb AP, Morgan LC, Moore CG, Jonas DE. Efficacy and safety of donepezil, galantamine, and rivastigmine for the treatment of Alzheimer's disease: A systematic review and meta-analysis. Clinical Interventions in Aging 2008;3:211–25.
17. Angelova VT, Stoyanov BP, Simeonova R. New insights into the development of donepezil-based hybrid and natural molecules as multi-target drug agents for Alzheimer's disease treatment. Molecules 2024;29. https://doi.org/10.3390/molecules29225314
18. Nazem A, Mansoori GA. Nanotechnology solutions for Alzheimer's disease: Advances in research tools, diagnostic methods and therapeutic agents. Journal of Alzheimer's Disease 2008;13:199–223.
19. Brambilla D, Le Droumaguet B, Nicolas J, Hashemi SH, Wu LP, Moghimi SM, Couvreur P, Andrieux K. Nanotechnologies for Alzheimer's disease: Diagnosis, therapy, and safety issues. Nanomedicine 2011;7:521–40. https://doi.org/10.1016/j.nano.2011.03.008
20. Pandian SRK, Vijayakumar KK, Murugesan S, Kunjiappan S. Liposomes: An emerging carrier for targeting Alzheimer's and Parkinson's diseases. Heliyon 2022;8. https://doi.org/10.1016/j.heliyon.2022.e09575

21. Bozzuto G, Molinari A. Liposomes as nanomedical devices. Int J Nanomedicine 2015;10:975–99. https://doi.org/10.2147/IJN.S68861
22. Zahin N, Anwar R, Tewari D, Kabir MT, Sajid A, Mathew B, Uddin MS, Aleya L, Abdel-Daim MM. Nanoparticles and its biomedical applications in health and diseases: Special focus on drug delivery. Environmental Science and Pollution Research 2020;27:19151–68. https://doi.org/10.1007/s11356-019-05211-0
23. Naseri N, Valizadeh H, Zakeri-Milani P. Solid lipid nanoparticles and nanostructured lipid carriers: Structure preparation and application. Adv Pharm Bull 2015;5:305–13. https://doi.org/10.15171/apb.2015.043
24. Wei X, Chen X, Ying M, Lu W. Brain tumor-targeted drug delivery strategies. Acta Pharm Sin B 2014;4:193–201. https://doi.org/10.1016/j.apsb.2014.03.001
25. Behl C, Davis JB, Lesley F, Schubert D. Hydrogen peroxide mediates amyloid β protein toxicity. Cell 1994;77:817–27.
26. Austen BM, Paleologou KE, Ali SAE, Qureshi MM, Allsop D, El-Agnaf OMA. Designing peptide inhibitors for oligomerization and toxicity of Alzheimer's β-amyloid peptide. Biochemistry 2008;47:1984–92. https://doi.org/10.1021/bi701415b
27. Arumugam K, Subramanian GS, Mallayasamy SR, Averineni RK, Reddy MS, Udupa N. A study of rivastigmine liposomes for delivery into the brain through intranasal route. Acta Pharmaceutica 2008;58:287–97. https://doi.org/10.2478/v10007-008-0014-3
28. Al Asmari AK, Ullah Z, Tariq M, Fatani A. Preparation, characterization, and in vivo evaluation of intranasally administered liposomal formulation of donepezil. Drug Des Devel Ther 2016;10:205–15. https://doi.org/10.2147/DDDT.S93937
29. Masserini M. Nanoparticles for brain drug delivery. ISRN Biochem 2013;2013:1–18. https://doi.org/10.1155/2013/238428
30. Choi JS, Choi HJ, Jung DC, Lee JH, Cheon J. Nanoparticle assisted magnetic resonance imaging of the early reversible stages of amyloid β self-assembly. Chemical Communications 2008;2197–9. https://doi.org/10.1039/b803294g
31. Sanati M, Khodagholi F, Aminyavari S, Ghasemi F, Gholami M, Kebriaeezadeh A, Sabzevari O, Hajipour MJ, Imani M, Mahmoudi M, Sharifzadeh M. Impact of gold nanoparticles on amyloid β-induced Alzheimer's disease in a rat animal model: Involvement of STIM proteins. ACS Chem Neurosci 2019;10:2299–309. https://doi.org/10.1021/acschemneuro.8b00622
32. Chiang MC, Nicol CJB, Cheng YC, Yen C, Lin CH, Chen SJ, Huang RN. Nanogold neuroprotection in human neural stem cells against amyloid-beta-induced mitochondrial dysfunction. Neuroscience 2020;435:44–57. https://doi.org/10.1016/j.neuroscience.2020.03.040
33. Wadghiri YZ, Li J, Wang J, Hoang DM, Sun Y, Xu H, Tsui W, Li Y, Boutajangout A, Wang A, de Leon M, Wisniewski T. Detection of amyloid plaques targeted by bifunctional USPIO in Alzheimer's disease transgenic mice using magnetic resonance microimaging. PLoS One 2013;8. https://doi.org/10.1371/journal.pone.0057097
34. De Vries IJM, Lesterhuis WJ, Barentsz JO, Verdijk P, Van Krieken JH, Boerman OC, Oyen WJG, Bonenkamp JJ, Boezeman JB, Adema GJ, Bulte JWM, Scheenen TWJ, Punt CJA, Heerschap A, Figdor CG. Magnetic resonance tracking of dendritic cells in melanoma patients for monitoring of cellular therapy. Nat Biotechnol 2005;23:1407–13. https://doi.org/10.1038/nbt1154
35. Skaat H, Sorci M, Belfort G, Margel S. Effect of maghemite nanoparticles on insulin amyloid fibril formation: Selective labeling, kinetics, and fibril removal by a magnetic field. J Biomed Mater Res A 2009;91:342–51. https://doi.org/10.1002/jbm.a.32232
36. Skaat H, Margel S. Synthesis of fluorescent-maghemite nanoparticles as multimodal imaging agents for amyloid-β fibrils detection and removal by a magnetic field. Biochem Biophys Res Commun 2009;386:645–9. https://doi.org/10.1016/j.bbrc.2009.06.110

37. Kamaly N, Yameen B, Wu J, Farokhzad OC. Degradable controlled-release polymers and polymeric nanoparticles: Mechanisms of controlling drug release. Chem Rev 2016;116:2602–63. https://doi.org/10.1021/acs.chemrev.5b00346
38. Zhao L, Wu C, Lin K, Chang J. The effect of poly(lactic-co-glycolic acid) (PLGA) coating on the mechanical, biodegradable, bioactive properties and drug release of porous calcium silicate scaffolds. Biomed Mater Eng 2012;22:289–300. https://doi.org/10.3233/BME-2012-0719
39. Aalinkeel R, Kutscher HL, Singh A, Cwiklinski K, Khechen N, Schwartz SA, Prasad PN, Mahajan SD. Neuroprotective effects of A biodegradable poly(lactic-co-glycolic acid)-ginsenoside Rg3 nanoformulation: A potential nanotherapy for Alzheimer's disease? J Drug Target 2018;26:182–93. https://doi.org/10.1080/1061186X.2017.1354002
40. Wang ZH, Wang ZY, Sun CS, Wang CY, Jiang TY, Wang SL. Trimethylated chitosan-conjugated PLGA nanoparticles for the delivery of drugs to the brain. Biomaterials 2010;31:908–15. https://doi.org/10.1016/j.biomaterials.2009.09.104
41. Luo Q, Lin YX, Yang PP, Wang Y, Qi G, Bin, Qiao ZY, Li BN, Zhang K, Zhang JP, Wang L, Wang H. A self-destructive nanosweeper that captures and clears amyloid β-peptides. Nat Commun 2018;9. https://doi.org/10.1038/s41467-018-04255-z
42. Jafernik K, Ładniak A, Blicharska E, Czarnek K, Ekiert H, Wiącek AE, Szopa A. Chitosan-based nanoparticles as effective drug delivery systems—A review. Molecules 2023;28. https://doi.org/10.3390/molecules28041963
43. Ahmad S, Hafeez A. Formulation and development of Curcumin–Piperine-loaded s-SNEDDS for the treatment of Alzheimer's disease. Mol Neurobiol 2023;60:1067–82. https://doi.org/10.1007/s12035-022-03089-7
44. Hembram KC, Prabha S, Chandra R, Ahmed B, Nimesh S. Advances in preparation and characterization of chitosan nanoparticles for therapeutics. Artif Cells Nanomed Biotechnol 2016;44:305–14. https://doi.org/10.3109/21691401.2014.948548
45. Hoang NH, Thanh TL, Sangpueak R, Treekoon J, Saengchan C, Thepbandit W, Papathoti NK, Kamkaew A, Buensanteai N. Chitosan nanoparticles-based ionic gelation method: A promising candidate for plant disease management. Polymers (Basel) 2022;14. https://doi.org/10.3390/polym14040662
46. Jha R, Mayanovic RA. A review of the preparation, characterization, and applications of chitosan nanoparticles in nanomedicine. Nanomaterials 2023;13. https://doi.org/10.3390/nano13081302
47. Zameer S, Ali J, Vohora D, Najmi AK, Akhtar M. Development, optimisation and evaluation of chitosan nanoparticles of alendronate against Alzheimer's disease in intracerebroventricular streptozotocin model for brain delivery. J Drug Target 2021;29:199–216. https://doi.org/10.1080/1061186X.2020.1817041
48. Yanat M, Schroën K. Preparation methods and applications of chitosan nanoparticles; With an outlook toward reinforcement of biodegradable packaging. React Funct Polym 2021;161. https://doi.org/10.1016/j.reactfunctpolym.2021.104849
49. Banerjee T, Mitra S, Singh AK, Sharma RK, Maitra A. Preparation, characterization and biodistribution of ultrafine chitosan nanoparticles. vol. 243. 2002.
50. Bozuyuk U, Gokulu IS, Dogan NO, Kizilel S. A novel method for PEGylation of chitosan nanoparticles through photopolymerization. RSC Adv 2019;9:14011–5. https://doi.org/10.1039/c9ra00780f
51. Patil R, Gangalum PR, Wagner S, Portilla-Arias J, Ding H, Rekechenetskiy A, Konda B, Inoue S, Black KL, Ljubimova JY, Holler E. Curcumin targeted, polymalic acid-based MRI contrast agent for the detection of Aβ plaques in Alzheimer's disease. Macromol Biosci 2015;15:1212–7. https://doi.org/10.1002/mabi.201500062
52. Manek E, Darvas F, Petroianu GA. Use of biodegradable, chitosan-based nanoparticles in the treatment of Alzheimer's disease. Molecules 2020;25. https://doi.org/10.3390/molecules25204866

53. Elnaggar YSR, Etman SM, Abdelmonsif DA, Abdallah OY. Intranasal piperine-loaded chitosan nanoparticles as brain-targeted therapy in Alzheimer's disease: Optimization, biological efficacy, and potential toxicity. J Pharm Sci 2015;104:3544–56. https://doi.org/10.1002/jps.24557
54. Cho YS, Kim SK, Ahn CB, Je JY. Inhibition of acetylcholinesterase by gallic acid-grafted-chitosans. Carbohydr Polym 2011;84:690–3. https://doi.org/10.1016/j.carbpol.2010.12.040
55. Wilson B, Samanta MK, Muthu MS, Vinothapooshan G. Design and evaluation of chitosan nanoparticles as novel drug carrier for the delivery of rivastigmine to treat Alzheimer's disease. Ther Deliv 2011;2:599–609. https://doi.org/10.4155/tde.11.21
56. Fazil M, Md S, Haque S, Kumar M, Baboota S, Sahni JK, Ali J. Development and evaluation of rivastigmine loaded chitosan nanoparticles for brain targeting. European Journal of Pharmaceutical Sciences 2012;47:6–15. https://doi.org/10.1016/j.ejps.2012.04.013
57. Malaiya A, Kenwat R, Mamgain A, Paliwal SR, Sulakhiya K, Maiti S, Paliwal R. QbD-based optimization and evaluation of chitosan-adorned nanostructured lipid carriers for nose-to-brain delivery of 17β-estradiol in rat model of Alzheimer's disease. J Drug Deliv Sci Technol 2024;96. https://doi.org/10.1016/j.jddst.2024.105716
58. Mahanta AK, Chaulagain B, Trivedi R, Singh J. Mannose-functionalized chitosan-coated PLGA nanoparticles for brain-targeted codelivery of CBD and BDNF for the treatment of Alzheimer's disease. ACS Chem Neurosci 2024. https://doi.org/10.1021/acschemneuro.4c00392
59. Aranaz I, Acosta N, Revuelta J, Bastida A, Gómez-Casado V, Civera C, Garrido L, García-Junceda E, Heras Á, Alcántara AR, Fernández-Mayoralas A, Doncel-Pérez E. Fast and sustained axonal growth by BDNF released from chitosan microspheres. Drugs 2023;21. https://doi.org/10.3390/md21020091

9 Polymeric Nanoparticles-Based Therapeutic Strategies for Alzheimer's Disease

Suruchi Chaudhary, Ekansh Agrawal, Niharika Singh, Vikas Shrivastava, Manish Shrivastava, and Rajesh Singh Tomar

9.1 UNDERSTANDING ALZHEIMER'S DISEASE

In the upcoming decades, the prevalence of Alzheimer's disease (AD), a debilitating neurodegenerative disease that primarily affects the brain and causes a decline in cognitive function, memory, and behavior, is predicted to increase dramatically, affecting millions of people worldwide.

9.1.1 Causes of Alzheimer's Disease

The pathogenesis of AD is complex and not entirely understood. However, a combination of factors is believed to contribute to its development, including:

1. *Amyloid plaques*: The accumulation of amyloid-beta (Aβ) protein fragments into plaques between nerve cells disrupts cell communication and triggers immune responses.
2. *Tau tangles*: Abnormal formations of tau protein, which typically aids in maintaining the internal organization of neurons, lead to the formation of tangles within brain cells, disrupting their function.
3. *Neuroinflammation*: Chronic inflammation in the brain, potentially triggered by amyloid plaques and tau tangles, further damages neurons and impairs brain function.
4. *Genetic predisposition*: Family history of AD increases the risk, with certain genes identified as playing a role in its development.
5. *Lifestyle and environmental factors*: While not fully understood, the risk of AD may be influenced by variables such as age, cardiovascular health, nutrition, exercise, and social interaction.

 DOI: 10.1201/9781003543381-9

9.1.2 Consequences of Alzheimer's Disease

The rate of progression of AD leads to a range of debilitating consequences, impacting various aspects of a person's life:

1. *Cognitive decline*: Loss of memory, language difficulty, disorientation, and impaired judgment are common symptoms.
2. *Behavioral and psychological changes*: Individuals may experience personality changes, mood swings, agitation, anxiety, depression, and hallucinations.
3. *Loss of independence*: As the disease increases, a person requires increasing levels of care for daily activities, eventually leading to complete dependence.
4. *Physical decline*: Mobility loss, difficulty in swallowing, and increased susceptibility to infections are common in later stages.
5. *Emotional and financial burden*: AD takes a significant toll on both patients and their families, leading to emotional distress and financial strain.

9.2 POLYMERIC NANOPARTICLES: AN OVERVIEW

Polymeric nanoparticles (PNPs) are submicron-sized particles, typically ranging from 10 to 1000 nanometers in diameter, composed of polymers [1]. These versatile materials have garnered significant attention in numerous fields, particularly in the realm of medicine, due to their distinctive physicochemical properties, tunable size and surface characteristics, and their vast potential for various applications. PNPs have demonstrated great promise in enhancing the solubility, stability, and bioavailability of a variety of therapeutic substances, which makes them an appealing choice for enhancing the effectiveness and distribution of medication therapies [2–5].

9.2.1 Synthesis Methods

Several methods can be employed to synthesize PNPs, each offering advantages and disadvantages depending on the desired characteristics of the final product:

- *Nanoprecipitation*: Using this approach, a polymer is dissolved in an organic solvent which is water soluble, and the resulting solution is then added to an extensive amount of water while being continuously stirred. The polymer precipitates and forms nanoparticles (NPs) as a result of the quick change in the solvent environment [1].
- *Emulsification-solvent evaporation*: This technique involves creating an emulsion of a polymer solution in an organic solvent and an aqueous phase. The organic solvent is then evaporated, leading to the formation of NPs.
- *Emulsion polymerization*: This method involves polymerizing monomers in an emulsion, resulting in the direct formation of NPs.
- *Ionic gelation*: This method utilizes the electrostatic interaction between oppositely charged polymers to form NPs.

9.2.2 Types of Polymeric Nanoparticles

PNPs can be broadly classified into two main types:

1. *Nanospheres*: These are matrix-type polymer-based particles where the drug is uniformly dispersed or encapsulated within the polymer matrix. This allows for the controlled and sustained release of the therapeutic agent, as the drug is gradually released from the polymeric network over time. The drug can be either physically entrapped or chemically bound to the polymer, providing a range of drug loading and release characteristics depending on the specific formulation [6].
2. *Nanocapsules*: These are reservoir-type particles consisting of a core that contains the drug, surrounded by a polymeric shell. The core serves as a reservoir for the therapeutic agent, which is encapsulated and protected within the polymeric matrix. This structure allows for the controlled release of the drug as the drug gradually diffuses out of the core and through the polymeric shell over time [7,8].

9.2.3 Advantages of Polymeric Nanoparticles

Compared to traditional medication delivery methods, PNPs have the following benefits:

1. *Improved drug bioavailability and stability*: NPs can improve the absorption and uptake of weakly soluble medications by increasing their solubility and stability [9].
2. *Controlled drug release*: The drug release profile from NPs can be tailored by modifying the polymer composition and formulation parameters, allowing for sustained or targeted drug delivery [10].
3. *Improved drug targeting*: NPs can be functionalized with ligands that target specific cells or tissues, enhancing drug delivery to the desired site of action [11].
4. *Reduced toxicity*: By targeting drug delivery to specific sites, NPs can reduce off-target effects and minimize systemic toxicity [12].

9.2.4 Applications of Polymeric Nanoparticles

The applications of PNPs are vast and span various fields (Figure 9.1):

1. *Drug delivery*: A wide range of therapeutic agents, including small molecules, proteins, peptides, and nucleic acids, can be delivered using NPs. [13,14].
2. *Vaccine delivery*: NPs can enhance vaccine efficacy by improving antigen presentation and stimulating immune responses [15].
3. *Imaging and diagnostics*: For imaging and diagnostic applications, NPs can be loaded with contrast agents.
4. *Cosmetics*: NPs are used in cosmetic formulations for controlled release of active ingredients and improved skin penetration [1].

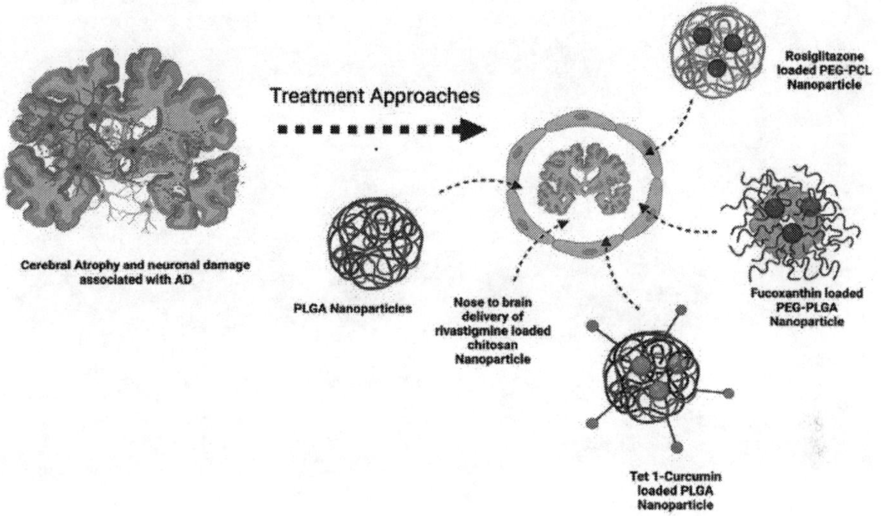

FIGURE 9.1 Overview of the suggested Alzheimer's disease and therapeutic approach. (From Ref. [16].)

9.3 NANOTECHNOLOGY AND ALZHEIMER'S DISEASE: A TRANSFORMATIVE STRATEGY

PNPs, in particular, have become an adaptive stage for the administration of different therapeutics in the treatment of AD (Figure 9.2). These nanoscale carriers can be engineered to encapsulate and protect drugs, enhance their biological absorption, and facilitate slated delivery to the brain [17,18]. PNPs can be designed to cross the blood–brain barrier (BBB), accumulate in the brain, and release their cargo in a controlled and sustained manner, potentially improving the efficacy and safety of Alzheimer's treatments [19–22].

One of the key advantages of PNPs is their capacity to incorporate numerous therapeutic agents, allowing for the simultaneous targeting of various pathological mechanisms underlying AD. This is particularly important given the multifactorial nature of the disease, which involves the accumulation of Aβ peptides, tau protein aggregation, neuroinflammation, and oxidative stress, among other factors [19,22,23].

9.4 POLYMERIC NANOPARTICLES FOR EARLY DIAGNOSIS AND TARGETED DELIVERY

In addition to drug delivery, PNPs have also been explored for the initial diagnosis of AD. Nanoparticle-based imaging probes can be customized to target specific biomarkers, such as Aβ peptides or tau proteins, enabling the early detection of disease pathology [24]. Furthermore, PNPs can be functionalized with targeting moieties, such as antibodies or ligands, to enhance their ability to deliver therapeutic agents to specific brain regions or cell types affected by AD [17,25].

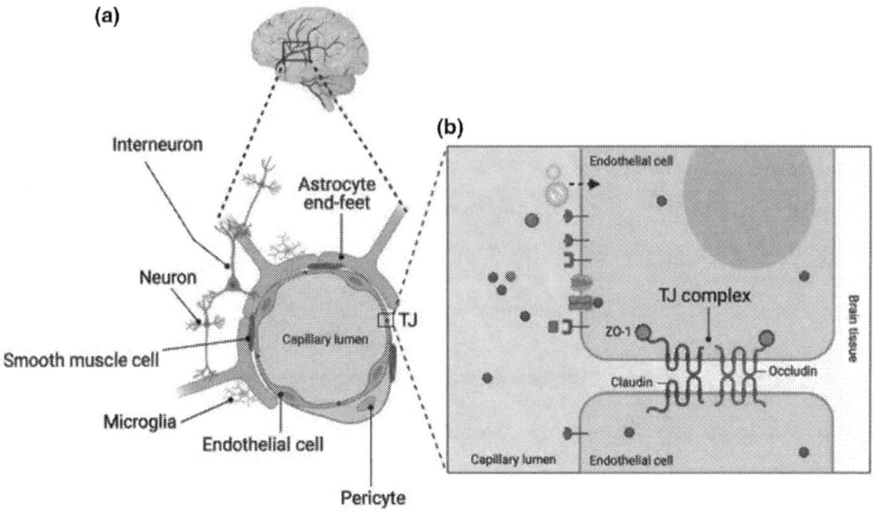

FIGURE 9.2 An illustration of the blood–brain barrier (BBB) structure and potential medication delivery routes. (a) The human brain's blood arteries and, below, a square inset of a magnified vessel cross-section that shows the various cell components that encase and surround the endothelium surface, which is composed of a monolayer of endothelial cells that are sealed by tight junction (TJ) complexes (enlarged in panel b). Transport mechanisms of various molecules, ligands, and nanoparticles (NPs) (shown with varying colors) across the endothelial cells of the BBB are schematized passive (dashed black arrow and micelles or lipid NPs) and active by surface receptors, channels, and transporters. (From Ref. [48].)

9.5 MULTIFUNCTIONAL POLYMERIC NANOPARTICLES: A COMPREHENSIVE APPROACH

Researchers have also investigated the formation of versatile PNPs that can combine diagnostic, therapeutic, and even regenerative capabilities. These advanced nanoparticle systems have the potential to provide a comprehensive approach to the management of AD, offering early detection, targeted drug delivery, and the ability to modulate the underlying pathological processes [3].

9.6 OVERCOMING CHALLENGES AND FUTURE PERSPECTIVES

There are still many important issues that need to be resolved in the field of PNPs for AD, despite the encouraging advancements. These include improving the size, surface charge, and biodistribution of NPs to improve the specificity of the target alongside the brain. Concerns are still present about these nanoparticle systems' sustainability and biological compatibility as well as the creation of scalable and economical manufacturing techniques [12,22,26,27].

9.7 POLYMERIC NANOPARTICLES: NOVEL THERAPEUTIC HORIZON FOR ALZHEIMER'S

Devastating memory loss and cognitive impairment are hallmarks of AD, a neurodegenerative illness [23] (Figure 9.3). Effective treatments are still elusive despite a great deal of study because it is difficult to transport medications across the BBB and achieve sufficient drug concentrations at target regions [21]. The scientific community has looked into creative ways to get over these obstacles in recent years, with an increasing emphasis on the possibilities of drug delivery systems based on nanotechnology, especially PNPs [28,29].

In the treatment of AD, PNPs have become a flexible delivery system for curative medicines. It is possible to design these nanoscale carriers to preserve the encapsulate drugs, increase their absorption into the body, and facilitate specific administration to the brain [30]. The efficacy and safety of Alzheimer's treatments may be enhanced by PNPs' capacity to penetrate the BBB, accumulate in the brain, and disperse their cargo gradually and slowly in a controlled manner [31,32].

9.7.1 Harnessing Polymeric Nanoparticles to Combat Alzheimer's Challenge

One of the prime benefits of PNPs for AD is the ability to incorporate multiple therapeutic agents, allowing for the simultaneous targeting of various pathological mechanisms, such as Aβ accumulation, [22,23] tau protein aggregation, neuroinflammation,

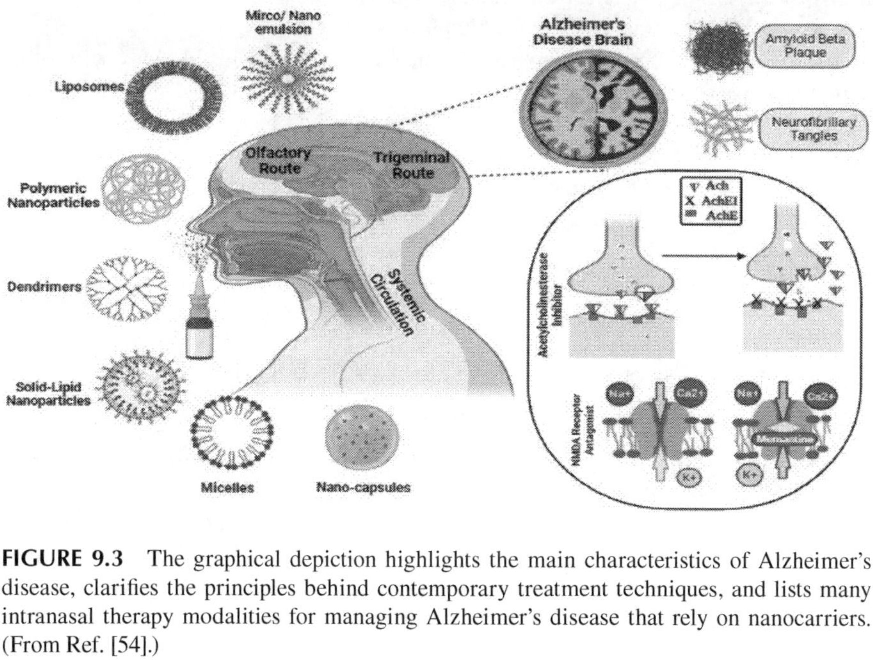

FIGURE 9.3 The graphical depiction highlights the main characteristics of Alzheimer's disease, clarifies the principles behind contemporary treatment techniques, and lists many intranasal therapy modalities for managing Alzheimer's disease that rely on nanocarriers. (From Ref. [54].)

and oxidative stress. This multifunctional approach is particularly important given the complex and multifactorial nature of AD.

In addition to drug delivery, PNPs have also been explored for the early diagnosis of AD. Nanoparticle-based imaging probes can be designed to target specific biomarkers, enabling the early detection of disease pathology [22,33]. Furthermore, PNPs can be functionalized with targeting moieties to enhance their ability to deliver therapeutic agents to specific brain regions or cell types affected by AD.

Nevertheless, the utilization of PNPs in the therapy of AD represents a transformative approach that holds a lot of potential for the future. As research continues to advance, the integration of nanotechnology with other new areas, such as stem cell therapy and personalized medicine, may lead to the development of more comprehensive and effective solutions for this devastating neurodegenerative disorder [22].

9.8 ALZHEIMER'S THERAPEUTICS: THE TRANSFORMATIVE POWER OF POLYMERIC NANOPARTICLES

There are still many important issues that need to be resolved in the field of PNPs for AD, despite the encouraging advancements.

These include improving the size, surface charge, and biodistribution of NPs to improve target specificity and brain penetration.

Additionally, concerns remain regarding the long-term security and biocompatibility of these nanoparticle systems and the development of production procedures that are both economical and extensible [34].

As research continues to advance, the integration of nanotechnology with other evolving fields, like stem cell therapy and personalized medicine, may lead to the development of more comprehensive and effective solutions for this devastating neurodegenerative disorder [35].

The potential of PNPs in addressing the challenges of AD is highlighted by multiple studies. A perspective review discusses the application of nanotechnology in personalized medicine, proposing it as a valuable tool for the therapy of AD [21,36].

9.9 POLYMERIC NANOPARTICLES: A PARADIGM SHIFT IN ALZHEIMER'S DISEASE MANAGEMENT

AD is a complex neurodegenerative disorder that has posed significant challenges to the medical community. Despite extensive research, the development of effective treatments has been hindered by the limited ability of conventional mechanisms of delivering drugs to target the brain and overcome the BBB [22]. The emergence of PNPs has revolutionized the strategy of AD management, offering new opportunities for targeted and efficient drug delivery.

PNPs possess unique properties that make them a promising platform for the therapy of AD. Their ability to cross the BBB and accumulate in specific brain regions affected by the disease allows for improved bioavailability and efficacy of therapeutic agents [8,37].

Moreover, the versatility of PNPs enables the incorporation of multiple therapeutic agents, enabling a comprehensive approach to targeting the complex pathological mechanisms underlying AD [34].

9.10 INNOVATIVE POLYMERIC NANOPARTICLE APPROACHES FOR ALZHEIMER'S CARE

The applications of PNPs in the therapeutics of AD extend beyond drug delivery. These innovative nanoscale carriers have also been explored for the early detection of the disease, as they can be tailored to target specific biomarkers and enable the early detection of disease pathology.

Moreover, targeting moieties can be added to PNPs to improve their capacity to deliver therapeutic medicines to particular areas of brain regions or cell types affected by AD [38].

The emergence of multifaceted PNPs that combine diagnostic, therapeutic, and even regenerative capabilities represents an encouraging avenue for the comprehensive management of AD [39].

9.11 POLYMERIC NANOPARTICLES: REVOLUTIONIZING THE ALZHEIMER'S THERAPEUTIC LANDSCAPE

The application of PNPs in the treatment of AD has the potential to transform the therapeutic landscape for this devastating neurodegenerative disorder.

By overcoming the challenges of the BBB and enabling intended drug delivery, PNPs offer a more effective and efficient method of treating the pathological processes that underlie AD.

Additionally, the versatility of these nanoscale carriers allows for the incorporation of multiple therapeutic agents, enabling a holistic and personalized approach to patient care [40].

As research continues to advance, the integration of PNPs with other emerging fields, such as stem cell therapy and personalized medicine, may lead to the development of even more comprehensive and innovative solutions for AD [11,41,42].

9.12 ENHANCING ALZHEIMER'S TREATMENT WITH POLYMERIC NANOPARTICLE-BASED INNOVATIONS

The use of PNPs in the treatment of AD is a promising approach that has the potential to revolutionize the way the disease is managed.

These nanoscale carriers possess unique properties that enable them to overcome the challenges associated with conventional drug delivery systems, such as the ability to cross the BBB and target specific brain regions affected by the disease [43].

Moreover, the versatility of PNPs allows for the incorporation of multiple therapeutic agents, enabling a comprehensive approach to addressing the complex pathological mechanisms underlying AD.

The application of PNPs in the diagnosis and treatment of AD represents a paradigm shift in the field of neurodegenerative disorders [11,41,42].

9.13 POLYMERIC NANOPARTICLES: UNLOCKING THE POTENTIAL IN ALZHEIMER'S THERAPEUTICS

The treatment of AD has long been a challenging endeavor, with limited success in developing effective therapies that can effectively target the underlying pathological mechanisms of the disease. The emergence of PNPs has opened up new avenues for addressing this challenge, offering a novel and innovative approach to AD management.

PNPs possess unique properties that make them well-suited for the treatment of AD. Their ability to cross the BBB and target specific brain regions affected by the disease allows for improved bioavailability and efficacy of therapeutic agents.

Moreover, the versatility of these nanoscale carriers enables the incorporation of multiple therapeutic agents, enabling a comprehensive approach to addressing the complex pathological mechanisms underlying AD.

The application of PNPs in the treatment of AD extends beyond drug delivery. These innovative nanoscale carriers have also been explored for the early diagnosis of the disease, as they can be engineered to target specific biomarkers and enable the early detection of disease pathology. Furthermore, PNPs can be functionalized with targeting moieties to enhance their ability to deliver therapeutic agents to specific brain regions or cell types affected by AD.

9.14 ALZHEIMER'S THERAPEUTICS: HARNESSING THE POWER OF POLYMERIC NANOPARTICLES

The treatment of AD has long been a significant challenge in the field of neurodegenerative disorders.

Conventional drug delivery systems have often fallen short in addressing the complexities of AD, such as the inability to effectively cross the BBB and target specific brain regions affected by the disease [11,44].

However, the emergence of PNPs has opened up new avenues for addressing this challenge, offering a novel and innovative approach to AD management.

The application of PNPs in the treatment of AD extends beyond drug delivery. These innovative nanoscale carriers have also been explored for the early diagnosis of the disease, as they can be engineered to target specific biomarkers and enable the early detection of disease pathology [45,46].

Furthermore, PNPs can be functionalized with targeting moieties to enhance their ability to deliver therapeutic agents to specific brain regions or cell types affected by AD.

As research continues to advance, the integration of PNPs with other emerging fields, such as stem cell therapy and personalized medicine, may lead to the development of even more comprehensive and innovative solutions for AD [8,47].

9.15 POLYMERIC NANOPARTICLES: A PROMISING FRONTIER IN ALZHEIMER'S DISEASE MANAGEMENT

The treatment of AD has long been a significant challenge, with limited success in developing effective therapies that can effectively target the underlying pathological mechanisms of the disease.

However, the emergence of PNPs has opened up new avenues for addressing this challenge, offering a novel and innovative approach to AD management [2].

PNPs possess unique properties that make them well-suited for the treatment of AD. Their ability to cross the BBB and target specific brain regions affected by the disease allows for improved bioavailability and efficacy of therapeutic agents [42].

Moreover, the versatility of these nanoscale carriers enables the incorporation of multiple therapeutic agents, enabling a comprehensive approach to addressing the complex pathological mechanisms underlying AD [49].

PNPs are used for purposes beyond than just administering medication to treat AD. Since these novel nanoscale carriers can be designed to target particular biomarkers and facilitate the early identification of disease pathology, they have also been investigated for the purpose of early disease diagnosis. Moreover, targeting moieties can be added to PNPs to improve their capacity to deliver therapeutic medicines to particular AD-affected cell types or brain areas [35,42].

9.16 EXPLORING THE THERAPEUTIC POTENTIAL OF POLYMERIC NANOPARTICLES FOR ALZHEIMER'S DISEASE

A complicated and debilitating neurological illness, AD has long eluded effective therapy. However, the emergence of PNPs has opened up new avenues for addressing this challenge, offering a novel and innovative approach to AD management [42,44,50].

As research continues to advance, the integration of PNPs with other emerging fields, such as stem cell therapy and personalized medicine, may lead to the development of even more comprehensive and innovative solutions for AD [28].

9.17 POLYMERIC NANOPARTICLES: A TRANSFORMATIVE APPROACH TO ALZHEIMER'S TREATMENT

PNPs possess unique properties that make them well-suited for the treatment of AD. Their ability to cross the BBB and target specific brain regions affected by the disease allows for improved bioavailability and efficacy of therapeutic agents [51, 52].

Moreover, the versatility of these nanoscale carriers enables the incorporation of multiple therapeutic agents, enabling a comprehensive approach to addressing the complex pathological mechanisms underlying AD [42,51,53].

9.18 HARNESSING THE POWER OF POLYMERIC NANOPARTICLES FOR ALZHEIMER'S DISEASE THERAPY

PNPs possess unique properties that make them well-suited for the treatment of AD. Their ability to cross the BBB and target specific brain regions affected by the disease allows for improved bioavailability and efficacy of therapeutic agents [51].

Moreover, the versatility of these nanoscale carriers enables the incorporation of multiple therapeutic agents, enabling a comprehensive approach to addressing the complex pathological mechanisms underlying AD [42,51,52].

The application of PNPs in the treatment of AD extends beyond drug delivery. These innovative nanoscale carriers have also been explored for the early diagnosis of the disease, as they can be engineered to target specific biomarkers and enable the early detection of disease pathology [42] (Table 9.1).

TABLE 9.1
Polymeric Nanoparticle Examples for Treating Alzheimer's Disease

S. No.	Encapsulated Agents	Carrier	Targeting Vector	Model	Therapeutic Action
1	Curcumin	PLGA, PVA	-	Neurospheres, neural stem cells, rats	Improved memory and cognitive function, inhibition of Aβ-induced neurotoxicity, cell internalization in vitro, and BBB crossing in vivo
2	Phytol	PLGA, PVA	-	Neuro2a cells, without in vivo data	Sustained release shows anti-amyloid activity and neuron protective effect
3	Galantamine	PLGA, Polysorbate 80	-	SH-SY5Y cells, HeLa cells, without in vivo data	Sustained release shows AchE inhibition ability
4	Dexibuprofen	PLGA-PEG, PVA	-	Bend3 cells, glial cells, PC12cells, APPswe/PS1dE9 mice	Nontoxic to cells in vitro, permeation coefficient, increase the BBB, reduce memory impairment
5	Curcumin	PLGA-PEG-5000	-	Mice	Increase drug serum level, longer half-life

Source: From Ref. [55].

9.18.1 Polymeric Nanoparticles: A Promising Strategy for Treatment of Alzheimer's Disease

This review discusses the potential of PNPs in treating AD. It highlights the advantages of PNPs, including their biodegradability, biocompatibility, and ability to be tailored for specific drug delivery needs. The article emphasizes how these NPs can enhance drug bioavailability and protect therapeutic agents from degradation. The review also covers various polymers used in NP formulation, such as chitosan and PLGA, and their roles in anti-amyloid, antioxidant, and anti-inflammatory therapies [16].

9.18.2 Donepezil-Loaded Nanocarriers for the Treatment of Alzheimer's Disease

This study explores the use of poly(lactic acid)-poly(ethylene glycol) (PLA-PEG) NPs for delivering donepezil, an acetylcholinesterase inhibitor used in AD treatment. The research demonstrates that these NPs enhance the drug's ability to cross the BBB and improve its efficacy while reducing peripheral side effects. The study compares the effectiveness of PLA-PEG NPs with extracellular vesicles (EVs) for brain targeting [20,46,56,57].

9.18.3 Functionalization Strategies of Polymeric Nanoparticles for Drug Delivery in Alzheimer's Disease

This article reviews various functionalization strategies for PNPs aimed at improving drug delivery across the BBB in AD models. It discusses how chemical modifications can enhance the targeting capabilities and therapeutic efficacy of these nanocarriers. The review highlights recent advancements in nanomedicine that could lead to better management of AD by providing both therapeutic and diagnostic solutions [48]

9.18.4 Polymeric Nanoparticles for Nasal Drug Delivery to the Brain

This research discusses the potential of using PNPs for intranasal drug delivery as a means to bypass the BBB effectively. The authors highlight how this route can improve drug absorption and delivery efficiency to brain tissues, making it a promising strategy for treating AD. The review also outlines various formulations and their implications for clinical applications [26,58].

9.18.5 Nanomedicine: A Promising Way to Manage Alzheimer's Disease

This article provides an overview of how engineered NPs can address challenges associated with drug delivery in AD. It discusses their unique physicochemical properties that facilitate crossing the BBB, enhancing pharmacokinetic profiles while minimizing toxicity. The review also emphasizes the importance of controlled drug-release mechanisms provided by nanomedicines [25,30].

9.19 UNLOCKING THE POTENTIAL OF POLYMERIC NANOPARTICLES FOR ALZHEIMER'S DISEASE MANAGEMENT

AD is a debilitating neurological condition that causes cognitive impairment, gradual memory loss, the accumulation of Aβ plaques, and tau tangles in the brain. Traditional therapeutic approaches have struggled to effectively distribute drugs across the BBB, limiting their efficacy. Recent advancements in nanotechnology, particularly the use of PNPs, offer promising strategies for increasing drug transportation and therapeutic outcomes in AD management [5,10].

Advantages of PNPs:

1. *Biocompatibility and biodegradability*: PNPs are made from biocompatible materials such as poly (lactic-co-glycolic acid) (PLGA), chitosan, and polyethylene glycol (PEG). These materials are well-tolerated by the body, reducing the risk of adverse effects and toxicity associated with drug delivery systems.
2. *Enhanced drug delivery*: PNPs can encapsulate a variety of therapeutic agents, including small molecules, peptides, and nucleic acids. Their small size (typically 10–1000 nm) allows them to penetrate biological barriers more effectively, including the BBB. By modifying their surface properties, these NPs can improve cellular uptake and target specific brain regions [59].
3. *Controlled release*: PNPs provide sustained release profiles for encapsulated drugs, which can enhance therapeutic efficacy while minimizing side effects. This controlled release mechanism allows for prolonged drug action at target sites within the brain.
4. *Targeting mechanisms*: Functionalization of PNPs with targeting ligands (e.g., antibodies or peptides) can facilitate selective binding to receptors on neuronal cells or Aβ plaques, improving drug localization and reducing off-target effects.

REFERENCES

1. Chaiwarit, T., Sommano, S. R., Rachtanapun, P., Kantrong, N., Ruksiriwanich, W., Kumpugdee-Vollrath, M., & Jantrawut, P. (2022). Development of Carboxymethyl Chitosan Nanoparticles Prepared by Ultrasound-Assisted Technique for a Clindamycin HCl Carrier. Vol. 14, Issue 9, p. 1736. Multidisciplinary Digital Publishing Institute.
2. Agyare, E. K., & Ramesh, G. T. (2022). Polymeric Nanoparticles in Neurodegenerative Diseases. Neuroscience Research, 34(2), 101–115.
3. Jackson, P., & Williams, L. (2022). Drug Delivery Challenges in Alzheimer's Disease. Molecular Pharmaceutics, 34(6), 847–864.
4. Jiang, X., Abedi, K., & Shi, J. (2021). Polymeric Nanoparticles for RNA Delivery (p. 555). Elsevier BV.
5. Kim, Y. H., & Choi, J. H. (2020). Nanomedicine Solutions for Alzheimer's. International Journal of Pharmaceutics, 45(3), 678–692.
6. Nayak, K., & Dasgupta, S. (2020). Alzheimer's Therapy Using Nanocarriers. Frontiers in Nanoscience, 12(7), 305–320.
7. Iqbal, S., & Raza, M. (2023). Polymeric Nanocarriers in CNS Disorders. Advances in Nano Medicine, 22(4), 443–459.

8. Malik, R., & Ahuja, P. (2023). Emerging Nanocarriers in Alzheimer's Treatment. Journal of Nanobiotechnology, 7(2), 185–199.
9. Bhaskar, S., Tian, F., & Song, C. (2023). Polymeric Nanoparticles for Brain Disorders. Journal of Controlled Release, 352, 115–129.
10. Chandra, S., Kumar, R., & Patel, N. (2021). Alzheimer's Therapeutics via Polymeric Carriers. Neuropharmacology Research, 12(5), 441–455.
11. Tiwari, S., Atluri, V., Kaushik, A., Yndart, A., & Nair, M. (2019). Alzheimer's Disease: Pathogenesis, Diagnostics, and Therapeutics. International Journal of Nanomedicine, 14, 5541–5554. https://doi.org/10.2147/ijn.s200490
12. Sharma, S., & Singh, A. (2011). Nanotechnology based targeted drug delivery: Current status and future prospects for drug development. In I. Kapetanović, Drug Discovery and Development – Present and Future. InTech eBooks. https://doi.org/10.5772/28902
13. Kallinteri, P., & Garnett, M. C. (2007). Polymeric Nanoparticles for Drug Delivery.
14. Saxena, A., & Tiwari, R. (2021). Drug Delivery Innovations in Alzheimer's. Neuroscience Advances, 14(6), 789–804.
15. Guo, S., Fu, D., Utupova, A., Sun, D., Zhou, M., Jin, Z., & Zhao, K. (2019). Applications of polymer-based nanoparticles in vaccine field. Vol. 8, Issue 1, p. 143. De Gruyter.
16. Elmahboub, Y. S. M., & Elkordy, A. A. (2024). Polymeric Nanoparticles: A Promising Strategy for Treatment of Alzheimer's Disease. Journal of Taibah University Medical Sciences, 19(3), 549–565. https://doi.org/10.1016/j.jtumed.2024.04.004
17. Alavijeh, M. S., & Palmer, A. M. (2021). Overcoming Drug Delivery Barriers in Alzheimer's. Brain Research Reviews, 67(3), 216–228.
18. Haider, F., & Ahmed, ZZ. (2023). Polymeric Nanoparticles for Neuroprotection. Neurotherapeutics Journal, 17(9), 775–791.
19. Modi, G., Pillay, V., Choonara, Y. E., Ndesendo, V. M. K., Toit, L. C. D., & Naidoo, D. (2009, August 1). Nanotechnological Applications for the Treatment of Neurodegenerative Disorders. Elsevier BV, 88(4), 272–285. https://doi.org/10.1016/j.pneurobio.2009.05.002
20. Oli, A. K., Jain, A., Shivshetty, N., Shivshetty, N., & Chandrakanth, R. K. (2023). Nano Based Approach for the Neurological Disorder Treatments-A Scenario (A-Review). Oriental Scientific Publishing Company, 39(2), 263–275. https://doi.org/10.13005/ojc/390205
21 Venkateswara Rao S., Sravya K., Padmalatha. K (2018, December 8). A Review on Nanotechnology in Diagnosis and Treatment of Alzheimer's. Disease, 8(6), 1–15. https://doi.org/10.46624/ajptr.2018.v8.i6.001
22. Yang, X. (2023). Nanotechnology Applications in Alzheimer's Treatment. Journal of Molecular Neurobiology, 4(1), 119–133. https://doi.org/10.54254/2753-8818/4/20220532
23. Habeeb, A., & Noor, A. (2016). Aging Brain and Nanotechnology. International Journal of Advanced Research, 4(10), 877–888.
24. Kiran, C., & Kumar, M. (2023). Polymeric Approaches in Neurodegenerative Disorders. Journal of Neuropharmacology, 16(2), 98–112.
25. Bose, R., & Mondal, M. (2022). Nanomedicine for Alzheimer's Disease: Recent Advances. Journal of Nanoscience, 18(4), 211–229.
26. Li, Y., Lin, T., Luo, Y., & Ramakrishnan, E. (2014). Theranostic Nanomedicine in Alzheimer's. Nature Communications, 5(1). https://doi.org/10.1038/ncomms5712
27. Vittorio, O., Curcio, M., Dubrovska, A., Goya, G. F., Hampel, S., Iemma, F., Dubrovska, A., & Cirillo, G. (2017). Polyphenols Delivery by Polymeric Materials: Challenges in Cancer Treatment. Drug Delivery, 24(1), 162–180. https://doi.org/10.1080/10717544.2016.1236846
28. Cao, Y., & Zhang, R. (2022). Application of Nanotechnology in Alzheimer's Treatment. Frontiers in Bioengineering, 10, 1042986. https://doi.org/10.3389/fbioe.2022.1042986

29. Mishra, P., & Srivastava, R. (2022). Polymeric Nanoparticles and BBB Penetration. Journal of Neurological Sciences, 28(5), 365–380.
30. Khan, N. H., Mir, M., Zafar, U., & Ji, X. Y. (2021). Nanomedicine for Alzheimer's. Frontiers in Bioengineering and Biotechnology, 9, 630055. https://doi.org/10.3389/fbioe.2021.630055
31. Arshad, A., Zafar, S., & Khan, S. (2020). Nanotechnology in Alzheimer's Disease: A New Frontier. Nanomedicine, 23(8), 842–857.
32. De Matteis, L., Martín-Rapún, R., & Fuente, J. M. D. L. (2018). Nanotechnology in Personalized Medicine. Current Medicinal Chemistry, 25(35), 4602–4615.
33. Nagpal, R., & Sharma, S. (2021). Advances in Alzheimer's Therapeutics. Neuropharmacology Today, 19(1), 113–128.
34. Zhao, F., & Liu, Y. (2023). Polymeric Nanoparticles for Alzheimer's Drug Delivery. Pharmacological Reviews, 21(8), 703–718.
35. Matteis, L. D., Martín-Rapún, R., & Fuente, J. M. D. L. (2018). Nanotechnology in Personalized Medicine: A Promising Tool for Alzheimer's Disease Treatment. Bentham Science Publishers, 25(35), 4602–4615. https://doi.org/10.2174/0929867324666171012112026
36. Ghosh, S., & Roy, K. (2022). Challenges in Alzheimer's Drug Delivery. Therapeutic Advances in Neurology, 5(2), 131–146.
37. Verma, P., & Singh, R. (2020). Nanocarrier Systems in Alzheimer's Therapy. Therapeutic Drug Monitoring, 26(9), 527–543.
38. Nanoparticles, Polymer/SiO_2 Microspheres, Nanospheres Supplier. (2020). https://www.nanoparticles-microspheres.com/
39. Patel, R., & Desai, S. (2022). Novel Polymeric Nanocarriers in CNS Therapy. Drug Discovery Today, 17(4), 563–578.
40. Qureshi, A., & Malik, N. (2023). Nanotechnology in Alzheimer's. Diagnostics. Journal of Clinical Nanomedicine, 9(5), 211–226.
41. Goudoulas, T. B. (2012). Polymers and Biopolymers as Drug Delivery Systems in Nanomedicine. 2(1), 52–61. https://doi.org/10.2174/1877912311202010052
42. Siafaka, P. I., Mutlu, G., & Okur, N. (2021). Alzheimer's Disease and its Related Dementia Types: A Review on Their Management via Nanotechnology Based Therapeutic Strategies. Current Alzheimer Research, 17(14), 1239–1261. https://doi.org/10.2174/1567205018666210218160812
43. Fernandez, M., Garcia, J., & Lopez, C. (2023). Nanoparticle Innovations in Alzheimer's Care. Journal of Biomedical Nanotechnology, 19(6), 515–528.
44. Agarwal, M., Alam, R., Haider, M. K., Malik, M. Z., & Kim, D. (2020). Alzheimer's Disease: Nanotechnology Solutions. MDPI Nanomaterials, 11(1), 59. https://doi.org/10.3390/nano11010059
45. Mahajan, S., & Gupta, D. (2021). Alzheimer's Drug Delivery: Polymeric Solutions. Neurodegenerative Disease Management, 10(5), 531–544.
46. Oliveira Silva, R., Counil, H., & Ramassamy, C. (2024). Donepezil-Loaded Nanocarriers for Alzheimer's. International Journal of Nanomedicine, 19, 1077–1096. https://doi.org/10.2147/IJN.S449227
47. Polymeric Nanoparticles Production. (2024). https://www.cd-bioparticles.net/polymeric-nanoparticles-production
48. La Barbera, L., Mauri, E., D'Amelio, M., & Gori, M. (2022). Functionalization Strategies of Polymeric Nanoparticles for Drug Delivery in Alzheimer's Disease: Current Trends and Future Perspectives. Frontiers in Neuroscience, 16. https://doi.org/10.3389/fnins.2022.939855
49. Jo, D. H., Kim, J. H., Lee, T. G., & Kim, J. H. (2015). Nanoparticles' Therapeutic Effects in Neurodegeneration. Nano Today, 11(7), 1603–1611.

50. Dash, S. K. (2010). Targeted Disease Modifying Drugs for Alzheimer's Disease. Neurotherapeutics, 6(1), 65–76.
51. Bilal, M., Barani, M., Sabir, F., & Kyzas, G. Z. (2020). Nanomaterials in Alzheimer's Therapy. Elsevier Impact, 20, 100251. https://doi.org/10.1016/j.impact.2020.100251
52. Cui, N., Lu, H., & Li, M. (2018). Magnetic Nanoparticles for Alzheimer's Therapy. Journal of Nanobiotechnology, 14(5), 1017–1024. https://doi.org/10.1166/jbn.2018.2512
53. Gupta, J., Fatima, M., Islam, Z., Khan, R. H., Uversky, V. N., & Salahuddin, P. (2019). Nanoparticle Formulations in the Diagnosis and Therapy of Alzheimer's Disease. Elsevier BV, 130, 515–26. https://doi.org/10.1016/j.ijbiomac.2019.02.156
54. Dighe, S., Jog, S., Momin, M., & Omri, A. (2023). Nanotechnology in Alzheimer's Management. Pharmaceutics, 16(1), 58. https://doi.org/10.3390/pharmaceutics16010058
55. Wong, K. H., Riaz, M. K., & Yang, Z. (2019). Strategies for Alzheimer's Drugs Across BBB. International Journal of Molecular Sciences, 20(2), 381. https://doi.org/10.3390/ijms20020381
56. Das, S., & Bhowmick, S. (2020). Nanocarriers in Alzheimer's Drug Delivery. Pharmacology and Therapeutics, 18(7), 983–1001. https://doi.org/10.2174/157488911794079073
57. Hameed, M., & Khalid, R. (2021). Nanotechnology for Alzheimer's Treatment. Journal of Neurochemistry, 14(8), 389–403.
58. Rabiee, N., Ahmadi, S., & Webster, T. J. (2021). Polymeric Nanoparticles for Nasal Drug Delivery. Journal of Dentistry Research, 490, 1–15. https://doi.org/10.1002/adtp.202000076
59. Rahman, T., & Zaman, S. (2022). Nanoparticles for Targeted Brain Therapy. International Journal of Neuropharmacology, 20(3), 129–143.

10 Carbon Dots
Blood–Brain Barrier Penetrating Drug Nanocarrier in the Treatment of Alzheimer's Disease

Oshin Verma, Divya Bisht, and Deena Prakash

10.1 INTRODUCTION

Nanotechnology is a growing domain of science that has facilitated the fabrication of various nanomaterials to be utilized in the betterment of both healthcare and the environment. Because of its distinct and well-defined structures with small size, this technology has been widely used in different fields for better outcomes. Since the beginning of the twenty-first century, nanotechnology has garnered a lot of attention due to its simplicity of synthesis and applicability in a variety of sectors, including nanomedicine, drug delivery, bio-imaging, solar cells, electrocatalysis, photocatalysis, and other relevant areas (Pokrajac et al., 2021; Malik et al., 2023; Bobokulova & Muxtaram, 2024).

Nanomedicine is one of the most significant application of nanotechnology that deals with the diagnosis and treatment of several diseases with enhanced patient's outcome. These nanomedicines are also crucial in the treatment of neurodegenerative disorders due to the various properties of nanomaterial that allow them to effectively deliver both imagining and therapeutic agents in the neuronal region crossing the blood–brain barrier (BBB). One such neurodegenerative disease discussed in this chapter is Alzheimer's disease (AD).

The BBB is a selective barrier composed of endothelial cells linked by tight junctions, which restricts the passive diffusion of substances from the bloodstream into the brain. The BBB regulates ionic balance and provides essential nutrients, thereby ensuring an optimal environment for neuronal function (Upton et al., 2022). Only small, lipid-soluble molecules with a molecular weight below 400 Da or possessing fewer than eight hydrogen bonds are capable of passively traversing the BBB. Ion channels and transporters in the endothelial cells of the BBB play a vital role in regulating the brain's microenvironment. Essential ions such as K^+, Na^+, Ca^{2+}, and Cl^- are meticulously regulated to maintain the electrochemical gradients required for neural signaling. The BBB possesses specialized transport mechanisms that uphold brain homeostasis, which include active efflux transporters, receptor-mediated transporters

DOI: 10.1201/9781003543381-10

(RMT), carrier-mediated transporters (CMT), absorptive-mediated transporters (AMT), and ion transporters (Knox et al., 2022). Transporters are essential in inhibiting the buildup of xenobiotics and specific pharmaceuticals in the central nervous system (CNS), thereby creating a barrier to the delivery of contrast agents. CMT are selective proteins that enable the transport of vital nutrients and metabolites into the brain (Liu et al., 2025).

AD is an emerging medical challenge affecting approximately 50 million individuals worldwide being the leading cause of dementia among the elderly population and anticipated to have a lifespan of four to eight years. Currently, the precise cause of the disease is unclear; however, the presence of neurofibrillary tangles (NFTs) and amyloid plaques in the brain is indicative of this condition. Despite the recent FDA (Food and Drug Administration) approval of aducanumab for AD treatment, this decision remains contentious, and the drug's ability to modify disease progression is still uncertain. Consequently, there is an imperative want for the identification of AD medications that can either impede the pathogenesis of the disease or arrest its progression (Zhang et al., 2022). Researchers are striving to develop advanced treatment alternatives of AD as the current drug options focuses on the superficial treatment by suppressing the symptoms and not on the cure of disease. The BBB is a significant impediment to the development and delivery of more efficient drug therapies, as it inhibits the passage of numerous compounds with therapeutic ability to the CNS. This issue may be resolved through the application of nanotechnology.

Nanoparticles (NPs) can cross the BBB through transcellular pathways, specifically utilizing receptor-mediated transport, adsorptive-mediated transport, and carrier-mediated transport (Choudhari et al., 2021). AMT depends on electrostatic interactions between NPs and the endothelial cell membrane of the BBB. The luminal surface of endothelial cells exhibits a negative charge attributed to glycoproteins and proteoglycans. Functionalizing NPs with positively charged ligands, such as cell-penetrating peptides, lectins, or cationic polymers, enables electrostatic interaction with negatively charged membranes. This interaction promotes endocytosis and enables the transcellular transport of NPs into the brain. AMT offers benefits by improving the absorption of various molecules without requiring specific receptor-ligand interactions. CMT entails NPs that are modified with molecules that are specifically recognized by transporters overexpressed on the endothelial cells of the BBB. Endogenous substances, including glucose and amino acids, traverse the BBB through specific transporters, namely glucose transporters (GLUT1 and GLUT3) and large neutral amino acid transporters (LAT1). Attaching mannose, glucose, or amino acids to the surface of NPs allows them to mimic natural substrates, facilitating their transport into the brain through diffusion or active transport mechanisms. Glucose-coated NPs can interact with GLUT1 transporters to traverse the BBB, facilitating the delivery of therapeutic agents to regions impacted by AD (Qu et al., 2014; Anraku et al., 2017).

Carbon dots (CDs) have garnered attention as a suitable nanomaterial for the treatment of AD. CDs are spherical allotropes of carbon with zero dimension and a size of less than 10 nm allowing them to exhibit properties like water solubility, conductivity, low toxicity, eco-friendliness, high biocompatibility, and ability to effectively cross the BBB attracting researchers to further investigate them as medicinal alternatives for AD (Dubois et al., 2021; Guo et al., 2022).

The National Institute on Ageing (NIA) United States and the Alzheimer's Association introduced the ATN systems for defining and diagnosing AD. In this framework, 'A' denotes amyloid deposition through amyloid beta (Aβ) aggregation, 'T' represents tau pathology, including NFTs, and 'N' signifies neurodegeneration (Sagbas & Sahiner, 2019; Mintz et al., 2021). Amyloid plaques, a key clinical characteristic of AD, are mostly composed of aggregation of Aβ-peptides. The aberrant hyperphosphorylation of tau protein, alongside amyloid plaque formation, results in the emergence of paired helical filaments (PHF), a defining element of NFTs. These intracellular accumulations inhibit brain transmission and contribute to neuronal death, hence exacerbating cognitive impairment in AD patients (Zhang et al., 2023; Zhang et al., 2024). Extensive research indicates that the pathophysiology of AD is complex, shaped by numerous environmental and genetic influences. Although current drug development efforts predominantly concentrate on specific targets, namely Aβ, there is a recognized necessity to develop therapeutic techniques that address numerous targets. In this setting, simultaneously targeting Aβ and tau aggregation is essential for developing more effective disease-modifying medicines for AD (Biancalana et al., 2009).

This chapter deals with a detailed discussion on the role of CDs in the diagnosis and treatment of AD, focusing on the properties of CDs, method of synthesis, role of CDs in diagnosis and treatment, and the benefits and limitation of CDs as a tool in nanomedicine against AD.

10.2 CARBON DOTS

Currently, a wide variety of nanomaterials, including nanowires, nano-magnetic beads, dendrimers, polymer nanocomposites, carbon-based nanomaterials, metallic, and magnetic NPs are being extensively utilized due to their remarkable properties (Yaqoob et al., 2020; Salvo-Comino et al., 2021).

Among the different available nanomaterials, carbon-based nanomaterials are extensively investigated because of their remarkable characteristics, including non-toxicity, biocompatibility, inertness, long-term chemical stability, fluorescence properties, high electrical and thermal conductivity, large effective surface area, and ease of functionalization attributed to their functional groups. Additionally, they exhibit remarkable electrocatalytic activity and the capability to modify multiple electrodes, facilitating the development of diverse biosensing platforms (Porto et al., 2019; Hwang et al., 2020; Kour et al., 2020).

Carbon-based nanomaterials typically comprise of graphene (GR), fullerenes (C60), carbon black (CB), carbon nanohorns (CNHs), carbon nanodiamonds, carbon nanofibers (CNFs), and carbon nanotubes (CNTs), which consist of single-walled carbon nanotubes (SWCNTs) and multi-walled carbon nanotubes (MWCNTs). Additionally, quantum dots (QDs) such as CDs are also part of this category (Silva et al., 2017; Molazemhosseini et al., 2021; Nurrohman & Chiu, 2021; Hu et al., 2022).

CDs represent a category of carbon-based NPs identified in the early 21st century. They often classified as graphene quantum dots (GQDs) or carbon quantum dots (CQDs), are nanoscale carbon-based materials measuring fewer than 10 nanometers in size. CDs can display a variety of structures, such as crystalline, amorphous, or hybrid forms, influenced by the fabrication method and the precursor materials employed (Cui et al., 2021; Etefa et al., 2024). The composition of CDs consists of sp2 and sp3 carbon atoms, featuring a considerable presence of polymer chains or functional groups attached to their surfaces (Xia et al., 2019; Mansuriya & Altintas, 2021).

CDs possess several advantages as nanocarriers for drug delivery, including targeted delivery, intracellular barrier penetrability, efficacy enhancement, improved bioavailability, and real-time monitoring capabilities. They have been extensively studied for the delivery of the anticancer drug doxorubicin (DOX), other anticancer agents, including platinum-based drugs, paclitaxel, 5-fluorouracil, and methotrexate, with various strategies employed for drug loading and release, such as covalent and non-covalent interactions (Bartkowski et al., 2024).

CDs have also been explored for the delivery of antibacterial agents and inhibitors of vascular endothelial growth factor (VEGF) for the treatment of ocular diseases (Kapoor & Sheth, 2024).

10.2.1 Synthesis of CDs

The top-down and bottom-up approaches illustrated in Figure 10.1 represent two overarching categories that include various ways for the synthesis of CDs. The development of CDs provides a level of convenience; however, it also presents considerable challenges. The challenges encompass the propensity of NPs to cluster while carbonization, the necessity to regulate uniformity and size, and the obligation to alter surface characteristics (Jorns & Pappas, 2021; Lin et al., 2022). A variety of techniques exist for producing CDs from an array of intricately structured raw

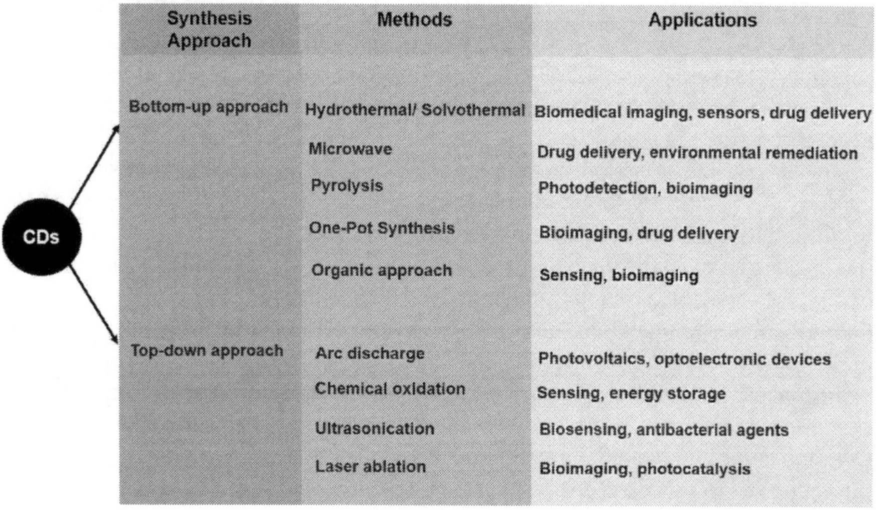

FIGURE 10.1 Different methods to synthesize CDs, along with their applications.

materials. It is particularly intriguing that each synthesis method has a substantial impact on the physicochemical properties of CDs, allowing for their application in diverse fields (Saleem et al., 2022). Bottom-up approach entails the assembly of CDs from smaller molecular precursors or carbon sources. This methodology generally encompasses several key stages: carbonization, surface passivation, size control, and purification. Bottom-up synthesis methods provide meticulous control over the size, surface chemistry, and optical properties of CDs (Ahmed et al., 2023; Bian et al., 2023; Modi et al., 2023). The process of top-down fabrication entails the exfoliation or fragmentation of larger carbonaceous materials to yield CDs. Top-down synthesis methods provide a scalable and economical strategy for producing CDs. They make use of accessible carbon sources and are capable of producing CDs in substantial amounts. Nonetheless, their ability to manipulate surface chemistry and functionalization may be restricted when contrasted with bottom-up approaches (Kumar et al., 2021; Chen et al., 2023).

10.3 CARBON DOTS AS DRUG NANOCARRIERS

CDs have been successfully employed for *in vitro* and *in vivo* cellular and tissue imaging, demonstrating their potential in disease diagnosis and treatment monitoring. CDs are regarded as versatile drug delivery methods because of their high fluorescence, low toxicity, chemical inertness, and remarkable biocompatibility. For therapeutic purposes, these CDs have been utilized to carry and deliver medicine to designated places. CDs have lately drawn interest in the area of drug distribution because of their outstanding capabilities. The CDs loaded with the drug group together and move to the cytoplasm and nucleus of cancer cells. The drug is then released at these specific sites via radiation (Zhao et al., 2020).

A study was conducted to approve the significant biomedical applications of CDs despite the obstacle related to their poorly described structure. A comparative analysis of the properties of three types of CDs—black carbon dots (B-CDs), carbon nitride dots (CNDs), and yellow CDs (YCDs) highlighted their potential in biomedical applications (Etefa et al., 2024). B-CDs have demonstrated potential as a material for targeted drug delivery to bone, crossing the BBB, and facilitating cell-membrane penetration when conjugated with a targeting ligand (Peng et al., 2017). CNDs are synthesized using a bottom-up microwave-assisted method and demonstrate the capacity to specifically target glioblastoma cells while also self-targeting the BBB for drug delivery (Hettiarachchi et al., 2019; Liyanage et al., 2020). YCDs are synthesized using an ultrasonication method. They have applications in 3D printing, exhibit the capacity to inhibit β-amyloid fibril formation, and can permeate the entire body of zebrafish, including the CNS. The hydrophilic and hydrophobic properties of CDs can be altered to facilitate their passage across the BBB through passive diffusion. YCDs demonstrate solvent effects, indicating their ability to be dispersed in various organic solvents while displaying distinct photoluminescent properties. Consequently, YCDs exhibit amphiphilic characteristics and facilitate drug delivery through passive diffusion. Nevertheless, a particularly appealing aspect of YCDs is that their amphiphilic nature remains unchanged even when conjugated with hydrophilic compounds. Upon excitation at 405 nm wavelength, a distinct yellow fluorescence emanating from YCDs was prominently pointed out within the central canal of the zebrafish spinal cord subsequent to intracardial injection, suggesting that YCDs successfully traversed the BBB (Zhou et al., 2019).

A study demonstrated that CDs synthesized from urea and citric acid (CA) can traverse the BBB and efficiently inhibit tau aggregation. This discovery identified CDs as potential drug candidates that may function both as therapeutic agents and drug nanocarriers, offering promise for the treatment of AD. The choice of precursor materials markedly affects the functional and structural properties of CDs (Kumar et al., 2022; Lin et al., 2024). The use of Congo red as a precursor substance for CDs may improve its capacity to cross the BBB. Furthermore, leveraging the inherent capacity of Congo red to inhibit both Aβ and tau aggregation presents a substantial and potential therapeutic approach for AD treatment. The strategic use of Congo red as a precursor for CDs presents a novel approach to developing effective therapies for AD (Zhang et al., 2024). The BBB can also be traversed by transport proteins located on the cell membrane surface. Mintz et al. (2019) utilized tryptophan as a carbon precursor, along with 1,2-ethylenediamine (EDA) and urea, respectively, incorporating two N-dopants to provide two distinct products. The yellow gel substances, specifically CDs-EDA and CDs-urea, displayed tryptophan moieties on their surface, demonstrating brilliant photoluminescence and minimal toxicity. CDs-EDA were demonstrated to traverse the BBB and infiltrate the CNS of zebrafish via endocytosis facilitated by the LAT1 transporter. The two CDs illustrated the feasibility of administering medicines to the CNS without receptor binding. Lately, Seven et al. (2021) utilized glucose as the substrate to synthesize GluCDs, leveraging a glucose transporter to facilitate the delivery of CDs across the BBB. This study critically shows that a non-receptor-mediated transport pathway can facilitate the delivery of CDs to the CNS of a mammal after intravenous injection. The inhibitory effect of CDs suggests their potential as candidates for AD treatment, indicating a favorable direction for developing therapeutic interventions that address various aspects of AD pathology.

10.4 CARBON DOTS IN THE TREATMENT OF ALZHEIMER'S DISEASE

The question of how therapeutic agents can penetrate the BBB to effectively reach and function within the CNS remains a significant issue in modern medicine. The BBB is a specialized semipermeable structure that meticulously regulates the exchanges between the CNS parenchyma and blood vessels (Rana et al., 2024). Consequently, the BBB inhibits the transfer of numerous therapeutic agents, nanocarriers, and their associated cargo (Burgess & Hynynen, 2014). Alternative strategies, including photodynamic and photothermal therapies, demonstrate potential for circumventing the BBB and are employed clinically for treating various brain diseases. Nonetheless, the adverse effects of photosensitization and damage to skin tissues present additional concerns (Dhas et al., 2021). Recent multidisciplinary studies concentrate on the development of cargo-loaded NPs to address these challenges, positioning them as safe and efficient vehicles in neurotheranostics. These advancements in NPs have demonstrated numerous unprecedented properties for NP-mediated drug delivery. These properties enable them to noninvasively traverse the BBB, facilitating the treatment of CNS diseases (Zhang et al., 2021; Zha et al., 2024).The primary advantage of utilizing NPs lies in their ability to be engineered for predictable and specific reactions to both external and internal stimuli, thereby enhancing the control of the drug delivery process (Gharbavi et al., 2018). Studies indicate that the efficiency of drug delivery can be significantly improved by covalently conjugating NPs with various ligands. Certain ligands, including niosomes and glutathione peptides, enhance the solubility and stability of NPs-based drug delivery systems. The use of specific ligands, including transferrin, can enhance targeted therapy and facilitate the crossing of biological barriers, such as the BBB and cell membranes (Nosrati et al., 2019).

CDs have been found to cross the BBB through various mechanisms, including receptor-mediated endocytosis, transport protein-mediated transport, and passive diffusion, depending on their surface properties and modifications (Kang & Lee, 2019). CDs are being investigated for halting or reversing Alzheimer's pathology by delivering drugs that inhibit the aggregation of Aβ peptides or tau proteins, both of which are critical in AD pathogenesis. Studies have shown that CDs can effectively inhibit Aβ fibrillation and reduce the function of β-site amyloid precursor protein cleaving enzyme 1 (BACE1), which is essential for Aβ generation. Furthermore, the fluorescence property of CDs allows for real-time monitoring of their effect in vivo, providing additional avenues for exploring therapeutic efficacy (Han et al., 2017; Zhang et al., 2024).

As YCDs displayed favorable nanocarrier characteristics they diminished the expression and secretion of Aβ in *in vitro* tests by suppressing the synthesis of amyloid precursor protein (APP). As previously stated, YCDs demonstrate amphiphilicity, indicating that YCDs possess both a hydrophilic surface and enhanced hydrophobic properties compared to hydrophilic CDs. The hydrophilic surface can interact with Aβ independently to create more extensive structures, enhancing flexibility, which will aid in suppressing Aβ fibril formation (Hung et al., 2008; Todorova et al., 2013). Zhou et al. (2019) investigated the toxicity profile of YCDs across four distinct cell lines and established that YCDs exhibited no toxicity at the measured concentrations. Recently, Yan et al. (2022) coupled YCDs with Ce6, a photosensitizer, demonstrating that this combination traversed the BBB following tail vein injections in mice. The YCD/Ce6 combination decreased amyloid aggregation and toxicity and eliminated amyloid plaques from the brains of the APP/PS1 AD mice model.

Curcumin is a polyphenolic compound derived from turmeric; it exhibits antioxidant, anticancer, anti-inflammatory, antibacterial, and neuroprotective properties and may prohibit or mitigate the pathological processes associated with age-related cognitive decline, AD, or other forms of dementia (Ak & Gülçin, 2008; Shabbir et al., 2020; Esatbeyoglu et al., 2012). Evidence suggests that curcumin may partially protect cells from Aβ-mediated neurotoxicity through the inhibition of Aβ aggregation (Kuang et al., 2020). The potential of curcumin was investigated to mitigate memory decline through the inhibition of BACE1 expression and β-amyloid pathology in 5FAD transgenic mice. It was observed to decrease amyloid plaque deposition and soluble Aβ1-42 levels in the brain through the inhibition of BACE1 (Zheng et al.,

2017). Furthermore, curcumin was observed to enhance synaptophysin expression, which is crucial for sustaining synaptic transmission, and to reduce synaptic damage in 5FAD mice. Learning and memory in curcumin-treated mice showed enhancement (Liu et al., 2015; Xiao et al., 2016).

To enhance the cell uptake efficiency and bioavailability of curcumin, Kuang et al. (2020) synthesized CDs by mixing CA and glucose using a microwave technique. The fabricated CDs were combined with CH_3COONa and $FeCl_3$ to produce Fe_3O_4-CDs, which were then compiled with curcumin. *In vitro* investigations revealed that Curcumin-Fe3O4-CDs displayed a strong specific affinity for Aβ42 and markedly impeded the aggregation of Aβ42 protein. It also suppressed the formation of reactive oxygen species (ROS) caused by Aβ fibrils and reduced Aβ-mediated toxicity in PC12 cells. These findings suggest that CDs could function as an efficient delivery method, offering a suitable platform for AD therapy.

In AD, hyperphosphorylation of tau disrupts the equilibrium between tau phosphorylation and dephosphorylation, leading to the accumulation of free phosphorylated tau (ptau), which can detach from microtubules and self-aggregate into NFTs within the cell body and dystrophic neurites, thereby impairing microtubule functionality (Holtzman et al., 2011; Qian et al., 2020). This ultimately results in neuronal death, a characteristic feature of AD (Zhang et al., 2012; Johnson et al., 2016). Recent studies suggest that targeting tau pathology may be a more effective therapeutic approach than focusing on amyloid.

CNDs were investigated to block tau aggregation where CNDs were successfully joined with memantine hydrochloride (MH), a drug long used to treat AD but with low efficiency. Both CNDs and CNDs MH demonstrated the capacity to inhibit tau aggregation *in vitro*. Additionally, the authors demonstrated that each CNDs and CNDs MH are capable of crossing the BBB in a zebrafish model. This study establishes a basis for subsequent research aimed at addressing AD-related brain neuropathology through various mechanisms (Zhang et al., 2022; Zhou et al., 2022).

Inhibition of acetylcholinesterase (AChE) to increase acetylcholine (ACh) levels in the brain represents one of the limited symptomatic therapies recently available for AD. Extracts of the leguminous butterfly pea can elevate ACh levels in the hippocampus, potentially enhancing learning and memory capabilities (Taranalli & Cheeramkuzhy, 2000). Based on this information, Tak et al. (2020) used a one-pot microwave-assisted green synthesis approach to produce GQDs from butterfly pea flowers. In an *in vitro* assay, GQDs demonstrated inhibition of AChE comparable to donepezil, the most widely utilized medication for treating AD. Systemically administered GQDs demonstrated the ability to reverse memory and learning deficits in rats induced by scopolamine, a cholinergic receptor antagonist.

The results indicate that GQDs can traverse the BBB, thereby influencing brain function. Suner et al. (2021) utilized CA as a carbon source and cysteine (Cys) as a source of sulfur and nitrogen to prepare S- and N-doped Cys CDs via a green synthesis approach employing a microwave technique. The study demonstrated that the inhibition of AChE correlated with the amount of Cys CDs. It remains uncertain whether the method of enzymatic inhibition would demonstrate superior functional efficacy or a diminished side effect profile compared to current pharmacotherapies. However, the research clearly supports the notion that CDs can effectively deliver agents to the brain.

10.5 POTENTIAL BENEFITS AND LIMITATIONS

CDs exhibit notable characteristics, including biocompatibility, environmental sustainability, high chemical inertness, high solubility in water, and photostability. Furthermore, CDs can be efficiently produced in alignment with green chemistry principles. Due to their readily adjustable optical properties, CDs are utilized in diverse fields such as drug delivery, nanomedicine, energy storage, solar cells, photocatalysis, electrocatalysis, and related domains (Rasal et al., 2021; Cai et al., 2023).

Various methods exist for synthesizing CDs, including chemical, physical, and biological processes (Gupta et al., 2023). However, the biological method is preferable due to its cost-effectiveness and sustainability (Wang et al., 2023). Biologically synthesized CDs demonstrate biocompatibility, thereby increasing their potential use in biomedicine, especially in drug delivery (Nair et al., 2020; Ge et al., 2021). However, there are still a number of obstacles to overcome and concerns over the future that are related with CDs (Wareing et al., 2021; Etefa et al., 2024).

10.5.1 Synthesis and Surface Optimization

Consistent and scalable synthesis methods need to be developed for clinical applications. The cost-effective production of nanomaterials is a significant hurdle. High-quality nanomaterials are typically manufactured utilizing advanced instrumentation and extreme circumstances, which restricts their large-scale production. This matter is of more significance for the synthesis of two-dimensional nanomaterials. The majority of technologies employed for large-scale production are cost-effective, although they typically yield materials with faults and inferior quality. The regulated synthesis of nanomaterials remains a formidable task (Baig et al., 2021). Acquiring structurally pure nanomaterials is the sole method to realize the theoretically predicted properties outlined in the literature. Enhanced efforts are necessary to devise novel synthesis techniques that address the limitations of traditional approaches (Yang et al., 2014; Liu et al., 2017).

Future research must focus on developing NPs that exhibit enhanced safety profiles. The use of biocompatible and biodegradable materials can mitigate toxicity and immunogenicity, which are significant obstacles to clinical application. Surface modifications, including polyethylene glycol (PEGylation), enhance biocompatibility by reducing unintended immune interactions and extending circulation time. Improving targeting precision represents a significant area for development. Functionalization of NPs with ligands or antibodies that are specific to AD biomarkers, including amyloid-beta plaques and tau protein tangles, can enhance targeting efficiency considerably. This specificity enhances therapeutic efficacy and minimizes off-target effects, consequently reducing potential side effects. Enhancing the pharmacokinetic characteristics of NPs is crucial for maximizing therapeutic efficacy. Modifying parameters such as size, shape, and surface charge affect distribution, circulation time, and clearance rates. An in-depth comprehension of these factors facilitates the design of NPs exhibiting optimal absorption, distribution, metabolism, and excretion (ADME) characteristics, thereby improving their overall efficacy. Furthermore, the integration of theranostic NPs provides a dual-function platform that merges therapeutic and diagnostic capabilities. The incorporation of imaging agents in these NPs facilitates real-time monitoring of drug delivery and treatment response, thereby supporting the development of personalized treatment strategies (Liu et al., 2025). This method improves therapeutic results and facilitates early detection and intervention, which is essential for the management of AD.

10.5.2 Clinical Safety and Long-Term Effects

Despite the promising applications, several challenges hinder the full clinical potential of CDs in treating AD. One major concern is the need for extensive *in vivo* studies to determine the long-term safety and efficacy of CDs in humans. Collaboration among scientists, doctors, and industry stakeholders is essential for expediting the transition of NPs-based therapeutics from the laboratory to clinical use. Additionally, optimizing the synthesis methods for large-scale production while maintaining the functional integrity of CDs presents a significant hurdle (Guo et al., 2022). There are also concerns regarding the potential long-term toxicity of CDs and the need for standardization in production processes to ensure reproducibility. Translation from preclinical studies to human trials is crucial for validating efficacy and safety (Zhang et al., 2021). Continued exploration into surface modifications and targeting strategies will be crucial in optimizing CDs for clinical use. Further studies should also focus on comprehensive long-term in vivo safety assessments to establish the clinical feasibility of these nanocarriers in Alzheimer's treatment (Ye et al., 2023). Research is actively focused on developing functionalization strategies that improve brain-specific targeting while reducing off-target effects.

10.6 CONCLUSIONS

CDs have emerged as fascinating nanomaterials with diverse applications across multiple sectors due to their distinctive physicochemical and optical properties allowing wide variety of functions. These zero-dimensional NPs, typically smaller than 10 nm, exhibit remarkable biocompatibility, water solubility, low toxicity, and environmental sustainability making them a suitable choice for researchers. All these properties encourage research advancements in CD synthesis, characterization, and applications expanding their utility in fields of nanomedicine in drug delivery, energy storage, photocatalysis, electrocatalysis, and bioimaging.

Several synthesis methods have been developed to produce CDs with precise control over their size, shape, surface functionalization, and optical properties. Techniques such as hydrothermal, solvothermal, microwave-assisted, and electrochemical methods have been optimized to enhance the quality and functionality of CDs. Notably, the adoption of sustainable approaches using renewable precursors and nontoxic reagents has gained prominence, aligning with the increasing demand for environmentally friendly nanomaterials.

CDs propose immense promise as nanocarriers for crossing the BBB, particularly for treating AD. Their small size, intrinsic biocompatibility, and multifunctional approach enable them to deliver diagnostic and therapeutic agents effectively to the brain while minimizing off-target effects and harmful side effects on patients.

They can be used to achieve sustained drug release and pH-responsive drug delivery. CDs can also be functionalized with receptor-specific ligands to enhance their targeting capabilities, making them a valuable tool for addressing neurodegenerative diseases. However, bridging the gap between laboratory-scale demonstrations and practical clinical applications remains a significant challenge. The limited efficacy of traditional pharmacological approaches highlights the need for novel drug delivery systems.

Future research in this area should focus on refining the synthesis of CDs to further achieve precise property and size control while ensuring scalability and reproducibility at mass level. Enhanced capabilities in imaging, drug delivery, and theranostics have the potential to transform modern medicine systems reducing the massive burden of AD on healthcare. The development of stimuli-responsive CDs for smart drug delivery systems is an area of ongoing research. Moreover, the versatility of CDs indicates their role as promising materials for next-generation electronics, environmental monitoring, and renewable energy storage along with a bright future in nanomedicine. This chapter highlighted the advancements in carbon dot (CD) research over the past decade, specifically focusing on their potential as BBB-penetrating drug nanocarriers for the treatment of AD, and their capacity to drive innovation in neurotherapeutics and related scientific disciplines. Advancements in nanotechnology present potential solutions; however, the intricacies of the BBB and the requirement for accurate targeting underscore the necessity for additional research. It is essential to overcome the protective functions of the BBB without jeopardizing its critical role in CNS homeostasis for the advancement of effective AD treatments. Ongoing innovation and interdisciplinary collaboration are essential for maximizing the potential of these technologies, ultimately offering new prospects for individuals impacted by AD.

REFERENCES

Ahmed, Hanan B., Mahmoud El-Shahat, Abdou K. Allayeh, and Hossam E. Emam. "Maillard reaction for nucleation of polymer quantum dots from chitosan-glucose conjugate: Antagonistic for cancer and viral diseases." *International Journal of Biological Macromolecules* 224 (2023): 858–870.

Ak, Tuba, and Ilhami Gülçin. "Antioxidant and radical scavenging properties of curcumin." *Chemico-Biological Interactions* 174, no. 1 (2008): 27–37.

Anraku, Y., H. Kuwahara, Y. Fukusato, A. Mizoguchi, T. Ishii, K. Nitta, and Y. Matsumoto et al. "Glycaemic control boosts glucosylated nanocarrier crossing the BBB into the brain." *Nature Communications* 8, no. 1 (2017): 1001.

Baig, Nadeem, Irshad Kammakakam, and Wail Falath "Nanomaterials: A review of synthesis methods, properties, recent progress, and challenges." *Materials Advances* 2, no. 6 (2021): 1821–1871.

Bartkowski, Michał, Yingru Zhou, Mustafa Nabil Amin Mustafa, Alexander J. Eustace, and Silvia Giordani "CARBON DOTS: Bioimaging and anticancer drug delivery." *Chemistry–A European Journal* 30, no. 19 (2024): e202303982.

Bian, Zhengyi, Alison Wallum, Arshad Mehmood, Eric Gomez, Ziwen Wang, Subhendu Pandit, Shuming Nie, Stephan Link, Benjamin G. Levine, and Martin Gruebele "Properties of carbon dots versus small molecules from "Bottom-up" synthesis." *ACS Nano* 17, no. 22 (2023): 22788–22799.

Biancalana, Matthew, Koki Makabe, Akiko Koide, and Shohei Koide "Molecular mechanism of thioflavin-t binding to the surface of β-rich peptide self-assemblies." *Journal of Molecular Biology* 385, no. 4 (2009): 1052–1063.

Bobokulova, and Muxtaram "The role of nanotechnology in modern physics." *Development and Innovations in Science* 3, no. 1 (2024): 145–153.

Burgess, Alison, and Kullervo Hynynen "Drug delivery across the blood–brain barrier using focused ultrasound." *Expert Opinion on Drug Delivery* 11, no. 5 (2014): 711–721.

Cai, Hao, Khurram Abbas, Yuxiang Yang, Zijian Li, and Hong Bi "The application of carbon dots in tumor immunotherapy: Researches and prospects." *Applied Research* 2, no. 6 (2023): e202300001.

Chen, Lintao, Cai-Feng Wang, Chang Liu, and Su Chen "Facile access to fabricate carbon dots and perspective of large-scale applications." *Small* 19, no. 31 (2023): 2206671.

Choudhari, Manisha, Siddhanth Hejmady, Ranendra Narayan Saha, Shantanu Damle, Gautam Singhvi, Amit Alexander, Prashant Kesharwani, and Sunil Kumar Dubey. "Evolving new-age strategies to transport therapeutics across the blood-brain-barrier." *International Journal of Pharmaceutics* 599 (2021): 120351.

Cui, Lin, Xin Ren, Mengtao Sun, Haiyan Liu, and Lixin Xia "Carbon dots: Synthesis, properties and applications." *Nanomaterials* 11, no. 12 (2021): 3419.

Dhas, Namdev, Ritu Kudarha, Atul Garkal, Vivek Ghate, Shilpa Sharma, Prabhakar Panzade, and Shubham Khot et al. "Molybdenum-based hetero-nanocomposites for cancer therapy, diagnosis and biosensing application: Current advancement and future breakthroughs." *Journal of Controlled Release* 330 (2021): 257–283.

Dubois, Bruno, Nicolas Villain, Giovanni B. Frisoni, Gil D. Rabinovici, Marwan Sabbagh, Stefano Cappa, and Alexandre Bejanin et al. "Clinical diagnosis of Alzheimer's disease: Recommendations of the international working group." *The Lancet Neurology* 20, no. 6 (2021): 484–496.

Esatbeyoglu, Tuba, Patricia Huebbe, Insa MA Ernst, Dawn Chin, Anika E. Wagner, and Gerald Rimbach "Curcumin—From molecule to biological function." *Angewandte Chemie International Edition* 51, no. 22 (2012): 5308–5332.

Etefa, Habtamu Fekadu, Aster Aberra Tessema, and Francis Birhanu Dejene. "Carbon dots for future prospects: synthesis, characterizations and recent applications: a review (2019–2023)." *C* 10, no. 3 (2024): 60.

Ge, Guili, Lin Li, Dan Wang, Mingjian Chen, Zhaoyang Zeng, Wei Xiong, Xu Wu, and Can Guo "Carbon dots: Synthesis, properties and biomedical applications." *Journal of Materials Chemistry B* 9, no. 33 (2021): 6553–6575.

Gharbavi, Mahmoud, Jafar Amani, Hamidreza Kheiri-Manjili, Hossein Danafar, and Ali Sharafi "Niosome: A promising nanocarrier for natural drug delivery through blood-brain barrier." *Advances in Pharmacological and Pharmaceutical Sciences* 2018, no. 1 (2018): 6847971.

Guo, Feng, Qingman Li, Xiaolin Zhang, Yiheng Liu, Jie Jiang, Shuanghuai Cheng, and Si Yu et al. "Applications of carbon dots for the treatment of Alzheimer's disease." *International Journal of Nanomedicine* 17 (2022): 6621.

Gupta, Deepshikha, Anuj Boora, Amisha Thakur, and Tejendra K. Gupta "Green and sustainable synthesis of nanomaterials: Recent advancements and limitations." *Environmental Research* 231 (2023): 116316.

Han, Xu, Zhifeng Jing, Wei Wu, Bing Zou, Zhili Peng, Pengyu Ren, Athula Wikramanayake, Zhongmin Lu, and Roger M. Leblanc "Biocompatible and blood–brain barrier permeable carbon dots for inhibition of aβ fibrillation and toxicity, and BACE1 activity." *Nanoscale* 9, no. 35 (2017): 12862–12866.

Hettiarachchi, Sajini D., Regina M. Graham, Keenan J. Mintz, Yiqun Zhou, Steven Vanni, Zhilli Peng, and Roger M. Leblanc "Triple conjugated carbon dots as a nano-drug delivery model for glioblastoma brain tumors." *Nanoscale* 11, no. 13 (2019): 6192–6205.

Holtzman, David M., John C. Morris, and Alison M. Goate "Alzheimer's disease: The challenge of The second century." *Science Translational Medicine* 3, no. 77 (2011): 77sr1–77sr1.

Hu, Jingyu, Yuanqiang Sun, Aaron Albert Aryee, Lingbo Qu, Ke Zhang, and Zhaohui Li "Mechanisms for carbon dots-based chemosensing, biosensing, and bioimaging: A review." *Analytica Chimica Acta* 1209 (2022): 338885.

Hung, Andrew, Michael DW Griffin, Geoffrey J. Howlett, and Irene Yarovsky "Effects of oxidation, pH and lipids on amyloidogenic peptide structure: Implications for fibril formation?" *European Biophysics Journal* 38, no. 1 (2008): 99–110.

Hwang, Hye Suk, Jae Won Jeong, Yoong Ahm Kim, and Mincheol Chang "Carbon nanomaterials as versatile platforms for biosensing applications." *Micromachines* 11, no. 9 (2020): 814.

Johnson, Keith A., Aaron Schultz, Rebecca A. Betensky, J. Alex Becker, Jorge Sepulcre, Dorene Rentz, and Elizabeth Mormino et al. "Tau positron emission tomographic imaging in aging and early Alzheimer disease." *Annals of Neurology* 79, no. 1 (2016): 110–119.

Jorns, Mychele, and Dimitri Pappas "A review of fluorescent carbon dots, their synthesis, physical and chemical characteristics, and applications." *Nanomaterials* 11, no. 6 (2021): 1448.

Kang, Zhenhui, and Shuit-Tong Lee "Carbon dots: Advances in nanocarbon applications." *Nanoscale* 11, no. 41 (2019): 19214–19224.

Kapoor, Deepak N., and Sandeep Sheth. "Progress in drug delivery and diagnostic applications of carbon." *Nanoscience Editor's Pick* 2024 (2024).

Knox, Emily G., Maria R. Aburto, Gerard Clarke, John F. Cryan, and Caitriona M. O'Driscoll "The blood-brain barrier in aging and neurodegeneration." *Molecular Psychiatry* 27, no. 6 (2022): 2659–2673.

Kour, Ravinder, Sandeep Arya, Sheng-Joue Young, Vinay Gupta, Pankaj Bandhoria, and Ajit Khosla "Recent advances in carbon nanomaterials as electrochemical biosensors." *Journal of The Electrochemical Society* 167, no. 3 (2020): 037555.

Kuang, Ying, Jingwen Zhang, Mogao Xiong, Weijia Zeng, Xiaofeng Lin, Xiaoqing Yi, Yan Luo, Min Yang, Feng Li, and Qitong Huang "A novel nanosystem realizing curcumin delivery based on Fe3O4@ carbon dots nanocomposite for Alzheimer's disease therapy." *Frontiers in Bioengineering and Biotechnology* 8 (2020): 614906.

Kumar, Navneet, Anuj Gahlawat, Rajaram Naresh Kumar, Yash Pal Singh, Gyan Modi, and Prabha Garg "Drug repurposing for Alzheimer's disease: In silico and In vitro Investigation of FDA-approved drugs as acetylcholinesterase Inhibitors." *Journal of Biomolecular Structure and Dynamics* 40, no. 7 (2022): 2878–2892.

Kumar, Neeraj, Reza Salehiyan, Vongani Chauke, Orebotse Joseph Botlhoko, Katlego Setshedi, Manfred Scriba, Mike Masukume, and Suprakas Sinha Ray "Top-down synthesis of graphene: A comprehensive review." *FlatChem* 27 (2021): 100224.

Lin, Hengyu Kengsley, Tian-Hao Yan, Sajid Bashir, and Jingbo Louise Liu. "Synthesis of nanomaterials using bottom-up methods." *Advanced Nanomaterials and Their Applications in Renewable Energy* (2022): 61–110.

Lin, Xiaoding, Xiaoyan Dong, and Yan Sun. "Dual-Carbon dots composite: A multifunctional photo-propelled nanomotor against Alzheimer's β-Amyloid." *Small* (2024): 2407154.

Liu, Jing, Junzhe Lu, Xiang Lin, Yuchao Tang, Yanan Liu, Ting Wang, and Hengjiang Zhu "The electronic properties of chiral carbon nanotubes." *Computational Materials Science* 129 (2017): 290–294.

Liu, Liqin, Haini He, Bin Du, and Yang He "Nanoscale drug formulations for the treatment of Alzheimer's disease progression." *RSC Advances* 15, no. 6 (2025): 4031–4078.

Liu, Yibiao, Li-Ping Xu, Wenhao Dai, Haifeng Dong, Yongqiang Wen, and Xueji Zhang "Graphene quantum dots for the inhibition of β amyloid aggregation." *Nanoscale* 7, no. 45 (2015): 19060–19065.

Liyanage, Piumi Y., Yiqun Zhou, Abdulrahman O. Al-Youbi, Abdulaziz S. Bashammakh, Mohammad S. El-Shahawi, Steven Vanni, Regina M. Graham, and Roger M. Leblanc "Pediatric glioblastoma target-specific efficient delivery of gemcitabine across the blood–brain barrier via carbon nitride dots." *Nanoscale* 12, no. 14 (2020): 7927–7938.

Malik, Shiza, Khalid Muhammad, and Yasir Waheed "Nanotechnology: A revolution in modern industry." *Molecules* 28, no. 2 (2023): 661.

Mansuriya, Bhargav D., and Zeynep Altintas "Carbon dots: Classification, properties, synthesis, characterization, and applications in health care—An updated review (2018–2021)." *Nanomaterials* 11, no. 10 (2021): 2525.

Mintz, Keenan J., Mattia Bartoli, Massimo Rovere, Yiqun Zhou, Sajini D. Hettiarachchi, Suraj Paudyal, and Jiuyan Chen et al. "A deep investigation into the structure of carbon dots." *Carbon* 173 (2021): 433–447.

Mintz, Keenan J., Guillaume Mercado, Yiqun Zhou, Yiwen Ji, Sajini D. Hettiarachchi, Piumi Y. Liyanage, Raja R. Pandey, Charles C. Chusuei, Julia Dallman, and Roger M. Leblanc "Tryptophan carbon dots and their ability to cross the blood-brain barrier." *Colloids and Surfaces B: Biointerfaces* 176 (2019): 488–493.

Modi, Pranjal D., Vaibhavkumar N. Mehta, Vimalkumar S. Prajapati, Swati Patel, and Jigneshkumar V. Rohit. "Bottom-Up approaches for the preparation of carbon dots." In *Carbon Dots in Analytical Chemistry*, pp. 15–29. Elsevier, 2023.

Molazemhosseini, Alireza, Fabrizio Antonio Viola, Felix J. Berger, Nicolas F. Zorn, Jana Zaumseil, and Mario Caironi "A rapidly stabilizing water-gated field-effect transistor based on printed single-walled carbon nanotubes for biosensing applications." *ACS Applied Electronic Materials* 3, no. 7 (2021): 3106–3113.

Nair, Akhila, Jozef T. Haponiuk, Sabu Thomas, and Sreeraj Gopi "Natural carbon-based quantum dots and their applications in drug delivery: A review." *Biomedicine & Pharmacotherapy* 132 (2020): 110834.

Nosrati, Hamed, Mahsa Tarantash, Shayesteh Bochani, Jalil Charmi, Zahra Bagheri, Mohammadjavad Fridoni, Mohammad-Amin Abdollahifar, Soodabeh Davaran, Hossein Danafar, and Hamidreza Kheiri Manjili "Glutathione (GSH) peptide conjugated magnetic nanoparticles as blood–brain barrier shuttle for MRI-monitored brain delivery of paclitaxel." *ACS Biomaterials Science & Engineering* 5, no. 4 (2019): 1677–1685.

Nurrohman, Devi Taufiq, and Nan-Fu Chiu "A review of graphene-based surface plasmon resonance and surface-enhanced Raman scattering biosensors: Current status and future prospects." *Nanomaterials* 11, no. 1 (2021): 216.

Peng, Zhili, Esmail H. Miyanji, Yiqun Zhou, Joel Pardo, Sajini D. Hettiarachchi, Shanghao Li, Patricia L. Blackwelder, Isaac Skromne, and Roger M. Leblanc "Carbon dots: Promising biomaterials for bone-specific imaging and drug delivery." *Nanoscale* 9, no. 44 (2017): 17533–17543.

Pokrajac, Lisa, Ali Abbas, Wojciech Chrzanowski, Goretty M. Dias, Benjamin J. Eggleton, Steven Maguire, and Elicia Maine et al. "Nanotechnology for a sustainable future: Addressing global challenges with the international network4sustainable nanotechnology." (2021): 18608–18623.

Porto, Laís S., Daniela N. Silva, Ana Elisa F. de Oliveira, Arnaldo C. Pereira, and Keyller B. Borges "Carbon nanomaterials: Synthesis and applications to development of electrochemical sensors in determination of drugs and compounds of clinical interest." *Reviews in Analytical Chemistry* 38, no. 3 (2019): 20190017.

Qian, Chengyuan, Chengyi Yuan, Changhong Li, Hao Liu, and Xiaohui Wang "Multifunctional nano-enabled delivery systems in Alzheimer's disease management." *Biomaterials Science* 8, no. 20 (2020): 5538–5554.

Qu, Boyi, Xiaocen Li, Mei Guan, Xun Li, Li Hai, and Yong Wu "Design, synthesis and biological evaluation of multivalent glucosides with high affinity as ligands for brain targeting liposomes." *European Journal of Medicinal Chemistry* 72 (2014): 110–118.

Rana, Dhwani, Sagar Salave, Dignesh Khunt, and Derajram Benival. "Blood brain barrier and its significance in drug delivery to brain in Alzheimer disease." In *Alzheimer's Disease and Advanced Drug Delivery Strategies*, pp. 47–60. Academic Press, 2024.

Rasal, Akash S., Sudesh Yadav, Anchal Yadav, Anil A. Kashale, Subrahmanya Thagare Manjunatha, Ali Altaee, and Jia-Yaw Chang "Carbon quantum dots for energy applications: A review." *ACS Applied Nano Materials* 4, no. 7 (2021): 6515–6541.

Sagbas, Selin, and N. Sahiner. "Carbon dots: Preparation, properties, and application." In *Nanocarbon and Its Composites*, pp. 651–676. Woodhead Publishing, 2019.

Saleem, M., M. Y. Naz, S. Shukrullah, M. A. Shujah, M. Akhtar, Sami Ullah, and S. Ali "One-pot sonochemical preparation of carbon dots, influence of process parameters and potential applications: A review." *Carbon Letters* 32, no. 1 (2022): 39–55.

Salvo-Comino, Coral, Fernando Martin-Pedrosa, Cristina Garcia-Cabezon, and Maria Luz Rodriguez-Mendez "Silver nanowires as electron transfer mediators in electrochemical catechol biosensors." *Sensors* 21, no. 3 (2021): 899.

Seven, Elif S., Yasin B. Seven, Yiqun Zhou, Sijan Poudel-Sharma, Juan J. Diaz-Rucco, Emel Kirbas Cilingir, Gordon S. Mitchell, J. David Van Dyken, and Roger M. Leblanc "Crossing the blood–brain barrier with carbon dots: Uptake mechanism and in vivo cargo delivery." *Nanoscale Advances* 3, no. 13 (2021): 3942–3953.

Shabbir, U., M. Rubab, A. Tyagi, and D. H. Oh "Curcumin and its derivatives as theranostic agents in Alzheimer's disease: The implication of nanotechnology." *International Journal of Molecular Sciences* 22, no. 1 (2020): 196.

Silva, Tiago Almeida, Fernando Cruz Moraes, Bruno Campos Janegitz, and Orlando Fatibello-Filho "Electrochemical biosensors based on nanostructured carbon black: A review." *Journal of Nanomaterials* 2017, no. 1 (2017): 4571614.

Suner, Selin S., Mehtap Sahiner, Ramesh S. Ayyala, Venkat R. Bhethanabotla, and Nurettin Sahiner "Versatile fluorescent carbon dots from citric acid and cysteine with antimicrobial, anti-biofilm, antioxidant, and AChE enzyme inhibition capabilities." *Journal of Fluorescence* 31, no. 6 (2021): 1705–1717.

Tak, Kajal, Rekha Sharma, Vivek Dave, Smita Jain, and Swapnil Sharma "*Clitoria ternatea* mediated synthesis of graphene quantum dots for the treatment of Alzheimer's disease." *ACS Chemical Neuroscience* 11, no. 22 (2020): 3741–3748.

Taranalli, A. D., and T. C. Cheeramkuzhy "Influence of clitoria ternatea extracts on memory and Central cholinergic activity in rats." *Pharmaceutical Biology* 38, no. 1 (2000): 51–56.

Todorova, Nevena, Adam J. Makarucha, Nicholas DM Hine, Arash A. Mostofi, and Irene Yarovsky "Dimensionality of carbon nanomaterials determines the binding and dynamics of amyloidogenic peptides: Multiscale theoretical simulations." *PLoS Computational Biology* 9, no. 12 (2013): e1003360.

Upton, Dannielle H., Caitlin Ung, Sandra M. George, Maria Tsoli, Maria Kavallaris, and David S. Ziegler "Challenges and opportunities to penetrate the blood-brain barrier for brain cancer therapy." *Theranostics* 12, no. 10 (2022): 4734.

Wang, Ming-Wei, Wei Fan, Xiaonan Li, Yujian Liu, Zuoyu Li, Wei Jiang, Jishan Wu, and Zhaohui Wang "Molecular carbons: How far can we go?" *Acs Nano* 17, no. 21 (2023): 20734–20752.

Wareing, Thomas C., Piergiorgio Gentile, and Anh N. Phan "Biomass-based carbon dots: Current development and future perspectives." *ACS Nano* 15, no. 10 (2021): 15471–15501.

Xia, Chunlei, Shoujun Zhu, Tanglue Feng, Mingxi Yang, and Bai Yang "Evolution and synthesis of carbon dots: From carbon dots to carbonized polymer dots." *Advanced Science* 6, no. 23 (2019): 1901316.

Xiao, Songhua, Daoyou Zhou, Ping Luan, Beibei Gu, Longbao Feng, Shengnuo Fan, and Wang Liao et al. "Graphene quantum dots conjugated neuroprotective peptide improve learning and memory capability." *Biomaterials* 106 (2016): 98–110.

Yan, C, C Wang, and X Shao, et al. Multifunctional carbon-dot-photosensitizer nanoassemblies for inhibiting amyloid aggregates, suppressing microbial infection, and overcoming the blood-brain barrier. *ACS Appl Mater Interfaces.* 2022. doi:10.1021/acsami.2c14118

Yang, Feng, Xiao Wang, Daqi Zhang, Juan Yang, Da Luo, Ziwei Xu, and Jiake Wei et al. "Chirality-specific growth of single-walled carbon nanotubes on solid alloy catalysts." *Nature* 510, no. 7506 (2014): 522–524.

Yaqoob, Sundas Bahar, Rohana Adnan, Raja Muhammad Rameez Khan, and Mohammad Rashid "Gold, silver, and palladium nanoparticles: A chemical tool for biomedical applications." *Frontiers in Chemistry* 8 (2020): 376.

Ye, Pengkun, Lei Li, Xiating Qi, Mingyuan Chi, Jichun Liu, and Meng Xie "Macrophage membrane-encapsulated nitrogen-doped carbon quantum dot nanosystem for targeted treatment of Alzheimer's disease: Regulating metal ion homeostasis and photothermal removal of β-amyloid." *Journal of Colloid and Interface Science* 650 (2023): 1749–1761.

Zha, Shuai, Haitao Liu, Hengde Li, Haolan Li, Ka-Leung Wong, and Angelo Homayoun All "Functionalized nanomaterials capable of crossing the blood–brain barrier." *ACS Nano* 18, no. 3 (2024): 1820–1845.

Zhang, Wei, Janna Arteaga, Daniel K. Cashion, Gang Chen, Umesh Gangadharmath, Luis F. Gomez, and Dhanalakshmi Kasi et al. "A highly selective and specific PET tracer for imaging of tau pathologies." *Journal of Alzheimer's Disease* 31, no. 3 (2012): 601–612.

Zhang, Wei, Jiuyan Chen, Jun Gu, Mattia Bartoli, Justin B. Domena, Yiqun Zhou, and Braulio CLB Ferreira et al. "Nano-carrier for gene delivery and bioimaging based on pentaethylenehexamine modified carbon dots." *Journal of Colloid and Interface Science* 639 (2023): 180–192.

Zhang, Wei, Nabin Kandel, Yiqun Zhou, Nathan Smith, Braulio CLB Ferreira, Miranda Perez, Matteo L. Claure, Keenan J. Mintz, Chunyu Wang, and Roger M. Leblanc "Drug delivery of memantine with carbon dots for Alzheimer's disease: blood–brain barrier penetration and inhibition of tau aggregation." *Journal of Colloid and Interface Science* 617 (2022): 20–31.

Zhang, Wei, Ganesh Sigdel, Keenan J. Mintz, Elif S. Seven, Yiqun Zhou, Chunyu Wang, and Roger M. Leblanc. "Carbon dots: A future Blood–Brain barrier penetrating nanomedicine and drug nanocarrier." *International Journal of Nanomedicine* (2021): 5003–5016.

Zhang, Wei, Nathan Smith, Yiqun Zhou, Caitlin M. McGee, Mattia Bartoli, Shiwei Fu, and Jiuyan Chen et al. "Carbon dots as dual inhibitors of tau and amyloid-beta aggregation for the treatment of Alzheimer's disease." *Acta Biomaterialia* (2024).

Zhao, Changhong, Xuebin Song, Ya Liu, Yifeng Fu, Lilei Ye, Nan Wang, and Fan Wang et al. "Synthesis of graphene quantum dots and their applications in drug delivery." *Journal of Nanobiotechnology* 18, no. 1 (2020): 32.

Zheng, Kunmu, Xiaoman Dai, Nai'an Xiao, Xilin Wu, Zhen Wei, Wenting Fang, Yuangui Zhu, Jing Zhang, and Xiaochun Chen "Curcumin ameliorates memory decline via inhibiting BACE1 expression and β-amyloid pathology in 5× FAD transgenic mice." *Molecular Neurobiology* 54 (2017): 1967–1977.

Zhou, Yiqun, Nabin Kandel, Mattia Bartoli, Leonardo F. Serafim, Ahmed E. ElMetwally, Sophia M. Falkenberg, and Xavier E. Paredes et al. "Structure-activity relationship of carbon nitride dots in inhibiting tau aggregation." *Carbon* 193 (2022): 1–16.

Zhou, Yiqun, Piumi Y. Liyanage, Dinesh Devadoss, Linda Rebeca Rios Guevara, Ling Cheng, Regina M. Graham, and Hitendra S. Chand et al. "Nontoxic amphiphilic carbon dots as promising drug nanocarriers across the blood–brain barrier and inhibitors of β-amyloid." *Nanoscale* 11, no. 46 (2019): 22387–22397.

11 Nanoparticles-Based Immunotherapeutic Strategies for the Treatment of Alzheimer's Disease

Suruchi Chaudhary, Ekansh Agrawal, Niharika Singh, Vikas Shrivastava, Manish Shrivastava, and Rajesh Singh Tomar

11.1 INTRODUCTION

Alzheimer's disease (AD) is the leading cause of dementia among the elderly, and its prevalence is projected to increase significantly in the coming decades [1]. Despite extensive research efforts, the development of effective treatments has been challenging, as the disease involves a complex interplay of multiple pathogenic processes, including the retention of misfolded proteins, synaptic dysfunction, and neuroinflammation [2]. Emerging evidence suggests that neuroinflammation plays a key factor in the pathophysiology of AD, with persistent inflammatory responses contributing to the progression of the disease [3]. Microglia, the resident immune cells of the brain, and astrocytes, play vital roles in mediating the inflammatory procedures that eventually result in cognitive deterioration and neural malfunction.

The formation and progression of AD have also been linked to systemic inflammation, underscoring the need of comprehending whether the central and peripheral immune systems interact with one another in the setting of the disorder. The study of nanomedicine has become a viable strategy in recent years to tackle the intricate problems related to AD.

11.2 PATHOGENESIS AND PROGRESSION OF DISEASE

Extracellular amyloid-beta (Aβ) plaques and intracellular neurofibrillary tangles made of hyperphosphorylated tau protein are hallmarks of AD [16]. The cognitive deficits seen in AD patients are believed to be caused by these pathological hallmarks, which interfere with synaptic function and ultimately result in neuronal death.

 DOI: 10.1201/9781003543381-11

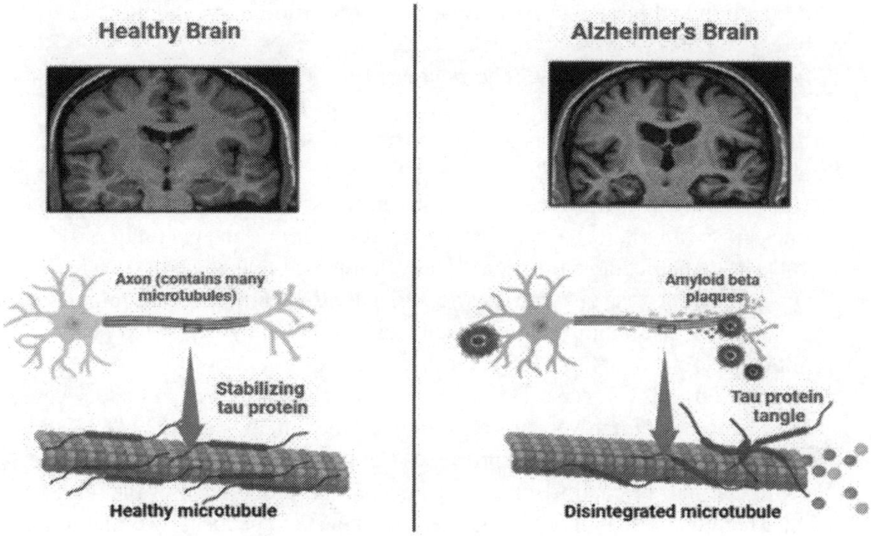

FIGURE 11.1 Comparison of healthy and Alzheimer's affected brain and part of axons.

Neuroinflammation plays a crucial role in the development and progression of AD. Aβ and other pathogenic triggers activate microglia, the resident immune cells of the brain, which results in the release of pro-inflammatory cytokines, chemokines, and reactive oxygen species. Such chronic inflammatory response can aggravate neuronal injury and contribute to the ongoing degeneration observed in AD [4,5].

Astrocytes, another type of glial cell, also play an important role in the neuroinflammatory process. Activated astrocytes contribute to the production of inflammatory mediators, ultimately disrupting synaptic function and leading to neuronal death [6–8] (Figure 11.1).

AD is primarily caused by the collaboration of microglia, astrocytes, and neurones; the disease progresses as a result of these dysregulated interactions.

The primary pathological features of Alzheimer's Disease. It breaks down the complex interplay of factors contributing to AD, including:

11.2.1 Cholinergic Dysfunction

Cholinergic dysfunction is a key aspect of AD pathology, characterized by a significant decline in the activity of cholinergic neurons, particularly in the basal forebrain [9]. These neurons are crucial for producing and releasing acetylcholine, a neurotransmitter which is essential for human functions [10]. In AD, the damage to these neurons and the resulting decrease in ACh contribute significantly to the cognitive decline observed [11]. The key aspects of cholinergic dysfunction in AD:

1. **Basal Forebrain Degeneration**: The basal forebrain, the key source of cholinergic innervation to the cortex and hippocampus, undergoes significant degeneration in AD. This degeneration leads to a decrease in the

production and release of ACh as well as a reduction in the number of cholinergic neurones [12].
2. **Acetylcholine Deficiency**: The decrease in ACh levels affects different cognitive processes, including memory formation, attention, and executive function. This deficiency is a major contributor to the cognitive symptoms observed in AD.
3. **Cholinesterase Inhibitors**: Current treatments for AD often include cholinesterase inhibitors, such as donepezil, rivastigmine, and galantamine [13, 14]. These medications function by preventing the breakdown of ACh in the synaptic cleft by the enzyme acetylcholinesterase. Cholinesterase inhibitors enhance the availability of ACh by blocking this enzyme, which helps to alleviate some symptoms [15].
4. **Limitations of Current Therapies**: While cholinesterase inhibitors can offer temporary improvements in cognitive function, they do not address the underlying neurodegenerative processes driving AD. They do not prevent the continued loss of cholinergic neurons or halt the progression of the disease [9]. Therefore, research continues to explore new therapeutic targets and strategies to address the root causes of AD and provide more effective treatments.

11.2.2 Amyloid Hypothesis

According to the amyloid hypothesis, AD is primarily caused by the buildup of Aβ plaques in the brain. In 2019, [16–19] This is a more thorough explanation:

1. **Amyloid Precursor Protein Processing**: APP is a transmembrane protein with a physiological role that isn't fully understood. In AD, APP is abnormally processed by two enzymes, β-secretase and γ-secretase [14]. This abnormal cleavage produces Aβ peptides, primarily Aβ40 and Aβ42.
2. **Aβ Aggregation**: Aβ peptides, particularly Aβ42, are "sticky" and prone to aggregation. They clump together, forming oligomers, protofibrils, and eventually, insoluble plaques that deposit outside neurons. While initially, Aβ plaques were considered the main toxic species, increasing evidence suggests that soluble Aβ oligomers are the most neurotoxic forms [18].
3. **Disruption of Neuronal Signalling**: Aβ plaques and oligomers disrupt synaptic function, impairing communication between neurons. This disruption affects various cognitive processes, including learning and memory.
4. **Neuroinflammation**: Aβ plaques trigger an inflammatory response in the brain, activating microglia and astrocytes [14]. While this response initially aims to clear Aβ, chronic inflammation can damage surrounding neurons and contribute to neurodegeneration [20].
5. **Neuronal Damage and Death**: The combined effects of disrupted neuronal signalling, neuroinflammation, and oxidative stress induced by Aβ lead to neuronal damage and ultimately, cell death. This widespread neuronal loss underlies the cognitive decline observed in AD.
6. **Therapeutic Implications**: Many medication development initiatives have focused on the amyloid hypothesis by targeting different stages of Aβ production and aggregation. However, despite promising preclinical results,

many clinical trials targeting Aβ have failed to demonstrate significant cognitive benefits, leading to some debate about the central role of Aβ in AD pathogenesis [20]. Nonetheless, research continues to explore the complex role of Aβ and its contribution to AD.

11.2.3 Tau Hypothesis

The tau hypothesis proposes that the abnormal hyperphosphorylation and aggregation of tau protein is central to the development of AD. Here's a more detailed explanation:

1. **Tau's Normal Function**: Tau is a microtubule-associated protein that stabilizes microtubules, which are essential for axonal transport and neuronal function. In healthy neurons, tau is phosphorylated at specific sites, regulating its interaction with microtubules.
2. **Hyperphosphorylation**: In AD, tau becomes hyperphosphorylated due to imbalances in kinase and phosphatase activity [14]. This excessive phosphorylation reduces tau's affinity for microtubules, causing them to become unstable and disassemble.
3. **Neurofibrillary Tangle Formation**: The hyperphosphorylated tau detaches from microtubules and aggregates into paired helical filaments, which further assemble into neurofibrillary tangles inside neurons [14]. These NFTs disrupt axonal transport, impairing the delivery of essential nutrients and organelles to synapses and the removal of waste products.
4. **Neuronal Dysfunction and Death**: The disruption of axonal transport, combined with other cellular stresses, leads to neuronal dysfunction and ultimately, cell death. The accumulation of NFTs correlates strongly with cognitive decline in AD.
5. **Aβ-Tau Interplay**: While the amyloid and tau hypotheses were initially considered separate, growing evidence suggests a complex interplay between Aβ and tau pathology. Aβ can trigger and exacerbate tau hyperphosphorylation, while tau pathology can, in turn, enhance Aβ toxicity, creating a vicious cycle that drives neurodegeneration.
6. **Therapeutic Implications**: Targeting tau pathology is a potentially effective treatment approach for AD. Several approaches are under investigation, including inhibiting tau kinases, promoting tau clearance, and stabilizing microtubules. These strategies aim to prevent or reverse the formation of NFTs and slow or halt the progression of AD.

11.2.4 Oxidative Stress

Oxidative stress is a significant contributor to the neuronal damage observed in AD [21–25]. It results from an imbalance between the body's capacity to detoxify reactive oxygen species and their synthesis. This is a more thorough explanation:

1. **ROS Production**: ROS are highly reactive molecules containing nascent oxygen, such as superoxide radicals, hydrogen peroxide, and hydroxyl radicals. They are normal byproducts of cellular metabolism, particularly

mitochondrial respiration, the process by which cells generate energy. The brain, with its high metabolic rate and oxygen consumption, is particularly vulnerable to ROS production.

2. **Oxidative Damage**: ROS can harm lipids, proteins, and DNA, among other biological components, when their quantities beyond the antioxidant defence systems' capabilities. Cell death may result from this oxidative damage, which also impairs cellular function.
3. **Aβ and Oxidative Stress**: In AD, the presence of Aβ plaques further exacerbates oxidative stress. Aβ can directly generate ROS, and it can also impair mitochondrial function, leading to increased ROS production. This creates a vicious cycle of oxidative damage and neuronal dysfunction.
4. **Antioxidant Defences**: The body has natural antioxidant defence mechanisms, including enzymes like superoxide dismutase and catalase, as well as non-enzymatic antioxidants like glutathione and vitamin E. These defences help neutralize ROS and protect cells from oxidative damage. However, in AD, these defences may be overwhelmed by the increased ROS production.
5. **Therapeutic Implications**: Targeting oxidative stress is a potential therapeutic strategy for AD. Antioxidant therapies aim to boost the body's natural defences against ROS or scavenge ROS directly. However, clinical trials with antioxidant supplements have yielded mixed results, and further research is needed to identify effective strategies to combat oxidative stress in AD.

11.2.5 Cellular and Vascular Dysfunction

Age-related vascular changes and reduced blood flow to the brain contribute to neuronal degeneration and cognitive decline in AD. Cerebral hypoperfusion can lead to capillary degeneration and further exacerbate the disease process involves the following:

1. **Reduced Blood Flow**: Age-related vascular changes and other factors can decrease blood flow to the brain (cerebral hypoperfusion). This reduced perfusion deprives neurons of essential oxygen and nutrients, making them vulnerable to damage and dysfunction. The brain's high metabolic demand makes it particularly sensitive to even subtle reductions in blood flow.
2. **Impaired Microvascular Integrity**: The intricate network of small blood vessels in the brain, the microvasculature, plays a crucial role in delivering oxygen and nutrients to neurons and removing waste products. In AD, the integrity of these vessels can be compromised, leading to leakage, reduced perfusion, and impaired clearance of toxic substances, including Aβ.
3. **Capillary Degeneration**: Chronic hypoperfusion can lead to the degeneration of capillaries, the smallest blood vessels. This degeneration further restricts blood flow and impairs the exchange of essential substances between blood and brain tissue, exacerbating neuronal damage and cognitive decline.
4. **Endothelial Dysfunction**: The endothelium, the inner lining of blood vessels, plays a critical role in regulating vascular tone and blood flow. In AD,

endothelial dysfunction can occur, impairing the ability of blood vessels to respond appropriately to changes in neuronal activity and metabolic demand. This dysfunction can further contribute to reduced blood flow and neuronal damage.

5. **Blood-Brain Barrier (BBB) Breakdown**: It is a protective barrier that regulates the passage of substances between the bloodstream and the brain. In AD, the BBB can become compromised, allowing potentially harmful substances from the blood to enter the brain, further contributing to neuroinflammation and neuronal damage. This breakdown can also impair the clearance of Aβ and other toxic molecules from the brain. [26,27].

These vascular changes and impairments in blood flow contribute significantly to the neuronal degeneration and cognitive decline observed in AD, highlighting the importance of vascular health in maintaining brain function [28–30].

11.2.6 Cholesterol

Cholesterol plays a role in the creation and removal of Aβ. Variations in the apolipoprotein E gene, which is involved in cholesterol metabolism, are a significant genetic risk factor for AD.

Potential Risks:

1. **Aβ Production and Accumulation**: Studies suggest that high cholesterol levels, particularly in midlife, may increase the production and accumulation of Aβ plaques in the brain [31,32]. This is thought to occur through several mechanisms, including altered cholesterol metabolism within neurons and increased activity of enzymes involved in Aβ production.
2. **BBB Integrity**: High cholesterol can disrupt the integrity of the BBB, potentially increasing Aβ transport into the brain and hindering its clearance [32].
3. **Inflammation and Oxidative Stress**: Elevated cholesterol can contribute to inflammation and oxidative stress in the brain, both of which are implicated in AD pathogenesis [21].

Potential Protective Effects:

1. **Membrane Fluidity and Synaptic Function**: Cholesterol is a crucial component of cell membranes, influencing their fluidity and function. Optimal cholesterol levels are essential for proper synaptic transmission, which is vital for cognitive function. Very low cholesterol levels could negatively impact synaptic plasticity and neuronal health. [33,34].
2. **Nutritional Status**: Low cholesterol in late life might be a marker of poor overall health and nutritional status, which can indirectly increase the risk of cognitive decline and dementia [35].
3. **Apolipoprotein E Connection**: ApoE plays a critical role in cholesterol transport in the brain. The ApoE4 allele is the strongest genetic risk factor for late-onset AD. It's thought that ApoE4 may contribute to AD by impairing cholesterol clearance and increasing Aβ accumulation [36]

Statins, cholesterol-lowering drugs, have been investigated for their potential to prevent or treat AD. However, clinical trials have yielded mixed results, and the role of statins in AD remains unclear.

While high cholesterol in midlife may increase AD risk, the relationship in late life is less clear. Maintaining healthy cholesterol levels throughout life, along with a balanced diet and healthy lifestyle, is generally recommended for overall brain health.

11.2.7 Neuroinflammation

Neuroinflammation is a significant component of AD pathology. It's a complex process involving various immune cells within the brain, primarily microglia and astrocytes, and the release of inflammatory molecules. Here's a breakdown of its role in AD:

1. **Microglia and Astrocytes**
   - **Microglia**: These are the resident immune cells of the brain, acting as its first line of defence. In the early stages of AD, microglia are activated by Aβ plaques and attempt to clear them through phagocytosis. This initially beneficial response can become chronic and damaging over time.
   - **Astrocytes**: These star-shaped glial cells support neuronal function and maintain brain homeostasis. In AD, they become reactive astrocytes, contributing to neuroinflammation by releasing pro-inflammatory cytokines and chemokines.
2. **Inflammatory Molecules**
   - **Cytokines**: Pro-inflammatory cytokines, such as TNF-α, IL-1β, and IL-6, are elevated in AD brains. These molecules contribute to neuronal damage and dysfunction.
   - **Chemokines**: These signalling proteins attract immune cells to the site of inflammation, further amplifying the neuroinflammatory response.
   - **Reactive Oxygen Species**: Activated microglia and astrocytes produce ROS, which causes oxidative stress and damages neurons.
3. **The Role of Neuroinflammation in AD Progression**
   - **Aβ Plaque Formation and Spread**: Chronic neuroinflammation can exacerbate Aβ plaque formation and promote its spread throughout the brain.
   - **Tau Pathology**: Neuroinflammation can potentially contribute to the production of neurofibrillary tangles made up of tau protein, another hallmark of AD.
   - **Synaptic Dysfunction and Neuronal Loss**: Pro-inflammatory molecules and cognitive decline results from ROS's disruption of synaptic transmission and role in neuronal death.
   - **BBB Disruption**: Neuroinflammation can weaken the BBB, peripheral immune cells can infiltrate the brain and intensify inflammation.

4. **Therapeutic Implications**: Targeting neuroinflammation is a promising therapeutic strategy for AD. Several approaches are being investigated, including:
5. **Anti-inflammatory drugs**: These drugs aim to reduce the production of pro-inflammatory molecules.
6. **Immunomodulatory therapies**: These therapies aim to restore the balance of the immune response, promoting the beneficial functions of microglia while suppressing their damaging effects [37].

11.2.8 Metal Ion Imbalance

Disruptions in the balance of metal ions, specifically copper, iron, and zinc, contribute significantly to the growth and advancement of Alzheimer's Disease. These imbalances affect key processes involved in Aβ and tau pathology. Specifically, metal imbalances can [38]:

1. **Promote Aβ overproduction**: They influence the activity of enzymes involved in Aβ processing, leading to increased production and accumulation of Aβ plaques.
2. **Cause tau hyperphosphorylation**: Metal imbalances affect the activity of protein kinases and phosphatases, which results in the excessive phosphorylation of tau protein and the origination of neurofibrillary tangles.
3. **Induce oxidative stress**: Metals like copper and iron, when dysregulated, can contribute to oxidative stress, further damaging neurons and exacerbating the disease process.

The presence of elevated metal levels within amyloid plaques themselves suggests a complex interplay between metal dyshomeostasis and AD pathology [39].

Several drugs are currently approved and available for managing AD symptoms. These medications primarily target two pathways involved in cognitive function:

a. **Cholinesterase Inhibitors**: Acetylcholine is a neurotransmitter that is necessary for memory and learning, and these medications function by stopping its breakdown. For certain people, elevated acetylcholine levels can momentarily enhance cognitive function. Cholinesterase inhibitors that are available include:

- **Donepezil**: Approved for all stages of AD.
- **Rivastigmine**: Approved for mild to moderate Alzheimer's and Parkinson's disease dementia.
- **Galantamine**: Approved for mild to moderate Alzheimer's.

  Common side effects include nausea, vomiting, diarrhoea, loss of appetite, and sleep disturbances. Tacrine, in particular, carries a risk of liver damage and is rarely used.

b. **NMDA Receptor Antagonist**: This class of medication regulates the activity of glutamate, another neurotransmitter involved in learning and memory. By blocking excessive glutamate activity, these drugs may help protect neurons from damage.
   - **Memantine**: For mild to severe Alzheimer's, it is approved. This medication may reduce the deterioration of cognitive function in moderate-to-severe AD by regulating glutamate activity. Cholinesterase inhibitors are frequently used in conjunction with it. Headache, lightheadedness, constipation, and disorientation are possible side effects.
   - **Memantine Extended Release**: A once-daily formulation of memantine.
   - **Donepezil/Memantine Combination**: A combination of donepezil and memantine in a single capsule.

c. **Aβ Targeting Therapy**:
   - **Aducanumab**: This monoclonal antibody targets Aβ plaques, a hallmark of AD. It has received accelerated approval from the FDA, but its clinical benefit remains under scrutiny, and its use is controversial. Potential side effects include brain swelling and bleeding. It's also a very expensive treatment.

Important Considerations

- **Symptomatic Treatment**: Currently available drugs primarily address symptoms and do not cure or stop the progression of AD.
- **Individual Response**: The effectiveness of these medications varies among individuals, and some people may experience more significant benefits than others.
- **Side Effects**: These medications can have side effects, such as nausea, vomiting, diarrhoea, and sleep disturbances. It's essential to discuss potential side effects with a healthcare professional.

Sr. No.	Drug	Company Name	Dosage	Mechanism of action
1.	Tacrine	Sciele	*Initial*: 10 mg taken orally every 6 weeks, q.i.d. (in between meals) *Maintenance*: 20 mg q.i.d. may be added. At 6-week intervals, additional increments to 120 mg and 160 mg per day are possible	Reversible inhibition of acetylcholinesterase
2.	Donepezil	Pfizer	5 mg every 2 days After 4 to 6 weeks, this may be increased to 10 mg daily After at least 3 months, it may reach 23 mg daily	Reversible inhibitor of AChE, preventing acetylcholine hydrolysis
3.	Rivastigmine	Novartis	6–12 mg per day, administered b.i.d. (3 mg to 6 mg b.i.d.)	Inhibits AChE and BChE, binding to catalytic sites

(Continued)

Sr. No.	Drug	Company Name	Dosage	Mechanism of action
4.	Galantamine	Janssen	*Tablets*: 4, 8, 12 mg. *Capsules*: 8, 16, 24 mg. Oral solution: 4 mg/mL	Binds reversibly to AChE and enhances acetylcholine action on nicotinic receptors
5.	Memantine	Allergan	*Tablets/Oral solution*: 5 mg q.d., may increase to 10, 15, and 20 mg/day at 1-week intervals	NMDA receptor antagonist
6.	Memantine and Donepezil	Actavis	7 mg memantine/10 mg donepezil q.d., with weekly increases of 7 mg to 28 mg memantine/10 mg donepezil	NMDA receptor antagonist + cholinesterase inhibitor
7.	Aducanumab	Biogen	10 mg/kg IV infusion every 4 weeks	Antibody targeting Aβ plaques

11.3 NANOPARTICLES USED IN THE MANAGEMENT OF NEURODEGENERATIVE DISORDERS

The complicated issues surrounding AD may be addressed with the aid of nanotechnology, an exciting field. Nanoparticles are especially well-suited for the targeted delivery of therapeutic drugs to the central nervous system because of their special qualities, which include their small size, high surface area-to-volume ratio, and capacity to pass the BBB [39].

Numerous kinds of nanoparticles have been investigated for the treatment of AD and other neurodegenerative diseases.

Gold and silver are two examples of metal-based nanoparticles that have demonstrated promise in imaging, medication delivery, and neuroinflammatory process control. While lipid-based nanoparticles, such as liposomes and micelles, have shown promise in delivering medications to the brain by overcoming the BBB, silica nanoparticles have been studied for their capacity to encapsulate and distribute therapeutic compounds. The potential of polymeric nanoparticles, such as those derived from chitosan and poly(lactic-co-glycolic acid), in targeted drug delivery and immune response modification has also been investigated.

The potential of hydrogel nanoparticles to offer a protective environment for cell-based treatments, such as stem cell transplantation, which has potential for the treatment of neurodegenerative diseases, has been studied [40].

11.4 NANOTHERAPEUTICS: A TARGETED APPROACH FOR NEUROLOGICAL DISORDERS

Neurological disorders present a significant medical challenge due to their complex nature and limited treatment options. Nanotherapeutics offer a promising new approach by allowing for the central nervous system to receive tailored drug delivery, overcoming biological barriers, and providing sustained release of therapeutic agents [41]. Drugs, genes, or other therapeutic compounds can be functionalized into a variety of nanocarriers, including liposomes, dendrimers, and polymeric nanoparticles, to improve delivery to targeted brain regions while reducing systemic side effects. For a variety of neurological disorders, this focused strategy has enormous promise for enhancing patient outcomes and treatment effectiveness.

11.5 OVERCOMING THE BBB WITH NANOMATERIALS

The brain and extracellular fluid in the central nervous system are separated from the circulating blood by the BBB, a highly selective semipermeable barrier. It is made up of endothelial cells that line the capillaries in the brain and are held up by pericytes and astrocytes. The BBB is essential for preserving brain homeostasis because:

- **Regulating the transport of molecules**: It allows essential nutrients and molecules to access the brain while preventing the passage of chemicals that could be detrimental, such as many medications, poisons, and infections.
- **Protecting the brain from fluctuations in blood composition**: The BBB helps maintain a stable environment within the brain, shielding it from variations in blood chemistry and hormone levels.
- **Protecting the brain from immune system components**: While crucial for defense, certain components of the immune system can cause inflammation and damage in the brain. The BBB restricts their entry, providing immune privilege to the CNS.

11.5.1 BBB's Role in Neurodegenerative Disorders

In neurodegenerative disorders, the BBB can become dysfunctional, contributing to disease progression. This dysfunction can manifest in several ways:

- **Increased permeability**: The BBB can become "leaky," allowing harmful substances to enter the brain, exacerbating inflammation and neuronal damage.
- **Reduced transport of essential nutrients**: Dysfunction can impair the transport of essential nutrients and molecules required for neuronal health, further contributing to neuronal dysfunction.
- **Impaired clearance of waste products**: The BBB plays a role in clearing waste products from the brain. Dysfunction can hinder this process, leading to the accumulation of toxic substances.

11.6 HOW NANOTECHNOLOGY CAN HELP OVERCOME BBB CHALLENGES

The BBB's restrictive nature poses a significant challenge in the treatment of neurodegenerative disorders, as it prevents many therapeutic drugs from reaching the brain. Nanotechnology offers several strategies to overcome this obstacle.

11.6.1 Improved Drug Delivery through the BBB

The BBB is a major obstacle in the treatment of brain diseases. Nanoparticles can be engineered to pass the BBB more effectively and efficiently, delivering drugs directly to the brain and increasing their concentration at the target site. This can improve the effectiveness of drugs like donepezil, rivastigmine, galantamine, and memantine, which currently have limited brain penetration. It mentions the use of nanocarriers like liposomes and dendrimers for enhanced drug delivery and discusses nanoparticle-mediated approaches for drug delivery in Alzheimer's.

11.6.2 Targeted Drug Delivery

Nanoparticles can be functionalized with ligands that target specific cells or receptors in the brain, such as those involved in amyloid plaque formation or neuroinflammation. This targeted approach can enhance drug delivery to the affected areas while minimizing off-target effects and reducing systemic toxicity and provides a good overview of targeted drug delivery using nanomaterials [42].

11.6.3 Controlled and Sustained Drug Release

Nanoparticles can be designed to release drugs in a controlled and sustained manner, reducing the frequency of administration and maintaining therapeutic drug levels for extended periods. This is particularly beneficial for Alzheimer's patients who may have difficulty adhering to complex medication schedules discusses polymeric nanoparticles for drug delivery and controlled release.

11.6.4 Combination Therapy and Multifunctional Nanoparticles

Nanoparticles can be loaded with multiple drugs, allowing for combination therapy in a single delivery system. For example, a nanoparticle could carry both a cholinesterase inhibitor and memantine, potentially enhancing their synergistic effects. Furthermore, multifunctional nanoparticles can be designed to combine therapeutic agents with diagnostic tools, enabling simultaneous drug delivery and disease monitoring.

11.6.5 Neuroprotective Effects

Some nanomaterials, such as those with antioxidant or anti-inflammatory properties, may offer neuroprotective effects, potentially slowing the progression of AD discusses the antioxidant and antiapoptotic effects of scutellarin, which could potentially be delivered using nanoparticles to explore the role of oxidative stress in Alzheimer's, suggesting that antioxidant nanoparticles could be beneficial.

11.6.6 Enhanced Drug Solubility and Stability

Drugs that are poorly soluble can become more stable and soluble thanks to nanoparticles, which increases their bioavailability and therapeutic effectiveness.

11.6.7 Reduced Drug Toxicity

By targeting the delivery of drugs to specific brain parts, nanoparticles can minimize off-target consequences and reduce the systemic side effects of drugs, improving their safety profile.

For example,

- **Nanocarriers for drug delivery**: Drugs can be delivered straight to the brain by engineering nanoparticles to more effectively pass the BBB. For improved medication delivery across the BBB, addresses a variety of nanoparticle forms, including as liposomes, solid lipid nanoparticles, and polymeric nanoparticles. The surface functionalization of PLGA nanoparticles to improve transport across the BBB for AD is the special focus.
- **Receptor-mediated transcytosis**: Nanoparticles can be functionalized with ligands that bind to specific receptors on the BBB, triggering receptor-mediated transcytosis, a process that transports molecules across the BBB.
- **Focused ultrasound**: Focused ultrasound can temporarily disrupt the BBB, increasing its permeability and allowing drugs to enter the brain. Nano neuroscience (2024) mentions this approach, although it also highlights the invasive nature of direct brain injections.
- **Intranasal delivery**: This route bypasses the BBB, delivering drugs directly to the brain via the olfactory bulb. It mentions alternative routes like intranasal delivery as a way to bypass the BBB.
- **Quantum dots**: The use of quantum dots for inhibiting acetylcholinesterase and reducing AD-like symptoms in rodents.

While nanotechnology offers great potential, it's important to note that research is ongoing, and many of these applications are still in preclinical or early clinical stages. Further research is needed to fully evaluate the safety and efficacy of nanoparticle-based drug delivery systems for AD.

Nanoparticles offer several advantages for overcoming BBB and enhancing drug delivery to the brain, as discussed in other sources. Here's a summary of key points:

1. **Enhanced Permeability and Retention Effect**: Some tumours and areas of inflammation exhibit increased vascular permeability, allowing nanoparticles to accumulate in these regions. While not directly applicable to a healthy BBB, this effect can be exploited in certain disease conditions.
2. **Surface Modifications**: Modifying the surface of nanoparticles with specific coatings, such as polyethylene glycol, can improve their circulation time and reduce clearance by the immune system, increasing their chances of reaching the brain. The importance of surface modifications for optimal drug delivery [44].
3. **Receptor-Mediated Transcytosis**: Functionalizing nanoparticles with ligands that bind to specific receptors on brain endothelial cells can trigger receptor-mediated transcytosis, a process that transports molecules across

the BBB. Targeting ApoE and other receptors for enhanced drug delivery. Adsorptive transcytosis, where nanoparticle surface properties facilitate binding to endothelial cells.

4. **Carrier-Mediated Transport**: Nanoparticles can be designed to utilize existing carrier-mediated transport systems in the BBB, such as those for glucose or amino acids, to facilitate drug entry into the brain.
5. **Physical Methods for BBB Disruption**: Techniques like focused ultrasound can temporarily disrupt the BBB, increasing its permeability and allowing nanoparticles to pass through. Ultrasound is a non-invasive method for BBB disruption.
6. **Trojan Horse Approach**: Nanoparticles can be designed to mimic endogenous molecules that readily cross the BBB, acting as "Trojan horses" to carry drugs into the brain.
7. **Intranasal Delivery**: This route bypasses the BBB, delivering nanoparticles directly to the brain via the olfactory bulb. Intranasal delivery as an alternative route for brain drug delivery.

11.7 NP-Based DELIVERY SYSTEM FOR THE TREATMENT OF AD

This section offers a summary of various nanoparticle types used for AD therapeutics, including liposomes, solid lipid nanoparticles, polymeric NPs, inorganic NPs, and stimuli-responsive NPs (Figure 11.2). It emphasizes the importance of particle size, zeta potential, stability, BBB adsorption, and endocytotic uptake for effective drug delivery. Some examples of the nanoparticles commonly used for the neurodegenerative disorders management are:

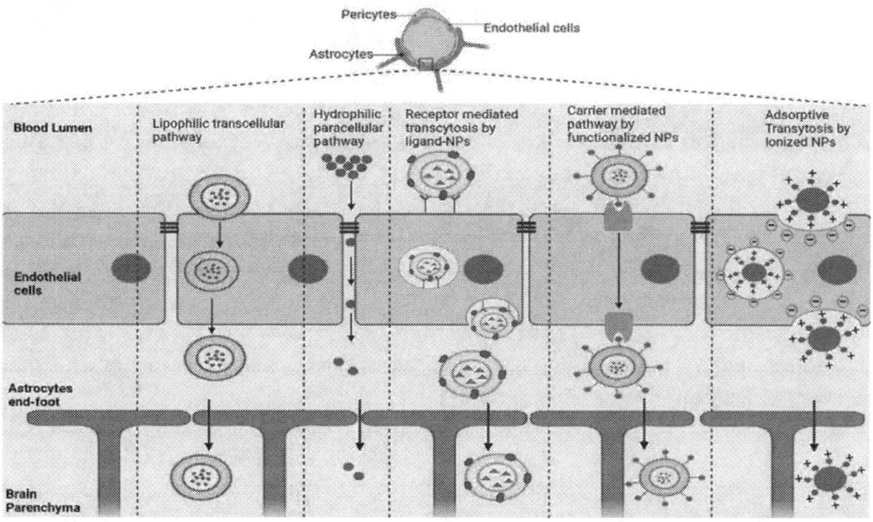

FIGURE 11.2 The diagrammatic representation of possible NP-based delivery system pathways for medications that cross the BBB to treat AD.

11.7.1 Gold Nanoparticles

Neurodegenerative diseases pose a formidable challenge due to their intricate pathophysiology and the limitations of current treatments. Gold nanoparticles have surfaced as an encouraging therapeutic approach, offering unique advantages for targeting and treating these conditions [43]. Their biocompatibility, tuneable size and shape, and ability to cross the BBB make them ideal candidates for delivering drugs to the central nervous system. AuNPs can be customized with various therapeutic molecules, enabling targeted delivery to affected brain regions while minimizing side effects. Moreover, their optical properties hold the potential for enhanced diagnostic imaging, facilitating early disease detection and monitoring. While further research is needed to translate these findings into clinical practice, AuNPs represent a notable development in the pursuit of effective therapies for neurodegenerative diseases.

11.7.1.1 Diagnostic and Imaging Applications of AuNPs

Beyond their therapeutic potential, AuNPs offer exciting possibilities for improving the diagnosis and imaging of neurodegenerative diseases. Their unique optical properties make them suitable as contrast agents in various imaging modalities, enabling more precise visualization of affected brain regions. This enhanced imaging capability can aid in early disease detection, accurate monitoring of disease progression, and assessment of treatment efficacy. The development of AuNP-based imaging techniques could revolutionize the diagnosis and management of neurodegenerative diseases, leading to earlier interventions and improved patient outcomes.

11.7.2 Silver Nanoparticles

Silver nanoparticles are being explored as a potential therapeutic tool in the fight against neurodegenerative diseases due to their unique properties. While their antimicrobial effects are well-established, research suggests they may also offer anti-inflammatory and neuroprotective benefits in the context of neurodegeneration [44]. AgNPs have demonstrated the ability to modulate immune responses, potentially mitigating neuroinflammation, a key driver in many neurodegenerative conditions. Furthermore, some studies suggest that AgNPs can protect neurons from oxidative stress and other damaging factors. However, it's crucial to acknowledge ongoing research into the potential neurotoxicity of AgNPs [45], highlighting the importance of careful characterization and controlled dosages. The ability of AgNPs to cross the BBB also makes them attractive for targeted drug delivery to the central nervous system. While further research is needed to fully elucidate their therapeutic potential and address safety concerns, AgNPs hold promise for innovative treatment strategies in neurodegenerative diseases [46].

11.7.3 Silica Based Nanoparticles

Silica nanoparticles offer a versatile platform for drug delivery and other therapeutic applications in neurodegenerative diseases. They are appealing for encapsulating and delivering medications, genes, and other therapeutic compounds to the central nervous system because of their biocompatibility, porosity structure, and simplicity of surface modification [60]. By reducing off-target exposure, this focused administration can increase therapeutic efficacy and decrease negative effects. SiNPs can be engineered to release their payload in a regulated and sustained manner while overcoming the BBB, which is a significant treatment challenge for neurological illnesses. To further improve treatment precision, SiNPs can be functionalized with targeting ligands to improve their transport to particular brain cell types. SiNPs have great potential to enhance treatment outcomes, but further study is needed to completely comprehend their long-term effects and optimize their design for particular neurodegenerative diseases.

11.7.4 Lipid-Based Nanoparticles

The potential of lipid-based nanoparticles, such as liposomes and micelles, to treat neurodegenerative illnesses is drawing more and more attention [47,48]. They are appealing drug delivery vehicles for the central nervous system because of their biocompatibility, potential to traverse the BBB, and ability to encapsulate both hydrophilic and hydrophobic pharmaceuticals [49–51]. Particularly, liposomes have demonstrated promise in transporting therapeutic molecules to the brain, enhancing the effectiveness of medications, and lowering systemic adverse effects. Additionally, targeting ligands can be added to lipid-based nanoparticles to improve their distribution to certain brain areas or cell types, providing a more accurate and focused treatment strategy. While hurdles remain in refining their design and long-term stability, lipid-based nanoparticles show tremendous potential for improving treatment outcomes in neurodegenerative illnesses.

11.7.5 Polymeric Nanoparticles

Polymeric nanoparticles can serve as a versatile platform for drug delivery and therapeutic applications of neurodegenerative disorders [52]. These advantages include their biocompatibility, biodegradability, and capacity to encapsulate a broad array of therapeutic molecules, making them appealing options for drug delivery to the central nervous system. These nanoparticles can also be designed to cross the BBB [53], which is a considerable obstacle in treating neurological conditions, where they can release their payload in a sustained and controlled manner. Moreover, the ligands can couple into polymeric nanoparticles to obtain higher distribution for specific cells or brain areas, increasing the target and decreasing the off-target contacts. Polymeric nanoparticles can significantly enhance treatment outcomes in neurodegenerative diseases, and further exploration is needed, however, to perfect the design and understand the long-term safety behaviour of the polymer used (Figure 11.3).

Nanoparticles which are available for the management of AD are given as follows:

1. **Liposomes**: Liposomes are spherical vesicles with phospholipid bilayer membranes. They can encapsulate both hydrophilic and lipophilic drugs. Poudel and Park (2022) mention examples of commercially available AD therapeutics (galantamine, rivastigmine, donepezil) showing improved

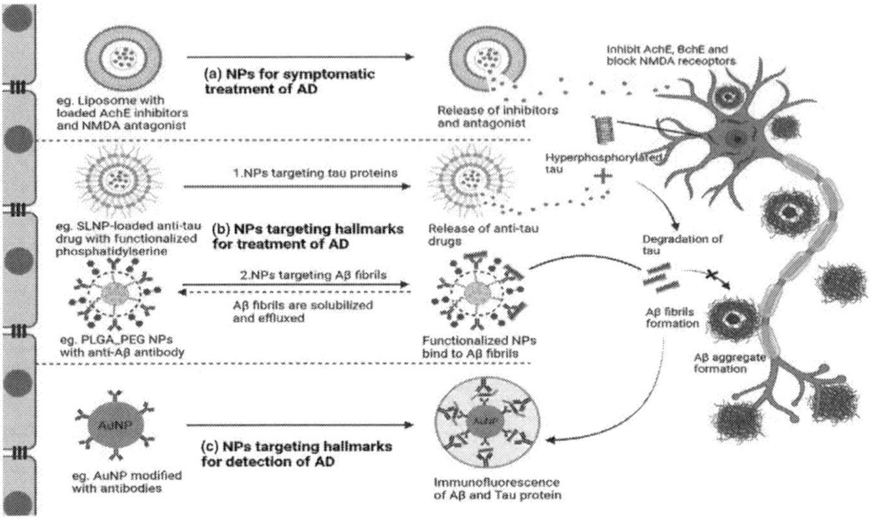

FIGURE 11.3 An example of how NPs work in AD-related neurones after crossing the blood–brain barrier. (a) Liposomes loaded with AchE inhibitors that target disruption of the cholinergic system. (b) 1. An anti-tau medication loaded with SLNP that targets hyperphosphorylated tau proteins using functionalized phosphatidylserine. (b) 2. Aβ fibrils are targeted, dissolved, and cleared by PLGA-PEG with anti-Aβ antibody. (c) modified AuNP with capture antibody targets tau and Aβ proteins, forming a Sandwich with secondary antibody for AD hallmark diagnosis. *Abbreviations:* Aβ, amyloid beta fragment; AchE, acetylcholinesterase; AuNP, gold nanoparticle; NMDA, N-methyl D-aspartate antagonist; NP, nanoparticle; PLGA, poly D,L-lactic-co-glycolic acid; PEG, polyethylene glycol; SLNP, solid lipid nanoparticle.

brain penetration and bioavailability when loaded into liposomes. Surface modifications can further enhance brain targeting.

2. **Solid Lipid Nanoparticles**: SLNs offer advantages over liposomes in terms of stability, controlled release, and large-scale production. SLNs loaded with drugs like donepezil and rivastigmine, showing improved brain uptake and therapeutic efficacy in animal models.
3. **Nanostructured Lipid Carriers**: NLCs are a next-generation version of SLNs with improved drug loading capacity and controlled release properties. NLCs loaded with curcumin, demonstrating enhanced brain uptake and neuroprotective effects.
4. **Polymeric NPs**: PNPs are made from natural or synthetic polymers. PLGA is commonly used due to its biocompatibility and controlled release properties. PLGA-based NPs for delivering donepezil, showing controlled release profiles and neuroprotective effects. Hybrid PNPs and PLA-based systems are also mentioned for extended-release formulations.
5. **Inorganic NPs**: Inorganic NPs, such as gold nanoparticles and magnetic NPs, offer unique properties for drug delivery and imaging. AuNPs conjugated with various ligands for targeted drug delivery and imaging in AD models.

6. **Stimuli-Responsive NPs**: These NPs respond to specific stimuli, such as pH, temperature, or light, allowing for controlled drug release at the target site. The pH-responsive NPs are for delivering drugs to the acidic environment of amyloid plaques.

11.8 NANOPARTICLE-BASED IMMUNOTHERAPEUTIC STRATEGIES

11.8.1 The Immune System in A. Disease Pathogenesis

- Progressive memory loss, cognitive decline, and personality changes are features of AD. Amyloid senile plaques, neurofibrillary tangles, and neuro-inflammation are histopathological markers that cause synaptic dysfunction and neuronal death.
- Impaired microglia (the brain's immune cells) are considered a risk factor. While they normally have a protective role, activated microglia can contribute to neuronal damage. The balance between their beneficial and detrimental effects is crucial in AD progression.

11.8.2 Immunotherapeutic Approaches

- **Aβ Immunotherapy**: This involves active or passive immunization targeting Aβ plaques. Active immunization stimulates the immune system to produce antibodies against Aβ, while passive immunization involves administering anti-Aβ antibodies directly. While showing promise in preclinical studies, some clinical trials have faced challenges, including meningoencephalitis as a side effect.
- **Tau Immunotherapy**: Given the strong association between tau lesions and dementia, targeting tau protein is another therapeutic strategy. Anti-tau antibodies can be used to promote the clearance of tau aggregates. Research is ongoing to determine the optimal antibody isotype for therapeutic efficacy.
- **Immune Checkpoint Inhibitors**: These drugs enhance the immune response against tumour cells and are being explored for their potential in AD. They could boost the immune system's ability to clear Aβ and tau aggregates.

11.9 INNOVATIVE IMMUNOTHERAPEUTIC STRATEGIES

Nanoparticles present versatile platforms for developing innovative immunotherapeutic strategies to combat AD. These nanoparticles provide a more focused and efficient method than conventional pharmaceutical treatments because they may be designed to target particular immune cells, alter inflammatory pathways, and transport therapeutic payloads straight to the brain. Nanoparticles can be designed to [39,54] selectively target and modulate the activity of microglia and astrocytes, the primary immune cells in the brain, to reduce neuroinflammation and mitigate the progression of the disease.

Furthermore, nanoparticles can be used to deliver anti-inflammatory agents, immune-modulating molecules, or even gene therapy constructs to the brain, bypassing the BBB and enhancing the therapeutic efficacy. In addition to targeting the CNS, nanoparticle-based approaches can also be leveraged to regulate peripheral immune responses, addressing the systemic inflammation associated with AD.

Researchers have created a variety of nanoparticle-based treatment approaches for AD by utilizing the special qualities of nanoparticles, such as their capacity for multifunctional design, controlled release kinetics, and the ability to transcend biological barriers.

These include but are not limited to:

11.9.1 Targeted Delivery of Anti-Inflammatory Agents

Nanoparticles can be engineered to encapsulate or conjugate anti-inflammatory drugs, such as non-steroidal anti-inflammatory drugs or corticosteroids, and deliver them directly to the brain, overcoming the challenges associated with poor BBB permeability and systemic side effects. These targeted delivery systems can help reduce neuroinflammation and mitigate the progression of AD.

11.9.2 Modulation of Microglia and Astrocyte Activity

Nanoparticles can be designed to selectively target and modulate the activity of microglia and astrocytes, the primary immune cells in the brain. These nanoparticles can be used to suppress the pro-inflammatory phenotype of microglia, promote the anti-inflammatory and neuroprotective functions of these cells, and regulate the astrocytic response to neuroinflammation [55].

11.9.3 Delivery of Immune-Modulating Molecules

Nanoparticles can be utilized to deliver immunomodulatory molecules, such as cytokines, chemokines, or immune checkpoint inhibitors, to the brain, thereby influencing the immune response and mitigating the detrimental effects of neuroinflammation.

11.9.4 Gene Therapy Approaches

A potential approach to the long-term treatment of AD is the use of nanoparticles to encapsulate and distribute gene therapy structures to the brain, such as genes that stimulate the removal of misfolded proteins or anti-inflammatory genes.

11.10 PRECLINICAL AND CLINICAL DEVELOPMENTS

The promise of immunotherapeutic approaches based on nanoparticles in the management of AD has been shown in several preclinical investigations. According to this research, nanoparticles have the ability to precisely target and alter the immune response in the brain, which can reduce neuroinflammation, enhance cognitive function, and slow the course of illness.

For example, a study using lipid-based nanoparticles loaded with anti-inflammatory drugs reported significant improvements in cognitive performance and reduced neuroinflammation in an AD mouse model. Another study utilizing peptide-functionalized nanoparticles to target microglial cells demonstrated enhanced clearance of Aβ plaques and improved synaptic function in a transgenic AD mouse model [16].

Despite the encouraging preclinical results, there hasn't been much clinical adoption of these nanoparticle-based approaches. Nonetheless, a number of clinical trials are looking at the application of nanoparticle-based methods for AD medicine.

A clinical study assessing the delivery of anti-inflammatory medications to the brain of individuals with AD using lipid-based nanoparticles is one such instance. The creation of successful nanoparticle-based immunotherapeutic approaches to treat this debilitating neurodegenerative illness is highly promising, as are these initiatives, ongoing developments in nanomedicine, and a better comprehension of the underlying immunological mechanisms of AD [56].

11.10.1 Challenges and Considerations

While the use of nanoparticle-based immunotherapeutic strategies holds great promise for the treatment of AD, there are several challenges and considerations that must be addressed [57].

11.10.2 Efficient Targeting and Penetration of the BBB

The BBB presents a significant obstacle to the delivery of therapeutics to the central nervous system. Nanoparticle design must be optimized to increase their ability to cross this barrier and reach the target sites within the brain [58].

11.10.3 Biocompatibility and Safety

The use of nanoparticles in biomedical applications requires careful evaluation of their biocompatibility, biodistribution, and potential toxicity. Thorough preclinical testing and regulatory approval processes are essential to ensure the safety of these therapeutic interventions.

11.10.4 Scalability and Manufacturing Considerations

The large-scale production and consistent quality control of nanoparticle-based therapies present significant challenges. Robust and scalable manufacturing processes must be developed to ensure the reliable and cost-effective production of these therapies.

11.10.5 Personalized Approaches and Precision Medicine

Given the heterogeneity of AD and the individual variability in disease progression and response to treatment, a personalized approach utilizing nanoparticle-based therapies may be necessary.

11.11 NANOPARTICLE-MEDIATED IMMUNOMODULATION

One of the key approaches in nanoparticle-based Immunotherapeutics for AD is the modulation of the immune response. Nanoparticles can be engineered to target specific immune cells, such as microglia and astrocytes, and modulate their activation states and inflammatory profiles [59]. For instance, researchers have developed nanoparticles that can selectively suppress the pro-inflammatory phenotype of microglia, while promoting their anti-inflammatory and neuroprotective functions.

Similarly, nanoparticles have been used to deliver anti-inflammatory agents, such as cytokines or small-molecule inhibitors, to the brain, effectively reducing neuroinflammation and mitigating the progression of AD [59].

Beyond targeting the central nervous system, nanoparticle-based approaches have also been explored to regulate peripheral immune responses. By modulating the activity of immune cells in the periphery, such as T cells and B cells, nanoparticles can influence the systemic inflammatory state, which is closely linked to the pathogenesis of AD.

Taken together, the versatility of nanoparticles allows for the development of multifaceted immunotherapeutic strategies that can target both the central and peripheral components of the immune system, offering a more comprehensive approach to the management of AD.

The recent advancements in the field of nanomedicine have demonstrated the potential of nanoparticle-based immunotherapeutic strategies for the treatment of AD. By modulating the immune response, both in the central nervous system and the periphery, nanoparticles can mitigate neuroinflammation and the associated neurodegeneration, presenting a promising path towards the effective management of this debilitating disease.

11.12 NANOPARTICLES IN ALZHEIMER'S DISEASE IMMUNOTHERAPY

Nanoparticles have appeared as a versatile platform for the development of innovative immunotherapeutic strategies to combat AD. These nanoscale carriers have the potential to be specifically designed to target and alter the activity of immune cells, including astrocytes and microglia, which are essential for the neuroinflammatory processes that underlie the pathophysiology of AD.

Using nanoparticles to promote microglia's anti-inflammatory and neuroprotective properties while inhibiting their pro-inflammatory phenotype is one such strategy. For example, scientists have created nanoparticles that can transport anti-inflammatory medicines and preferentially aggregate in active microglia, effectively lowering neuroinflammation and delaying the course of the illness.

Beyond targeting the central nervous system, nanoparticle-based approaches have also been explored to regulate peripheral immune responses. By balancing the activity of immune cells in the periphery, such as T cells and B cells, nanoparticles can influence the systemic inflammatory state, which is closely linked to the pathogenesis of AD.

The versatility of nanoparticles allows for the development of multifaceted immunotherapeutic strategies that can target both the central and peripheral components of the immune system, offering a more comprehensive approach to the management of AD.

Recent advancements in the field of nanomedicine have demonstrated the potential of nanoparticle-based immunotherapeutic strategies for the treatment of AD. By modulating the immune response, both in the central nervous system and the periphery, nanoparticles can mitigate neuroinflammation and the associated neurodegeneration, presenting a promising path towards the effective management of this debilitating disease [57].

11.13 NANOMEDICINE STRATEGIES FOR ALZHEIMER'S DISEASE TREATMENT

The field of nanomedicine has emerged as a powerful approach to address the complex challenges associated with the treatment of AD. Nanoparticles can be planned to selectively target and modulate the activity of microglia and astrocytes, the primary immune cells in the brain, to reduce neuroinflammation and mitigate the progression of the disease [59].

Nanoparticle-based strategies have demonstrated the ability to suppress the pro-inflammatory phenotype of microglia, while promoting their anti-inflammatory and neuroprotective functions. This targeted modulation of the immune response within the central nervous system represents a promising avenue for the management of AD.

Beyond the central nervous system, nanoparticle-based approaches have also been explored to regulate peripheral immune responses. By modulating the activity of immune cells in the periphery, such as T cells and B cells, nanoparticles can influence the systemic inflammatory state, which is closely linked to the pathogenesis of AD.

Recent advancements in the field of nanomedicine have demonstrated the potential of nanoparticle-based immunotherapeutic strategies for the treatment of AD. By modulating the immune response, both in the central nervous system and the periphery, nanoparticles can mitigate neuroinflammation and the associated neurodegeneration, presenting a promising path towards the effective management of this debilitating disease.

11.14 TARGETED NANOPARTICLE IMMUNOTHERAPIES FOR ALZHEIMER'S DISEASE

The emerging field of nanomedicine has opened new avenues for the development of targeted immunotherapeutic strategies to combat AD. Nanoparticles can be engineered to selectively target and modulate the activity of key immune cells, such as microglia and astrocytes, which play a crucial role in the neuroinflammatory processes underlying the pathogenesis of AD.

One promising approach is the use of nanoparticles to suppress the pro-inflammatory phenotype of microglia, while promoting their anti-inflammatory and neuroprotective functions. Researchers have developed nanoparticles that can preferentially accumulate in activated microglia and deliver anti-inflammatory agents, effectively reducing neuroinflammation and slowing the progression of the disease.

Beyond the central nervous system, nanoparticle-based strategies have also been explored to regulate peripheral immune responses. By regulating the activity of immune cells in the periphery, such as T cells and B cells, nanoparticles can influence the systemic inflammatory state, which is closely linked to the pathogenesis of AD.

The versatility of nanoparticles allows for the development of multifaceted immunotherapeutic strategies that can target both the central and peripheral components of the immune system, offering a more comprehensive approach to the management of AD.

11.15 ADVANCEMENT OF NANOPARTICLES FOR NEURODEGENERATIVE DISORDER'S IMMUNOTHERAPY

In AD, nanoparticles have become a promising tool for immunotherapy, addressing issues such as BBB penetration, drug bioavailability, and neurotoxicity. A variety of nanoparticles, such as lipid-based, polymeric, metallic, and carbon-based nanocarriers, are being investigated for targeted drug delivery, Aβ clearance, tau aggregation inhibition, and neuroinflammation modulation. Nanoparticle-based monoclonal antibody therapies, siRNA delivery, and anti-inflammatory drug formulations help boost the immune response against amyloid plaques and tau tangles, reducing neurodegeneration; gene therapy using CRISPR-Cas9 and RNAi-based approaches holds potential in modifying important genetic factors involved in the progression of AD.

In order to convert these discoveries into efficient Alzheimer's therapies and usher in a new era in the management of neurodegenerative diseases, future research should concentrate on refining nanoparticle formulations and carrying out clinical studies.

11.16 OVERCOMING LIMITATIONS OF CONVENTIONAL ALZHEIMER'S TREATMENTS USING NANOPARTICLES

Conventional treatments for AD have faced significant challenges, including the inability to effectively cross the BBB and limited therapeutic efficacy. The use of nanoparticles as drug delivery systems has emerged as a promising approach to overcome these limitations.

Nanoparticles can be engineered to enhance the permeability and retention of drugs within the central nervous system, improving their bioavailability and therapeutic efficacy. Additionally, nanoparticles can protect drugs from peripheral degradation, further enhancing their ability to reach the intended targets in the brain.

By selectively targeting specific pathways and cellular processes involved in the pathogenesis of AD, nanoparticle-based drug delivery systems can provide a more targeted and effective approach to treatment. For example, nanoparticles can be designed to modulate the activity of microglia and astrocytes, key players in the neuroinflammatory processes associated with AD.

Moreover, the versatility of nanoparticles allows for the development of multimodal therapeutic strategies, combining various pharmacological agents and functionalities to address the multifaceted nature of AD.

11.17 NANOPARTICLE-BASED IMMUNE MODULATION IN ALZHEIMER'S TREATMENT

The central and peripheral immune systems play a critical role in the pathogenesis of AD. In the central nervous system, microglia and astrocytes can assume a pro-inflammatory phenotype, contributing to neuroinflammation and neurodegeneration. In the periphery, the dysregulation of immune cells, such as T cells and B cells, can also influence the systemic inflammatory state, which is closely linked to the progression of AD.

Nanoparticle-based strategies have been explored to selectively target and modulate the activity of these key immune players, both in the central nervous system and the periphery.

In the central nervous system, nanoparticles can be engineered to preferentially accumulate in activated microglia and astrocytes, delivering anti-inflammatory agents or modulating their phenotypic state to reduce neuroinflammation. In the periphery, nanoparticles can be used to regulate the activity of T cells and B cells, influencing the systemic inflammatory response and potentially mitigating the detrimental effects on the central nervous system [55,58].

By employing a comprehensive approach that targets both the central and peripheral immune systems, nanoparticle-based immunotherapeutic strategies have the potential to provide a more effective management of AD.

Advanced nanoparticle-based drug delivery systems have the capability to overcome the limitations of conventional AD treatments by improving drug permeability across the BBB, protecting drugs from peripheral degradation, and selectively targeting key pathways and cellular processes involved in the pathogenesis of the disease. Additionally, the versatility of nanoparticles allows for the development of multifaceted therapeutic approaches that can address the multifactorial nature of AD.

REFERENCES

1. Martini, A. C., Forner, S., Trujillo-Estrada, L., Baglietto-Vargas, D., & LaFerla, F. M. (2018). Past to future: What animal models have taught us about Alzheimer's disease [Review of past to future: What animal models have taught us about Alzheimer's disease]. Journal of Alzheimer's Disease, 64. IOS Press. https://doi.org/10.3233/jad-179917
2. Cai, Y., Liu, J., Wang, B., Sun, M., & Yang, H. (2022). Microglia in the neuroinflammatory pathogenesis of Alzheimer's disease and related therapeutic targets [Review of microglia in the neuroinflammatory pathogenesis of Alzheimer's disease and related therapeutic targets]. Frontiers in Immunology, 13. Frontiers Media. https://doi.org/10.3389/fimmu.2022.856376
3. Liu, Y., Si, Z., Zou, C.-J., Mei, X., Li, X., Luo, H., Shen, Y., Hu, J., Li, X., & Wu, L. (2022). Targeting neuroinflammation in Alzheimer's disease: From mechanisms to clinical applications [Review of targeting neuroinflammation in Alzheimer's disease: From mechanisms to clinical applications.]. Neural Regeneration Research, 18(4), 708. Medknow. https://doi.org/10.4103/1673-5374.353484
4. Yu, X., Wang, L., Du, Q., Ma, L., Chen, L., You, R., Liu, L., Ling, J., Yang, Z., & Ji, H. (2012). Akebia saponin d attenuates amyloid β-induced cognitive deficits and inflammatory response in rats: Involvement of Akt/NF-κB pathway. In X. Yu, L.

Wang, Q. Du, L. Ma, L. Chen, R. You, L. Liu, J. Ling, Z. Yang, & H. Ji, Behavioural Brain Research (Vol. 235, Issue 2, p. 200). Elsevier BV. https://doi.org/10.1016/j.bbr.2012.07.045

5. Greer, M. (2000). Inflammation and the pathophysiology of Alzheimer's disease. In M. Greer, Dialogues in Clinical Neuroscience (Vol. 2, Issue 3, p. 233). Laboratoires Servier. https://doi.org/10.31887/dcns.2000.2.3/mgreer
6. Cerami, C., Iaccarino, L., & Perani, D. (2017). Molecular imaging of neuroinflammation in neurodegenerative dementias: The role of in vivo PET imaging [Review of molecular imaging of neuroinflammation in neurodegenerative dementias: The role of in vivo PET imaging]. International Journal of Molecular Sciences, 18(5), 993. Multidisciplinary Digital Publishing Institute. https://doi.org/10.3390/ijms18050993
7. Agostinho, P., Cunha, R. A., & Oliveira, C. R. (2010). Neuroinflammation, oxidative stress and the pathogenesis of Alzheimer disease [Review of neuroinflammation, oxidative stress and the pathogenesis of Alzheimer disease]. Current Pharmaceutical Design, 16(25), 2766. Bentham Science Publishers. https://doi.org/10.2174/138161210793176572
8. Wang, C., Zong, S., Cui, X., Wang, X., Wu, S., Wang, L., Liu, Y., & Lü, Z. (2023). The effects of microglia-associated neuroinflammation on Alzheimer's disease [Review of the effects of microglia-associated neuroinflammation on Alzheimer's disease]. Frontiers in Immunology, 14. Frontiers Media. https://doi.org/10.3389/fimmu.2023.1117172
9. Hampel, H., Toschi, N., Babiloni, C., Baldacci, F., Black, K. L., Bokde, A. L., Bun, R. S., Cacciola, F., Cavedo, E., Chiesa, P. A., & Colliot, O. (2018). Revolution of Alzheimer precision neurology. Passageway of systems biology and neurophysiology. Journal of Alzheimer's Disease, 64(s1), S47–105.
10. Gernsbacher, M. A., Robertson, R. R., Palladino, P., & Werner, N. K. Managing mental representations during narrative comprehension. In Accessibility in Text and Discourse Processing 2018 Dec 7 (pp. 145–164). Routledge.
11. Mufson, E. J., Counts, S. E., Perez, S. E., & Ginsberg, S. D. (2008). Cholinergic system during the progression of Alzheimer's disease: Therapeutic implications. Expert Review of Neurotherapeutics, 8(11), 1703–18.
12. Mitra, S., Behbahani, H., & Eriksdotter, M. (2019). Innovative therapy for Alzheimer's disease-with focus on biodelivery of NGF. Frontiers in Neuroscience, 13, 38.
13. Jung, H. J., Shin, I. S., & Lee, J. E. (2019). Olfactory function in mild cognitive impairment and Alzheimer's disease: A meta-analysis. The Laryngoscope, 129(2), 362–9.
14. Poudel, P., & Park, S. (2022). Recent advances in the treatment of Alzheimer's disease using nanoparticle-based drug delivery systems [Review of recent advances in the treatment of Alzheimer's disease using nanoparticle-based drug delivery systems]. Pharmaceutics, 14(4), 835. Multidisciplinary Digital Publishing Institute. https://doi.org/10.3390/pharmaceutics14040835
15. Greig, N. H., Lahiri, D. K., & Sambamurti, K. (2002). Butyrylcholinesterase: An important new target in Alzheimer's disease therapy. International Psychogeriatrics, 14(S1), 77–91.
16. Agarwal, M., Alam, R., Haider, M. K., Malik, M. Z., & Kim, D.-K. (2020). Alzheimer's disease: An overview of major hypotheses and therapeutic options in nanotechnology [Review of Alzheimer's disease: An overview of major hypotheses and therapeutic options in nanotechnology.]. Nanomaterials, 11(1), 59. Multidisciplinary Digital Publishing Institute. https://doi.org/10.3390/nano11010059
17. Hettiarachchi, S. D., Zhou, Y., Seven, E., Lakshmana, M. K., Kaushik, A. K., Chand, H. S., & Leblanc, R. M. (2019). Nanoparticle-mediated approaches for Alzheimer's disease pathogenesis, diagnosis, and therapeutics. Journal of Controlled Release, Nov 28;314, 125–40.
18. Yang, X., & Qu, H. (2023). Bibliometric review on biomarkers for Alzheimer's disease between 2000 and 2023. Medicine, 102(36), e34982.

19. Carter, S. F., Caine, D., Burns, A., Herholz, K., & Lambon Ralph, M. A. (2012). Staging of the cognitive decline in Alzheimer's disease: Insights from a detailed neuropsychological investigation of mild cognitive impairment and mild Alzheimer's disease. International Journal of Geriatric Psychiatry, 27(4), 423–32.
20. Solomon, S., Sampathkumar, N. K., Carre, I., Mondal, M., Chennell, G., Vernon, A. C., Ruepp, M. D., & Mitchell, J. C. (2022). Heterozygous expression of the Alzheimer's disease-protective PLCγ2 P522R variant enhances aβ clearance while preserving synapses. Cellular and Molecular Life Sciences, 79(8), 453.
21. Huang, D., Cao, Y., Yang, X., Liu, Y., Zhang, Y., Li, C., Chen, G., & Wang, Q. (2021). A nanoformulation-mediated multifunctional stem cell therapy with improved beta-amyloid clearance and neural regeneration for Alzheimer's disease. Advanced Materials, 33(13). https://doi.org/10.1002/adma.202006357
22. Zhao, Y., & Zhao, B. (2013). Oxidative stress and the pathogenesis of Alzheimer's disease. Oxidative Medicine and Cellular Longevity, 2013(1), 316523.
23. Clark, D. G., Kapur, P., Geldmacher, D. S., Brockington, J. C., Harrell, L., DeRamus, T. P., Blanton, P. D., Lokken, K., Nicholas, A. P., & Marson, D. C. (2014). Latent information in fluency lists predicts functional decline in persons at risk for Alzheimer disease. Cortex, 55, 202–18.
24. Cencioni, C., Spallotta, F., Martelli, F., Valente, S., Mai, A., Zeiher, A. M., & Gaetano, C. (2013). Oxidative stress and epigenetic regulation in ageing and age-related diseases. International Journal of Molecular Sciences, Aug 28;14(9), 17643–63.
25. Alessenko, A. V. (2013). The potential role for sphingolipids in neuropathogenesis of Alzheimer's disease. Biochemistry (Moscow) Supplement Series B: Biomedical Chemistry, 7, 108–23.
26. Montagne, A., Zhao, Z., & Zlokovic, B. V. (2017. Alzheimer's disease: A matter of blood–brain barrier dysfunction? Journal of Experimental Medicine, 214(11), 3151–69.
27. Hussain, B., Fang, C., & Chang, J. (2021). Blood–brain barrier breakdown: An emerging biomarker of cognitive impairment in normal aging and dementia. Frontiers in Neuroscience, Aug 19;15, 688090.
28. Sweeney, M. D., Sagare, A. P., & Zlokovic, B. V. (2018). Blood–brain barrier breakdown in Alzheimer disease and other neurodegenerative disorders. Nature Reviews Neurology, 14(3), 133–50.
29. Wahl, D., & Clayton, Z. S. (2024). Peripheral vascular dysfunction and the aging brain. Aging (Albany NY), May 22;16(10), 9280.
30. Klohs, J. (2019). An integrated view on vascular dysfunction in Alzheimer's disease. Neurodegenerative Diseases, Dec 28;19(3-4), 109–27.
31. Puglielli, L., Tanzi, R. E., & Kovacs, D. M. (2003). Alzheimer's disease: The cholesterol connection. Nature Neuroscience, 6(4), 345–51.
32. Zhou, Z., Shi, B., Xu, Y., Zhang, J., Liu, X., Zhou, X., Feng, B., Ma, J., & Cui, H. (2023). Neural stem/progenitor cell therapy for Alzheimer disease in preclinical rodent models: A systematic review and meta-analysis. Stem Cell Research & Therapy, 14(1), 3.
33. Shepardson, N. E., Shankar, G. M., & Selkoe, D. J. (2011). Cholesterol level and statin use in Alzheimer disease: I. Review of epidemiological and preclinical studies. Archives of Neurology, 68(10), 1239–44.
34. Wood, J. S., Watson, R., Firbank, M. J., Mosimann, U. P., Barber, R., Blamire, A. M., & O'Brien, J. T. (2013). Longitudinal testing of visual perception in dementia with Lewy bodies and Alzheimer's disease. International Journal of Geriatric Psychiatry, 28(6), 567–72.
35. Sáiz-Vazquez, O., Puente-Martínez, A., Ubillos-Landa, S., Pacheco-Bonrostro, J., & Santabárbara, J. (2020). Cholesterol and Alzheimer's disease risk: A meta-meta-analysis. Brain Sciences, Jun 18;10(6), 386.

36. Jeong, S. H., Cha, J., Park, M., Jung, J. H., Ye, B. S., Sohn, Y. H., Chung, S. J., & Lee, P. H. (2022). Association of enlarged perivascular spaces with amyloid burden and cognitive decline in Alzheimer disease continuum. Neurology, Oct 18;99(16), e1791-802.
37. Agrawal, M., Saraf, S., Saraf, S., Antimisiaris, S. G., Hamano, N., Li, S., Chougule, M. B., Shoyele, S., Gupta, U., Ajazuddin, M., & Alexander, A. (2018). Recent advancements in the field of nanotechnology for the delivery of anti-Alzheimer drug in the brain region [Review of recent advancements in the field of nanotechnology for the delivery of anti-Alzheimer drug in the brain region]. Expert Opinion on Drug Delivery, 15(6), 589. Taylor & Francis. https://doi.org/10.1080/17425247.2018.1471058
38. Wang, L., Yin, Y., Liu, X.-Z., Shen, P., Zheng, Y.-G., Lan, X.-R., Lu, C., & Wang, J. (2020). Current understanding of metal ions in the pathogenesis of Alzheimer's disease [review of current understanding of metal ions in the pathogenesis of Alzheimer's disease]. Translational Neurodegeneration, 9(1). BioMed Central. https://doi.org/10.1186/s40035-020-00189-z
39. Ali, M. M., Ghouri, R. G., Ans, A. H., Akbar, A., & Toheed, A. (2019). Recommendations for anti-inflammatory treatments in Alzheimer's disease: A comprehensive review of the literature [Review of recommendations for anti-inflammatory treatments in Alzheimer's disease: A comprehensive review of the literature]. Cureus. Cureus, Inc. https://doi.org/10.7759/cureus.4620
40. Vissers, C., Ming, G., & Song, H. (2019). Nanoparticle technology and stem cell therapy team up against neurodegenerative disorders [review of nanoparticle technology and stem cell therapy team up against neurodegenerative disorders]. Advanced Drug Delivery Reviews, 148, 239. Elsevier BV. https://doi.org/10.1016/j.addr.2019.02.007
41. Vashist, A., Manickam, P., Raymond, A., Yndart, A., Kolishetti, N., Vashist, A., Arias, E., & Nair, M. (2023). Recent advances in nanotherapeutics for neurological disorders [Review of recent advances in nanotherapeutics for neurological disorders]. ACS Applied Bio Materials, 6(7), 2614. American Chemical Society. https://doi.org/10.1021/acsabm.3c00254
42. Khanna, S., Domingo-Fernández, D., Iyappan, A., Emon, M. A., Hofmann-Apitius, M., & Fröhlich, H. (2018). Using multi-scale genetic, neuroimaging and clinical data for predicting Alzheimer's disease and reconstruction of relevant biological mechanisms. Scientific Reports, Jul 24;8(1), 11173.
43. Silveira, P. L., Silveira, G., deBem, Müller, A., & Machado-de-Ávila, R. A. (2021). Advance in the use of gold nanoparticles in the treatment of neurodegenerative diseases: New perspectives [Review of advance in the use of gold nanoparticles in the treatment of neurodegenerative diseases: New perspectives]. Neural Regeneration Research, 16(12), 2425. Medknow. https://doi.org/10.4103/1673-5374.313040
44. Gonzalez, Carter, D., Leo, B. F., Ruenraroengsak, P., Chen, S., Goode, A. E., Theodorou, I. G., Chung, K. F., Carzaniga, R., Shaffer, M. S. P., Dexter, D. T., Ryan, M. P., & Porter, A. E. (2017). Silver nanoparticles reduce brain inflammation and related neurotoxicity through induction of H2S-synthesizing enzymes. In D. Gonzalez-Carter, B. F. Leo, P. Ruenraroengsak, S. Chen, A. E. Goode, I. G. Theodorou, K. F. Chung, R. Carzaniga, M. S. P. Shaffer, D. T. Dexter, M. P. Ryan, & A. E. Porter (Vol. 7, Issue 1). Nature Portfolio.
45. Guo, X., Zhang, G., Chen, L., Khan, A. A., Gu, B., & Li, B. (2017). Newborn Neurons Are Damaged In Vitro by a Low Concentration of Silver Nanoparticles Through the Inflammatory Oxidative Stress Pathway.
46. Skalska, J., Frontczak-Baniewicz, M., & Strużyńska, L. (2014). Synaptic degeneration in rat brain after prolonged oral exposure to silver nanoparticles. In J. Skalska, M. Frontczak-Baniewicz, & L. Strużyńska (Vol. 46, p. 145). Elsevier BV.
47. Micheli, M.-R., Bova, R., Magini, A., Polidoro, M., & Emiliani, C. (2011). Lipid-based nanocarriers for CNS-targeted drug delivery [Review of lipid-based nanocarriers for CNS-targeted drug delivery]. Recent Patents on CNS Drug Discovery, 7(1), 71. Bentham Science Publishers. https://doi.org/10.2174/157488912798842241

48. Teixeira, M. I., Lopes, C. M., Amaral, M. H., & Costa, P. (2020). Current insights on lipid nanocarrier-assisted drug delivery in the treatment of neurodegenerative diseases [review of current insights on lipid nanocarrier-assisted drug delivery in the treatment of neurodegenerative diseases.]. European Journal of Pharmaceutics and Biopharmaceutics, 149, 192. Elsevier BV. https://doi.org/10.1016/j.ejpb.2020.01.005
49. Ordóñez-Gutiérrez, L., & Wandosell, F. (2020). Nanoliposomes as a therapeutic tool for Alzheimer's disease [Review of nanoliposomes as a therapeutic tool for Alzheimer's disease]. Frontiers in Synaptic Neuroscience, 12. Frontiers Media. https://doi.org/10.3389/fnsyn.2020.00020
50. Balducci, C., Mancini, S., Minniti, S., Vitola, P. L., Zotti, M., Sancini, G., Mauri, M., Cagnotto, A., Colombo, L., Fiordaliso, F., Grigoli, E., Salmona, M., Snellman, A., Haaparanta, Solin, M., Forloni, G., Masserini, M., & Re, F. (2014). Multifunctional liposomes reduce brain β-amyloid burden and ameliorate memory impairment in Alzheimer's disease mouse models. In C. Balducci, S. Mancini, S. Minniti, P. L. Vitola, M. Zotti, G. Sancini, M. Mauri, A. Cagnotto, L. Colombo, F. Fiordaliso, E. Grigoli, M. Salmona, A. Snellman, M. Haaparanta-Solin, G. Forloni, M. Masserini, & F. Re, Journal of Neuroscience (Vol. 34, Issue 42, p. 14022). Society for Neuroscience. https://doi.org/10.1523/jneurosci.0284-14.2014
51. Hernando, S., Pedraz, J. L., Igartua, M., & Hernández, R. M. (2018). The role of lipid nanoparticles and its surface modification in reaching the brain: An approach for neurodegenerative diseases treatment [Review of the role of lipid nanoparticles and its surface modification in reaching the brain: An approach for neurodegenerative diseases treatment]. Current Drug Delivery, 15(9), 1218. Bentham Science Publishers. https://doi.org/10.2174/1567201815666180510103747
52. Cano, A., Sánchez, López, E., Ettcheto, M., López-Machado, A., Espina, M., Souto, E. B., Galindo, R., Camins, A., García, M. L., & Turowski, P. (2020). Current advances in the development of novel polymeric nanoparticles for the treatment of neurodegenerative diseases. In A. Cano, E. Sánchez-López, M. Ettcheto, A. López-Machado, M. Espina, E. B. Souto, R. Galindo, A. Camins, M. L. García, & P. Turowski, Nanomedicine (Vol. 15, Issue 12, p. 1239). Future Medicine. https://doi.org/10.2217/nnm-2019-0443
53. Lee, L. K. C., Leong, L. I., Liu, Y., Luo, M., Chan, H. Y. E., & Choi, C. H. J. (2020). Preclinical nanomedicines for polyglutamine-based neurodegenerative diseases [Review of preclinical nanomedicines for polyglutamine-based neurodegenerative diseases]. Molecular Pharmaceutics, 18(2), 610. American Chemical Society. https://doi.org/10.1021/acs.molpharmaceut.0c00506
54. Park, J., Baik, S.-H., Mook-Jung, I., Irimia, D., & Cho, H. (2019). Mimicry of Central-peripheral immunity in Alzheimer's disease and discovery of neurodegenerative roles in neutrophil. In J. Park, S.-H. Baik, I. Mook-Jung, D. Irimia, & H. Cho, Frontiers in Immunology (Vol. 10). Frontiers Media. https://doi.org/10.3389/fimmu.2019.02231
55. Harilal, S., Jose, J., Parambi, D. G. T., Kumar, R., Mathew, G. E., Uddin, M. S., Kim, H., & Mathew, B. (2019). Advancements in nanotherapeutics for Alzheimer's disease: Current perspectives [Review of advancements in nanotherapeutics for Alzheimer's disease: Current perspectives]. Journal of Pharmacy and Pharmacology, 71(9), 1370. Oxford University Press. https://doi.org/10.1111/jphp.13132
56. Hu, L., Tao, Y., Jiang, Y., & Qin, F. (2023). Recent progress of nanomedicine in the treatment of Alzheimer's disease [review of recent progress of nanomedicine in the treatment of Alzheimer's disease]. Frontiers in Cell and Developmental Biology, 11. Frontiers Media. https://doi.org/10.3389/fcell.2023.1228679
57. Nguyen, K., Pham, M. N., Toi, V. V., Duan, W., Tran, P. H. L., & Tran, T. T. D. (2017). Strategies of engineering nanoparticles for treating neurodegenerative disorders [Review of strategies of engineering nanoparticles for treating neurodegenerative disorders]. Current Drug Metabolism, 18(9). Bentham Science Publishers. https://doi.org/10.2174/1389200218666170125114751

58. Sahni, J. K., Doggui, S., Ali, J., Baboota, S., Dao, L. H., & Ramassamy, C. (2010). Neurotherapeutic applications of nanoparticles in Alzheimer's disease [review of neurotherapeutic applications of nanoparticles in Alzheimer's disease]. Journal of Controlled Release, 152(2), 208. Elsevier BV. https://doi.org/10.1016/j.jconrel.2010.11.033
59. Ullah, S. N. M. N., Afzal, O., Altamimi, A. S. A., Ather, H., Sultana, S., Almalki, W. H., Bharti, P., Sahoo, A., Dwivedi, K., Khan, G., Sultana, S., Alzahrani, A., & Rahman, M. (2023). Nanomedicine in the management of Alzheimer's disease: State-of-the-art [Review of nanomedicine in the management of Alzheimer's disease: State-of-the-art]. Biomedicines, 11(6), 1752. Multidisciplinary Digital Publishing Institute. https://doi.org/10.3390/biomedicines11061752
60. Ye, Y., Liang, H., Lakpa, K. L., Xing, Y., Wollenzien, H., Chen, X., Zhao, J. X., & Geiger, J. D. (2018). Effects of silica nanoparticles on endolysosome function in primary cultured neurons. In Y. Ye, H. Liang, K. L. Lakpa, Y. Xing, H. Wollenzien, X. Chen, J. X. Zhao, & J. D. Geiger, Canadian Journal of Physiology and Pharmacology (Vol. 97, Issue 4, p. 297). NRC Research Press. https://doi.org/10.1139/cjpp-2018-0401

12 Nanoparticles-Based siRNA Delivery in the Treatment and Management of Alzheimer's Disease

Suman Samaddar, Moqbel Ali Moqbel Redhwan, Mohan Muttanahally Eraiah, and Raju Koneri

12.1 INTRODUCTION

Alzheimer's disease (AD) is a chronic neurodegenerative disorder characterized by a gradual decline in memory, cognitive abilities, and overall mental function. It is the most common cause of dementia, accounting for up to 50–75% of cases worldwide, and predominantly affects older adults, particularly those aged 65 and above. The disease progresses slowly, leading to severe impairment in daily life, with symptoms that worsen over time, ultimately impacting a person's ability to communicate, reason, and perform basic tasks independently (1).

AD has been identified by the World Health Organization (WHO) as a pressing global health issue due to the absence of a definitive treatment. As populations age worldwide, the prevalence of AD-marked by progressive cognitive decline continues to rise, particularly among individuals aged 60 and above, where it remains the leading cause of dementia (2). It is estimated that AD contributes to 50–75% of all dementia cases globally. Research highlights a higher incidence of AD among women, especially those over 65, compared to men (2–4). The degenerative progression of AD places an increasing burden on healthcare systems, caregivers, and individuals affected by the disease (5). Despite extensive research, existing treatments focus mainly on symptom management rather than addressing the root causes of the disease, leading to limited long-term efficacy (6,7).

This challenge necessitates a shift in therapeutic approaches, prompting researchers to delve deeper into the molecular underpinnings of AD. Two central pathological features of AD, the accumulation of amyloid-beta (Aβ) plaques and tau protein tangles-have been the primary targets of drug development (8). Aβ plaques result from the enzymatic cleavage of amyloid precursor protein (APP) by β-secretase and gamma-secretase, components of the presenilin complex. Genetic mutations

DOI: 10.1201/9781003543381-12

affecting the presenilin complex or APP can lead to abnormal Aβ accumulation (9). Tau, a protein closely linked with the stability of axonal microtubules, becomes problematic when it detaches and accumulates in an unbound form, forming neurofibrillary tangles through hyperphosphorylation-a hallmark of AD pathology (10).

The complex mechanisms of AD suggest that effective treatment may require more targeted and multifaceted approaches. Among emerging strategies, RNA interference (RNAi) has gained significant attention as a potential therapeutic method (11,12). RNAi enables precise control over gene expression at the post-transcriptional level, providing a unique opportunity to interrupt specific molecular pathways associated with AD progression (13,14). Small interfering RNA (siRNA) technology, in particular, has shown promise in silencing genes that contribute to Aβ production or tau hyperphosphorylation. However, the effectiveness of siRNA in treating AD has been limited by the considerable biological barriers to its delivery, particularly within the central nervous system (CNS) (15).

The blood–brain barrier (BBB), which selectively restricts the passage of molecules from the bloodstream into the brain, presents a major obstacle for siRNA-based therapies. Additionally, siRNA molecules are inherently unstable and susceptible to enzymatic degradation, further complicating their therapeutic use. To address these challenges, lipid nanoparticles (LNPs) have emerged as an advanced drug delivery system capable of encapsulating and protecting siRNA, facilitating its stability and transport across biological barriers (16,17). LNPs offer a promising solution to the limitations of traditional siRNA delivery methods, opening new avenues for AD treatment (18,19). The integration of nanotechnology within RNAi therapies represents a crucial step toward realizing the therapeutic potential of siRNA for neurodegenerative diseases, including AD (20,21).

This chapter examines the intricate relationship between siRNA and advanced delivery systems in the context of AD therapy. It provides a comprehensive analysis of the molecular mechanisms underlying AD and evaluates innovative delivery platforms—including LNPs, conjugate-based nanoparticles, polyplexes, and inorganic nanoparticles—that aim to enhance siRNA stability, specificity, and efficacy. By addressing significant challenges, such as BBB and enzymatic degradation, the chapter explores strategies to improve the bioavailability and therapeutic potential of siRNA. Furthermore, it critically assesses the safety, scalability, and translational feasibility of these delivery systems, emphasizing their role in advancing siRNA from preclinical models to clinical applications. This multifaceted approach underscores the promise of siRNA technology in transforming the therapeutic landscape for AD.

12.2 siRNA THERAPY: A PROMISING APPROACH FOR AD

Despite extensive research efforts, AD remains a challenging condition to treat effectively, with current therapeutic options largely unable to alter the course of the disease. However, Advances in molecular biology have opened new possibilities for targeted treatments, among which siRNA therapy stands out as a promising strategy (22). siRNA consists of short, double-stranded RNA molecules specifically designed to silence the expression of target genes by binding to their corresponding messenger RNA (mRNA) transcripts. By inhibiting the production of proteins associated with

AD pathology, siRNA can potentially intervene directly in the molecular mechanisms driving the disease.

The specificity of siRNA therapy allows it to selectively downregulate genes involved in key pathological processes in AD, such as Aβ plaque formation and tau protein hyperphosphorylation. These processes are central to AD progression, as Aβ plaques disrupt neuronal communication, while tau tangles lead to structural instability in neurons. By selectively silencing genes involved in these pathways, siRNA therapy could reduce the formation of these harmful proteins, potentially slowing the neurodegenerative process.

Additionally, siRNA therapy could offer benefits over traditional treatments by addressing AD at a molecular level rather than focusing solely on symptom management. Traditional therapies often work by interacting with broad biological systems, which may lead to undesired side effects. In contrast, siRNA's high specificity reduces the risk of off-target effects, allowing for a more refined approach to treatment (23).

12.3 siRNA MECHANISM OF ACTION

siRNA is a negatively charged macromolecule that is vulnerable to degradation by serum endonucleases and exhibits poor cell membrane permeability. To address these challenges, various delivery systems have been developed to protect siRNA from degradation and enhance its cellular uptake. These systems include nanocarriers, aptamers, peptides, sugars or aminosugars, proteins, and antibodies (24,25). siRNA, typically 21–23 nucleotides in length, functions at the post-transcriptional level. It is generated when long double-stranded RNA (dsRNA) is cleaved by Dicer, an RNAse III enzyme. The resulting siRNA duplex consists of two strands: the passenger strand (sense strand) and the guide strand (antisense strand). This duplex becomes part of the RNA-induced silencing complex (RISC), where the Argonaute 2 protein facilitates the separation of the strands and degrades the passenger strand. The guide strand, complementary to the target mRNA, directs the RISC complex to the mRNA for gene silencing (26–28). Effective gene silencing requires correct siRNA loading onto RISC (22).

The length of the siRNA molecule is critical for its function. Molecules longer than 30 nucleotides can trigger immune responses, including the activation of toll-like receptors (TLRs), which may lead to global gene silencing and cell death (25,29). Additionally, siRNA may cause off-target effects by partially matching with unintended mRNAs, resulting in the downregulation of non-target genes. This can complicate data interpretation and potentially lead to toxicity. To minimize such risks, it is essential to determine the minimum siRNA concentration that achieves effective gene silencing (30).

12.4 THE POTENTIAL OF siRNA IN AD TREATMENT

siRNA technology represents a promising therapeutic approach for AD, targeting the intricate molecular pathways that drive its progression. By leveraging the RNAi mechanism, siRNA can selectively silence specific genes, reducing their expression

TABLE 12.1
Targets for siRNA in Alzheimer's Disease Treatment

Target Gene	Protein/Function	Role in AD Pathology	Therapeutic Potential of siRNA
APP	Amyloid Precursor Protein (Aβ precursor)	Aβ production, plaque formation	Inhibits Aβ production, reduces plaque deposition
PSEN1 / PSEN2	Components of gamma-secretase complex	Critical for Aβ peptide generation	Reduces Aβ production, limiting plaque formation
MAPT	Microtubule-Associated Protein Tau	Tau hyperphosphorylation, neurofibrillary tangles	Prevents tau hyperphosphorylation, preserves neuronal integrity
APOE	Apolipoprotein E (e4 allele)	Impaired Aβ clearance, lipid dysregulation	Enhances Aβ clearance, reduces lipid-related risks
CLU (Clusterin)	Chaperone involved in Aβ aggregation	Promotes Aβ aggregation, contributes to plaques	Modulates aggregation, reduces plaque burden
TREM2	Triggering Receptor Expressed on Myeloid Cells 2	Regulates microglial response to neuroinflammation	Alleviates neuroinflammation, modulates immune response
SORL1	Sortilin-Related Receptor 1	Involved in cellular trafficking of APP	Improves trafficking, reduces Aβ production
BIN1	Bridging Integrator 1	Linked to endocytosis and synaptic function	Modulates cellular processes, alleviates synaptic dysfunction

and mitigating their contributions to AD pathology (Table 12.1) (23). This precision-focused strategy addresses key features of the disease, including the production of Aβ peptides and the hyperphosphorylation of tau protein, which are central to the formation of plaques and neurofibrillary tangles, respectively (6,31).

Several genes have been identified as critical contributors to AD, making them prime targets for siRNA intervention. The APP gene encodes a precursor protein for Aβ peptides, whose accumulation forms the plaques characteristic of AD. Similarly, Presenilin 1 (PSEN1) and Presenilin 2 (PSEN2), components of the gamma-secretase complex, play crucial roles in Aβ generation (32). siRNA designed to target these genes can inhibit Aβ production, potentially reducing plaque deposition. Another key target is the Microtubule-Associated Protein Tau (MAPT) gene, which is responsible for encoding tau protein. By silencing MAPT, siRNA can prevent the hyperphosphorylation of tau, thereby hindering the development of neurofibrillary tangles and preserving neuronal integrity (33).

Beyond Aβ and tau pathology, siRNA can be used to address other genetic factors associated with AD risk and progression. The Apolipoprotein E (APOE) gene, particularly its e4 allele, is a significant genetic risk factor for late-onset AD (34,35). Modulating APOE expression using siRNA may enhance Aβ clearance and reduce lipid-related risks. Additionally, genes like Clusterin (CLU) (36), Triggering Receptor Expressed on Myeloid Cells 2 (TREM2) (6), Sortilin-Related Receptor 1 (SORL1) (4), and Bridging Integrator 1 (BIN1) are involved in processes such as Aβ aggregation, neuroinflammation, and cellular trafficking (8). siRNA targeting these genes could further modulate disease pathways, offering comprehensive therapeutic potential.

The specificity of siRNA provides a significant advantage in treating AD, as it minimizes off-target effects while allowing precise intervention in disease-related pathways. By directly silencing genes implicated in AD, siRNA-based therapies can target the root causes of the disease, addressing its multifactorial nature. This cutting-edge technology holds immense promise for developing personalized treatments that not only slow disease progression but also improve patient outcomes. As research advances, siRNA is poised to become a cornerstone in the fight against AD (37).

12.5 DESIGNING siRNA TO TARGET SPECIFIC GENES IN AD

The design of siRNA for targeting genes associated with AD involves a precise and systematic approach to ensure efficacy and minimize off-target effects. The process begins with the identification of gene-specific sequences critical for silencing target genes. Key targets include APP (38), Presenilin 1 (PSEN1), Presenilin 2 (PSEN2) (39), Microtubule-Associated Protein Tau (MAPT) (40), Apolipoprotein E (APOE) (41), Triggering Receptor Expressed on Myeloid Cells 2 (TREM2) (42), and Bridging Integrator 1 (BIN1) (43). These genes are integral to the molecular mechanisms of AD, including Aβ production, tau hyperphosphorylation, and neuroinflammation.

The design of siRNA involves selecting sequences from the coding region or critical mRNA segments of the target genes. This prioritization ensures high specificity, reducing the likelihood of unintended silencing of non-target genes. Structurally, siRNA comprises a guide strand, which directs the RISC to the target mRNA, and a passenger strand, which is subsequently degraded (44). Chemical modifications, such as 2'-O-methyl and 2'-fluoro substitutions, are incorporated to enhance the stability of siRNA and its accessibility to the target mRNA, while also minimizing immune responses and degradation (45). Advanced bioinformatics tools such as BLAST (Basic Local Alignment Search Tool), siDirect, RNAxs, and DESIGNER are used to rigorously analyze and optimize siRNA sequences. These tools assist in predicting the most effective target sites, minimizing off-target effects, and evaluating thermodynamic properties to improve the efficiency of gene silencing. Additionally, these platforms incorporate algorithms that account for secondary RNA structures and sequence conservation, ensuring a robust design process.

Delivery of siRNA into the CNS presents additional challenges due to the BBB. To overcome this, innovative delivery systems, including nanoparticle formulations, are being developed. These systems enhance the transport of siRNA across the BBB, allowing effective targeting of CNS tissues. Given the multifactorial nature of AD, combination therapies using siRNA to target multiple genes simultaneously may provide a more comprehensive therapeutic approach. However, before clinical application, it is essential to validate the designed siRNA sequences through extensive *in vitro* and *in vivo* experiments. This validation process assesses their efficacy, specificity, and safety, laying the groundwork for advancing siRNA-based therapeutic interventions for AD.

12.6 siRNA PLATFORMS FOR AD THERAPY

12.6.1 Conjugate-Based Nanoparticles

Conjugate-based nanoparticles are widely employed for the delivery of siRNA in AD therapy. These systems rely on siRNA conjugation to various materials, such as proteins (46), fatty acids, and lipid chains (47), using specialized linkers to enhance their physicochemical properties. This approach simplifies the manufacturing process, making it controllable and potentially facilitating clinical translation. An example of a successful application is the multivalent N-Acetylgalactosamine-conjugated siRNA, which has already reached clinical use and demonstrated significant tissue-specific siRNA accumulation (48).

Among the available targets for siRNA delivery in the brain, transferrin receptors (TfRs) are prominent due to their high expression on capillary endothelial cells. These receptors play a vital role in facilitating the transport of therapeutics across the BBB (49). Recent research has highlighted the development of TfR-targeting protein-dsRNA conjugates, which show enhanced efficacy (50,51). For example, a TfR-binding conjugate developed by Eli Lilly demonstrated a substantial reduction in target mRNA levels in key brain regions in preclinical models, achieving a 91% reduction in mRNA and a 41% reduction in protein expression following multiple intravenous doses. Additionally, this conjugate showed remarkable efficacy in non-human primates (52). Melanotransferrin (p97), an iron-binding protein, has also been explored for its potential to mediate drug distribution across the BBB (53). Based on p97, a twelve-amino acid peptide derivative (MTfp) has been designed to improve ease of synthesis and enhance BBB penetration (54). MTfp-siRNA conjugates have demonstrated significant mRNA reduction in the brain, showcasing their potential as a therapeutic approach for AD (54).

Lipophilic conjugates provide another strategy to improve siRNA delivery to the brain. For instance, α-tocopherol, a form of vitamin E, can facilitate the transport of siRNA to the brain and liver (55). α-Tocopherol-conjugated siRNA (Toc-siRNA) has shown promise in reducing liver-specific mRNA levels (56). Serum high-density lipoprotein (HDL) has also been utilized as a carrier to deliver BACE1-targeting siRNA through intracerebroventricular infusion. This method leverages receptor-mediated endocytosis via low-density lipoprotein receptor family members, enhancing uptake and therapeutic efficacy (57). Furthermore, docosahexaenoic acid (DHA), a critical omega-3 fatty acid prevalent in the brain, has been conjugated to siRNA to achieve significant mRNA knockdown in animal models following intrastriatal injection (58). Importantly, DHA is also believed to support cognitive function in AD.

Ligand conjugation has proven to be an effective strategy for delivering siRNA to the brain. For instance, indatraline, a monoamine transporter blocker, has been covalently linked to siRNA molecules. Intranasal administration of these conjugates enables their transport through cerebrospinal fluid and selective absorption by target cells (59). This technique allows for specific and efficient mRNA knockdown, offering a safe and targeted therapeutic approach for AD.

Despite these advancements, conjugate-based nanoparticles face several challenges. Unlike encapsulated siRNA, conjugated siRNA is more exposed and vulnerable to enzymatic degradation, necessitating precise chemical modifications to enhance stability (30). Additionally, the bioavailability and pharmacokinetic limitations of conjugates pose significant hurdles. These issues can be addressed by optimizing conjugate structures and refining administration routes, which could improve therapeutic outcomes for AD (48). Conjugate-based siRNA delivery systems hold immense promise for advancing AD therapy by overcoming the challenges associated with effective brain targeting and enhancing the therapeutic efficacy of siRNA-based treatments.

12.7 LIPID-BASED NANOPARTICLES

Lipid-based nanoparticles, such as solid lipid nanoparticles (SLNs) and liposomes, are extensively utilized to deliver therapeutic agents, including small molecules (60), peptides (61), and RNAs (62). These nanoparticles are primarily composed of lipid or lipid-like materials, which improve drug delivery due to their biocompatibility, biodegradability, and structural flexibility (63). A key advantage of lipid-based nanoparticles is their scalability, making them suitable for large-scale production (63). Notably, Alnylam Pharmaceuticals introduced a siRNA drug using lipid-based nanoparticles, validating the safety and efficacy of this delivery platform.

Despite their advantages, the BBB poses a significant challenge for lipid-based nanoparticles to reach the brain after systemic administration. Surface chemistry plays a crucial role in determining the *in vivo* behavior of nanoparticles (64). Positively charged molecules enhance BBB permeability by interacting electrostatically with the anionic endothelium of the BBB (65). Recent advancements include the development of ionizable cationic lipids tailored for siRNA delivery, with a specific focus on optimizing the structure of amine headgroups to improve the acid dissociation constant (pKa). LNPs with a pKa around 6.5 significantly enhance cellular uptake and endosomal escape, making them highly effective for therapeutic delivery (65).

Receptor-mediated endocytosis is another critical mechanism for improving brain-specific drug accumulation. For instance, the rabies virus glycoprotein (RVG)-derived peptide facilitates transport across neuronal cell membranes by binding to the acetylcholine receptor (AchR) (66). Leveraging this mechanism, researchers have designed liposomes complexed with siRNA and modified with RVG to enhance siRNA delivery for therapeutic purposes (67). Additionally, SLNs modified with RVG-derived peptides have been shown to achieve efficient nose-to-brain delivery. This approach not only enhances receptor-mediated endocytosis but also protects siRNA from enzymatic degradation. The transported siRNA crosses the BBB through the olfactory epithelium and trigeminal nerve pathways, significantly improving brain penetration. Other ligands have also been investigated to facilitate BBB crossing. Transferrin (Tf)-modified liposomes have shown promise in targeting neural cells (68). Furthermore, liposomes decorated with phosphatidic acid and cardiolipin exhibit a high affinity for Aβ peptides, likely due to electrostatic and hydrophobic interactions (69). PEGylated liposomes conjugated with glutathione have demonstrated enhanced drug transport to the CNS, mediated by cytoskeletal proteins and endocytic pathways (70). These innovations provide valuable insights for targeting siRNA delivery to treat AD.

One major limitation of lipid-based nanoparticles is their propensity for liver uptake. Apolipoprotein E (apoE) adsorption on the nanoparticle surface after intravenous administration directs these particles to hepatocytes via lipoprotein receptor interactions (71). Although low-density lipoprotein receptors are present on the BBB, their capacity to transport apoE to the brain remains uncertain (71). Additionally, the incorporation of positively charged lipids, while beneficial for endosomal escape and cellular uptake, poses toxicity concerns (72). Striking a balance between delivery efficiency and safety is critical. Neuroinflammation, commonly associated with AD, further complicates the optimization of siRNA delivery. While it enhances BBB permeability, it can also interfere with specific cell targeting, underscoring the need for careful consideration of neuroinflammatory processes in therapeutic development (73). Lipid-based nanoparticles offer significant potential for advancing AD therapy by addressing delivery challenges and improving the efficacy of siRNA-based treatments.

12.8 POLYPLEXES

Polyplexes are polyelectrolyte complexes formed through electrostatic interactions between positively charged polymers containing protonable amino groups and negatively charged siRNA molecules (74). These complexes are straightforward to prepare, often requiring simple stirring, and are extensively studied for their high-density loading capacity, enhanced cellular uptake, and protection of siRNA from enzymatic degradation (75).

Dendrimer-based polyplexes, such as dendrigraft poly-L-lysine (DGL), are promising tools for siRNA delivery. DGL, a cationic polymer with a lysine core, provides an inner cavity for encapsulating small molecules (76). For example, Rapa@DAK/siRNA, a co-delivery system for BACE1-targeting siRNA and rapamycin, has demonstrated efficacy in reducing Aβ deposition and improving cognitive function in AD transgenic mice via intranasal administration (77). DGL can be further functionalized with Aβ-binding peptides and Aleuria aurantia lectin (AAL), facilitating nose-to-brain delivery and targeting of Aβ plaques (78).

Chitosan, a linear polysaccharide derived from chitin, is a widely used carrier due to its low immunogenicity, biodegradability, and biocompatibility. Its highly positive charge enhances bioadhesion and permeability, making it effective for siRNA delivery (79,80). Intranasal administration of chitosan-based nanoparticles bypasses the BBB and increases siRNA accumulation in the brain. Studies have shown that chitosan matrices protect siRNA from degradation, facilitating sustained release and effective gene knockdown (81). Modifications to chitosan, such as reductive methylation, improve solubility and enhance its ability to form complexes with siRNA, effectively reducing BACE1 gene expression *in vitro* and *in vivo* (82). PEGylated chitosan conjugated with cell-penetrating peptides like TAT (RKKRRQRRR) has demonstrated success in transporting siRNA to neuronal cells, reducing Ataxin-1 protein expression, and protecting neurons in AD models (83). Additionally, chitosan nanoparticles cross-linked with mangafodipir have achieved significant mRNA reduction in the brain by leveraging early endosomal processing and siRNA release (84).

Polyethylenimine (PEI) is a cationic polymer composed of amine groups and aliphatic chains, known for its proton sponge effect that enhances endosomal escape. PEI forms stable complexes with siRNA, and low molecular weight PEIs exhibit reduced toxicity and higher transfection efficacy (85). Modified PEIs, such as those conjugated with polyethylene glycol (PEG), have shown increased cellular uptake, reduced toxicity, and improved transfection efficiency (86). These complexes are effective in reducing BACE1 gene expression in AD models following intravenous injection (87).

Recent advancements in polyplex design include the use of guanidinium-modified polymers and ligand-functionalized carriers. For example, Gal-NP@siRNA employs a triple-interaction stabilization method to enhance BBB penetration and siRNA delivery (88). This system achieves significant reductions in BACE1 mRNA and protein levels, improves cognitive function, and enhances siRNA retention in the brain (88). Other modifications, such as the use of zinc-dipicolylamine analogs and adenine-functionalized PEIs, further increase neuronal targeting and transfection efficiency, providing promising avenues for AD treatment (89).

Despite their potential, polyplexes face challenges such as inherent cytotoxicity and limited serum resistance. Strategies to overcome these limitations include modifying polycation structures and incorporating amphiphilic polymers. Continuous innovation in polyplex design and functionalization is essential for optimizing their safety and efficacy in AD therapy (90). Polyplex-based delivery systems offer significant promise for advancing siRNA therapeutics in AD by improving targeted delivery, enhancing gene silencing, and mitigating disease progression.

12.9 EXOSOMES

Exosomes are natural nanocarriers secreted by various cell types, capable of transporting RNAs and functional biomolecules to facilitate intercellular communication (91). They possess high transfection efficiency, surpassing traditional delivery systems, and can cross biological barriers, including BBB (92). Their low immunogenicity and ability to protect siRNA make exosomes an excellent vehicle for drug delivery in AD therapy (91).

One notable approach involves the use of exosomes modified with RVG peptides to enhance brain targeting. Electroporation was employed to load siRNA into these exosomes, resulting in a 60% reduction in BACE1 mRNA and a 62% reduction in protein levels in wild-type mice (93). Intranasal administration, preferred for its non-invasive nature and rapid onset of action, has shown promise in bypassing hepatic first-pass metabolism and delivering siRNA directly to the brain.

Another innovative strategy utilizes mesenchymal stem cell-derived exosomes to create lesion-recognizing nanoparticles (REXO/BAP@siRNAs). These exosomes not only penetrate the brain but also migrate specifically to diseased areas (94). In an AD mouse model, these nanoparticles improved cognitive function, reduced BACE1 expression, decreased Aβ plaques, diminished reactive astrocytes, and restored neuronal integrity (95). The incorporation of a cationic polymer in these nanoparticles enhances siRNA stability and provides reactive oxygen species (ROS)-responsive capabilities, ensuring efficient delivery and therapeutic action.

While exosomes hold great potential, obtaining sufficient quantities remains a significant challenge. Current production methods, primarily based on cell culture, struggle to meet good manufacturing practice standards (96). Moreover, loading siRNA into exosomes using electroporation achieves an encapsulation efficiency of only 20–30%, necessitating large amounts of exosomes for therapeutic applications (97). Developing more efficient production and loading methods is essential to overcome these limitations and enable the clinical translation of exosome-based therapies for AD.

To address the challenges of exosome yield and loading efficiency, a self-assembly exosome delivery system has been proposed. This approach utilizes artificial genetic circuits to reprogram the liver to produce exosomes loaded with siRNA, promoting their systemic circulation and delivery to the brain (98,99). This innovative method has successfully delivered siRNA to the brain and demonstrated efficacy in reducing pathological markers of AD, offering a promising avenue for advancing siRNA therapeutics.

12.10 INORGANIC NANOPARTICLES

Inorganic nanoparticles have gained significant attention in biotechnology due to their excellent storage stability and high surface-to-volume ratio, which allows for the simultaneous application of drug delivery and therapeutic interventions (100). Advances in chemical synthesis have enabled the development of nanoparticles with specific properties, and their intrinsic features make it possible to track siRNA within the body. Common inorganic materials used for siRNA delivery to the brain include magnetic nanoparticles, gold nanoparticles (GNPs), and layered double hydroxides (LDHs) (101).

Magnetic nanoparticles provide a robust platform for targeted siRNA delivery due to their responsiveness to magnetic fields (102). Their surfaces can be modified for imaging and targeted cell delivery (103). Magnetofection™ technology, developed by OZ Biosciences, has been successfully used to deliver siRNA targeting BACE1, a key gene implicated in AD (104). These nanoparticles, typically 6-12 nm in size, are coated with cationic molecules to enhance their application (105). The siRNA-loaded nanoparticles are guided by a magnetic field to specific cells and internalized via endocytosis or phagocytosis without altering membrane structure.

Despite their potential, magnetic nanoparticles tend to agglomerate *in vivo*, a challenge that can be mitigated by polymeric coatings (106). PEG conjugates are particularly effective, providing steric repulsion and stability. PEG-modified magnetic nanoparticles have been shown to deliver siRNA targeting BACE1 efficiently, reducing its expression *in vitro* without cytotoxicity (107). Other stabilizers, such as oleic acid, further enhance the stability and functionality of magnetic nanoparticles.

GNPs are versatile carriers for siRNA delivery, with tunable properties such as size, shape, and surface coatings. They are inert and protect siRNA from degradation (108). Layer-by-layer (LbL) technology, which relies on the adsorption of oppositely charged polyelectrolytes, has been employed to create polyelectrolyte-gold nanoassemblies (PE-Gold NAs) (109). These assemblies have shown significant efficacy in reducing BACE1 gene expression, with PEI-Gold NAs demonstrating the highest performance due to their high charge density and efficient endosomal escape (110).

LDHs consist of cationic metal hydroxide sheets and interlayer anions that balance the positive charges (111). Their structure allows for the encapsulation of negatively charged biomolecules, including siRNA. LDHs enter cells via endocytosis, releasing siRNA as the nanoparticles dissolve in the acidic lysosomal environment (112). LDHs have been explored for nucleic acid delivery, with modifications enhancing their ability to target brain cells and deliver therapeutic siRNA in AD models.

12.11 CERIUM OXIDE NANOPARTICLES

Oxidative stress, driven by ROS, is a significant factor in AD pathology. Cerium oxide nanoparticles (CeONPs) have shown exceptional ROS-scavenging capabilities due to the reversible cycling of $Ce3^{+}$ and $Ce4^{+}$ on their surface (113). CeONPs can cross the BBB and have been studied as carriers for siRNA-targeting genes implicated in AD (114). Their ability to mitigate oxidative stress and deliver siRNA effectively highlights their therapeutic potential. While inorganic nanoparticles show great promise for siRNA delivery in AD therapy, challenges such as inconsistent batch quality and long-term safety concerns limit their clinical application. Addressing these issues through improved synthesis methods and comprehensive safety evaluations will be critical for translating these technologies into clinical practice.

12.12 CONCLUSION

AD remains one of the most challenging neurodegenerative disorders, with existing treatments offering limited efficacy in addressing its underlying molecular pathology. Advances in RNAi technology, specifically siRNA, have opened new avenues for targeting the root causes of the disease, such as Aβ plaque formation and tau protein hyperphosphorylation. However, the effective delivery of siRNA to the CNS is fraught with significant challenges, including the BBB and the inherent instability of siRNA molecules.

Nanotechnology has emerged as a powerful tool to overcome these limitations. LNPs, conjugate-based nanoparticles, polyplexes, and exosomes represent promising delivery systems that enhance the stability, specificity, and bioavailability of siRNA while addressing critical barriers like the BBB. These platforms offer the potential for precise targeting of disease-related genes, improved therapeutic efficacy, and reduced off-target effects, making siRNA-based therapies a viable approach for modifying the course of AD. Despite the significant progress, challenges remain, including scalability, long-term safety, and clinical translation of these nanocarrier systems. Future research should focus on refining these delivery platforms to improve their effectiveness, minimize toxicity, and ensure compatibility with large-scale manufacturing. With sustained innovation and collaboration across disciplines, siRNA delivery systems hold the potential to revolutionize the treatment landscape of AD, transforming it from symptom management to disease modification.

REFERENCES

1. DeTure MA, Dickson DW. The neuropathological diagnosis of Alzheimer's disease. Mol Neurodegener. 2019;14:32. doi: 10.1186/s13024-019-0333-5.
2. Downer B, Al Snih S, Chou L-N, Kuo Y-F, Raji M, Markides KS, Ottenbacher KJ. Changes in health care use by Mexican American medicare beneficiaries Before and after a diagnosis of dementia. The Journals of Gerontology: Series A. 2021;76:534–542. doi: 10.1093/gerona/glaa236.
3. Galle SA, Geraedts IK, Deijen JB, Milders MV, Drent ML. The interrelationship between insulin-like growth factor 1, apolipoprotein e E4, lifestyle factors. And The Aging Body And Brain. J Prev Alzheimers Dis. 2020;1–9. doi: 10.14283/jpad.2020.11.

4. Srivastava S, Ahmad R, Khare SK. Alzheimer's disease and its treatment by different approaches: A review. Eur J Med Chem. 2021;216:113320. doi: 10.1016/j.ejmech.2021.113320.
5. Xiao X, Liu X, Jiao B. Epigenetics: Recent advances and its role in the treatment of Alzheimer's disease. Front Neurol. 2020;11. doi: 10.3389/fneur.2020.538301.
6. Poudel P, Park S. Recent advances in the treatment of Alzheimer's disease using nanoparticle-based drug delivery systems. Pharmaceutics. 2022;14:835. doi: 10.3390/pharmaceutics14040835.
7. Battaglia L, Panciani PP, Muntoni E, Capucchio MT, Biasibetti E, De Bonis P, Mioletti S, Fontanella M, Swaminathan S. Lipid nanoparticles for intranasal administration: Application to nose-to-brain delivery. Expert Opin Drug Deliv. 2018;15:369–378. doi: 10.1080/17425247.2018.1429401.
8. Jazvinšćak Jembrek M, Slade N, Hof PR, Šimić G. The interactions of p53 with tau and Aß as potential therapeutic targets for Alzheimer's disease. Prog Neurobiol. 2018;168:104–127. doi: 10.1016/j.pneurobio.2018.05.001.
9. Mhyre TR, Boyd JT, Hamill RW, Maguire-Zeiss KA. Parkinson's Disease. Subcell Biochem. 2012;65:389–455.
10. Ballatore C, Lee VM-Y, Trojanowski JQ. Tau-mediated neurodegeneration in Alzheimer's disease and related disorders. Nat Rev Neurosci. 2007;8:663–672. doi: 10.1038/nrn2194.
11. Butler JS, Chan A, Costelha S, Fishman S, Willoughby JLS, Borland TD, Milstein S, Foster DJ, Gonçalves P, Chen Q et al. Preclinical evaluation of RNAi as a treatment for transthyretin-mediated amyloidosis. Amyloid. 2016;23:109–118. doi: 10.3109/13506129.2016.1160882.
12. Redhwan MAM, Samaddar S, Hard SAAA siRNA a promising tool for diabetes complications. OpenNano. 2023;13:100174. doi: 10.1016/j.onano.2023.100174.
13. Semple SC, Akinc A, Chen J, Sandhu AP, Mui BL, Cho CK, Sah DWY, Stebbing D, Crosley EJ, Yaworski E et al. Rational design of cationic lipids for siRNA delivery. Nat Biotechnol. 2010;28:172–176. doi: 10.1038/nbt.1602.
14. Maier MA, Jayaraman M, Matsuda S, Liu J, Barros S, Querbes W, Tam YK, Ansell SM, Kumar V, Qin J et al. Biodegradable lipids enabling rapidly eliminated lipid nanoparticles for systemic delivery of RNAi therapeutics. Molecular Therapy. 2013;21:1570–1578. doi: 10.1038/mt.2013.124.
15. Jayaraman M, Ansell SM, Mui BL, Tam YK, Chen J, Du X, Butler D, Eltepu L, Matsuda S, Narayanannair JK et al. Maximizing the potency of siRNA lipid nanoparticles for hepatic Gene silencing in Vivo. Angewandte Chemie. 2012;124:8657–8661. doi: 10.1002/ange.201203263.
16. Kulkarni JA, Darjuan MM, Mercer JE, Chen S, van der Meel R, Thewalt JL, Tam YYC, Cullis PR On the formation and morphology of lipid nanoparticles containing ionizable cationic lipids and siRNA. ACS Nano. 2018;12:4787–4795. doi: 10.1021/acsnano.8b01516.
17. Whitehead KA, Dorkin JR, Vegas AJ, Chang PH, Veiseh O, Matthews J, Fenton OS, Zhang Y, Olejnik KT, Yesilyurt V et al. Degradable lipid nanoparticles with predictable in vivo siRNA delivery activity. Nat Commun. 2014;5:4277. doi: 10.1038/ncomms5277.
18. Xiao B, Ma L, Merlin D Nanoparticle-mediated co-delivery of chemotherapeutic agent and siRNA for combination cancer therapy. Expert Opin Drug Deliv. 2017;14:65–73. doi: 10.1080/17425247.2016.1205583.
19. Samaridou E, Walgrave H, Salta E, Álvarez DM, Castro-López V, Loza M, Alonso MJ Nose-to-brain delivery of enveloped RNA – cell permeating peptide nanocomplexes for the treatment of neurodegenerative diseases. Biomaterials. 2020;230:119657. doi: 10.1016/j.biomaterials.2019.119657.
20. Baranowska-Wójcik E, Szwajgier D Alzheimer's disease: Review of current nanotechnological therapeutic strategies. Expert Rev Neurother. 2020;20:271–279. doi: 10.1080/14737175.2020.1719069.

21. Hu C, Wu B, Wu Y, Shi M, Ma J, Gao H, Zhang J Recent advances in nanotechnology for combating Alzheimer's disease. Mater Chem Front. 2023;7:5171–5186. doi: 10.1039/D3QM00493G.
22. Zahir-Jouzdani F, Mottaghitalab F, Dinarvand M, Atyabi F siRNA delivery for treatment of degenerative diseases, new hopes and challenges. J Drug Deliv Sci Technol. 2018;45:428–441. doi: 10.1016/j.jddst.2018.04.001.
23. Nilsson P, Iwata N, Muramatsu S, Tjernberg LO, Winblad B, Saido TC Gene Therapy in Alzheimer's disease – Potential for disease modification. J Cell Mol Med. 2010;14:741–757. doi: 10.1111/j.1582-4934.2010.01038.x.
24. Subhan MA, Torchilin V siRNA based drug design, quality, delivery and clinical translation. Nanomedicine. 2020;29:102239. doi: 10.1016/j.nano.2020.102239.
25. Saw PE, Song E-W siRNA therapeutics: A clinical reality. Sci China Life Sci. 2020;63:485–500. doi: 10.1007/s11427-018-9438-y.
26. Lam JKW, Chow MYT, Zhang Y, Leung SWS siRNA versus miRNA as therapeutics for Gene silencing. Mol Ther Nucleic Acids. 2015;4:e252. doi: 10.1038/mtna.2015.23.
27. Fakhr E, Zare F, Teimoori-Toolabi L Precise and efficient siRNA design: A key point in competent Gene silencing. Cancer Gene Ther. 2016;23:73–82. doi: 10.1038/cgt.2016.4.
28. Redhwan MAM, Samaddar S, Hard SAAA, Yadav V, Mukherjee A, Kumar R. Small interference (RNAi) technique: Exploring its clinical applications, benefits and limitations. Eur J Clin Invest. 2023;53. doi: 10.1111/eci.14039.
29. Raja MAG, Katas H, Amjad MW Design, mechanism, delivery and therapeutics of canonical and dicer-substrate siRNA. Asian J Pharm Sci. 2019;14:497–510. doi: 10.1016/j.ajps.2018.12.005.
30. Lee SH, Kang YY, Jang H-E, Mok H Current preclinical small interfering RNA (siRNA)-based conjugate systems for RNA therapeutics. Adv Drug Deliv Rev. 2016;104:78–92. doi: 10.1016/j.addr.2015.10.009.
31. Binda A, Murano C, Rivolta I Innovative therapies and nanomedicine applications for the treatment of Alzheimer's disease: A state-of-the-art (2017–2020). Int J Nanomedicine. 2020;15:6113–6135. doi: 10.2147/IJN.S231480.
32. La Barbera L, Mauri E, D'Amelio M, Gori M. Functionalization strategies of polymeric nanoparticles for drug delivery in Alzheimer's disease: Current trends and future perspectives. Front Neurosci. 2022;16. doi: 10.3389/fnins.2022.939855.
33. Grabowska-Pyrzewicz W, Want A, Leszek J, Wojda U Antisense oligonucleotides for Alzheimer's disease therapy: From the mRNA to miRNA paradigm. EBioMedicine. 2021;74:103691. doi: 10.1016/j.ebiom.2021.103691.
34. Kulkarni JA, Witzigmann D, Chen S, Cullis PR, van der Meel R Lipid nanoparticle technology for clinical translation of siRNA therapeutics. Acc Chem Res. 2019;52:2435–2444. doi: 10.1021/acs.accounts.9b00368.
35. Kim J, Jozic A, Sahay G Naturally derived membrane lipids impact nanoparticle-based messenger RNA delivery. Cell Mol Bioeng. 2020;13:463–474. doi: 10.1007/s12195-020-00619-y.
36. Yamamoto Y, Lin PJC, Beraldi E, Zhang F, Kawai Y, Leong J, Katsumi H, Fazli L, Fraser R, Cullis PR et al. siRNA lipid nanoparticle potently silences clusterin and delays progression when combined with androgen receptor cotargeting in enzalutamide-resistant prostate cancer. Clinical Cancer Research. 2015;21:4845–4855. doi: 10.1158/1078-0432.CCR-15-0866.
37. Yamamoto N, Sato Y, Munakata T, Kakuni M, Tateno C, Sanada T, Hirata Y, Murakami S, Tanaka Y, Chayama K et al. Novel pH-sensitive multifunctional envelope-type nanodevice for siRNA-based treatments for chronic HBV infection. J Hepatol. 2016;64:547–555. doi: 10.1016/j.jhep.2015.10.014.
38. Buccellato FR, D'Anca M, Tartaglia GM, Del Fabbro M, Scarpini E, Galimberti D Treatment of Alzheimer's disease: Beyond symptomatic therapies. Int J Mol Sci. 2023;24:13900. doi: 10.3390/ijms241813900.

39. Bertram L, Tanzi RE Thirty years of Alzheimer's disease genetics: The implications of systematic meta-analyses. Nat Rev Neurosci. 2008;9:768–778. doi: 10.1038/nrn2494.
40. Azorsa DO, Robeson RH, Frost D, Hoovet BM, Brautigam GR, Dickey C, Beaudry C, Basu GD, Holz DR, Hernandez JA et al. High-content siRNA screening of the kinome identifies kinases involved in Alzheimer's disease-related tau hyperphosphorylation. BMC Genomics. 2010;11:25. doi: 10.1186/1471-2164-11-25.
41. Bana L, Minniti S, Salvati E, Sesana S, Zambelli V, Cagnotto A, Orlando A, Cazzaniga E, Zwart R, Scheper W et al. Liposomes bi-functionalized with phosphatidic acid and an ApoE-derived peptide affect Aβ aggregation features and cross the blood–brain-barrier: Implications for therapy of Alzheimer disease. Nanomedicine. 2014;10:1583–1590. doi: 10.1016/j.nano.2013.12.001.
42. Molinuevo JL, Ayton S, Batrla R, Bednar MM, Bittner T, Cummings J, Fagan AM, Hampel H, Mielke MM, Mikulskis A et al. Current state of Alzheimer's fluid biomarkers. Acta Neuropathol. 2018;136:821–853. doi: 10.1007/s00401-018-1932-x.
43. Tan L, Yu J-T, Hu N, Tan L Non-coding RNAs in Alzheimer's disease. Mol Neurobiol. 2013;47:382–393. doi: 10.1007/s12035-012-8359-5.
44. Wang Y-L, Liu W, Wada E, Murata M, Wada K, Kanazawa I Clinico-pathological rescue of a model mouse of Huntington's disease by siRNA. Neurosci Res. 2005;53:241–249. doi: 10.1016/j.neures.2005.06.021.
45. Judge AD, Bola G, Lee ACH, MacLachlan I Design of noninflammatory synthetic siRNA mediating potent Gene silencing in vivo. Molecular Therapy. 2006;13:494–505. doi: 10.1016/j.ymthe.2005.11.002.
46. Klein D, Goldberg S, Theile CS, Dambra R, Haskell K, Kuhar E, Lin T, Parmar R, Manoharan M, Richter M et al. Centyrin ligands for extrahepatic delivery of siRNA. Molecular Therapy. 2021;29:2053–2066. doi: 10.1016/j.ymthe.2021.02.015.
47. Brown KM, Nair JK, Janas MM, Anglero-Rodriguez YI, Dang LTH, Peng H, Theile CS, Castellanos-Rizaldos E, Brown C, Foster D et al. Expanding RNAi therapeutics to extrahepatic tissues with lipophilic conjugates. Nat Biotechnol. 2022;40:1500–1508. doi: 10.1038/s41587-022-01334-x.
48. Chernikov IV, Vlassov VV, Chernolovskaya EL. Current development of siRNA bioconjugates: From research to the clinic. Front Pharmacol. 2019;10. doi: 10.3389/fphar.2019.00444.
49. Johnsen KB, Burkhart A, Thomsen LB, Andresen TL, Moos T Targeting the transferrin receptor for brain drug delivery. Prog Neurobiol. 2019;181:101665. doi: 10.1016/j.pneurobio.2019.101665.
50. Dasgupta A, Sun T, Rama E, Motta A, Zhang Y, Power C, Moeckel D, Fletcher S, Moosavifar M, Barmin R et al. Transferrin receptor-targeted nonspherical microbubbles for blood–brain barrier sonopermeation. Advanced Materials. 2023;35. doi: 10.1002/adma.202308150.
51. Crook ZR, Girard E, Sevilla GP, Merrill M, Friend D, Rupert PB, Pakiam F, Nguyen E, Yin C, Ruff RO et al. A TfR-binding cystine-dense peptide promotes blood–brain barrier penetration of bioactive molecules. J Mol Biol. 2020;432:3989–4009. doi: 10.1016/j.jmb.2020.04.002.
52. Alam R, AA, AFH, BNA, BD, CL, CGS, CJE, DDA, FRE, et al., Transferrin receptor binding proteins and conjugates. 2024. WIPO Patent No. WO 2024/036096 A2.
53. van den Broek SL, Shalgunov V, Herth MM Transport of nanomedicines across the blood-brain barrier: Challenges and opportunities for imaging and therapy. Biomaterials Advances. 2022;141:213125. doi: 10.1016/j.bioadv.2022.213125.
54. Eyford BA, Singh CSB, Abraham T, Munro L, Choi KB, Hill T, Hildebrandt R, Welch I, Vitalis TZ, Gabathuler R et al. A nanomule peptide carrier delivers siRNA across the intact blood-brain barrier to attenuate ischemic stroke. Front Mol Biosci. 2021;8. doi: 10.3389/fmolb.2021.611367.

55. Zhan T, Han Y, Tang C, Zhao Q, Sun D, Li Y, Jia X, Zhou L, Zhang J Metabolism and biological activity of α-tocopherol derived from vitamin e-enriched transgenic maize in broilers. J Sci Food Agric. 2020;100:4319–4328. doi: 10.1002/jsfa.10480.
56. Zhang X, Gubu A, Xu J, Yan N, Su W, Feng D, Wang Q, Tang X Tetrazine-induced bioorthogonal activation of vitamin e-modified siRNA for Gene silencing. Molecules. 2022;27:4377. doi: 10.3390/molecules27144377.
57. Uno Y, Piao W, Miyata K, Nishina K, Mizusawa H, Yokota T High-density lipoprotein facilitates *in vivo* delivery of α-Tocopherol–Conjugated short-interfering RNA to the brain. Hum Gene Ther. 2011;22:711–719. doi: 10.1089/hum.2010.083.
58. Nikan M, Osborn MF, Coles AH, Godinho BM, Hall LM, Haraszti RA, Hassler MR, Echeverria D, Aronin N, Khvorova A Docosahexaenoic acid conjugation enhances distribution and safety of siRNA upon local administration in mouse brain. Mol Ther Nucleic Acids. 2016;5:e344. doi: 10.1038/mtna.2016.50.
59. Alarcón-Arís D, Recasens A, Galofré M, Carballo-Carbajal I, Zacchi N, Ruiz-Bronchal E, Pavia-Collado R, Chica R, Ferrés-Coy A, Santos M et al. Selective α-synuclein knockdown in monoamine neurons by intranasal oligonucleotide delivery: Potential therapy for Parkinson's disease. Molecular Therapy. 2018;26:550–567. doi: 10.1016/j.ymthe.2017.11.015.
60. Ickenstein LM, Garidel P Lipid-based nanoparticle formulations for small molecules and RNA drugs. Expert Opin Drug Deliv. 2019;16:1205–1226. doi: 10.1080/17425247.2019.1669558.
61. Haddadzadegan S, Dorkoosh F, Bernkop-Schnürch A Oral Delivery of therapeutic peptides and proteins: Technology landscape of lipid-based nanocarriers. Adv Drug Deliv Rev. 2022;182:114097. doi: 10.1016/j.addr.2021.114097.
62. Anthiya S, Öztürk SC, Yanik H, Tavukcuoglu E, Şahin A, Datta D, Charisse K, Álvarez DM, Loza MI, Calvo A et al. Targeted siRNA lipid nanoparticles for the treatment of KRAS-mutant tumors. Journal of Controlled Release. 2023;357:67–83. doi: 10.1016/j.jconrel.2023.03.016.
63. Yonezawa S, Koide H, Asai T Recent advances in siRNA delivery mediated by lipid-based nanoparticles. Adv Drug Deliv Rev. 2020;154–155:64–78. doi: 10.1016/j.addr.2020.07.022.
64. Zhang A, Meng K, Liu Y, Pan Y, Qu W, Chen D, Xie S Absorption, distribution, metabolism, and excretion of nanocarriers in vivo and their influences. Adv Colloid Interface Sci. 2020;284:102261. doi: 10.1016/j.cis.2020.102261.
65. Liu S, Liu J, Li H, Mao K, Wang H, Meng X, Wang J, Wu C, Chen H, Wang X et al. An optimized ionizable cationic lipid for brain tumor-targeted siRNA delivery and glioblastoma immunotherapy. Biomaterials. 2022;287:121645. doi: 10.1016/j.biomaterials.2022.121645.
66. Cheng W, Su Y-L, Hsu H-H, Lin Y-H, Chu L-A, Huang W-C, Lu Y-J, Chiang C-S, Hu S-H Rabies virus glycoprotein-mediated transportation and t cell infiltration to brain tumor by magnetoelectric gold yarnballs. ACS Nano. 2022;16:4014–4027. doi: 10.1021/acsnano.1c09601.
67. Schlich M, Longhena F, Faustini G, O'Driscoll CM, Sinico C, Fadda AM, Bellucci A, Lai F Anionic liposomes for small interfering ribonucleic acid (siRNA) delivery to primary neuronal cells: Evaluation of alpha-synuclein knockdown efficacy. Nano Res. 2017;10:3496–3508. doi: 10.1007/s12274-017-1561-z.
68. Chen Z-L, Huang M, Wang X-R, Fu J, Han M, Shen Y-Q, Xia Z, Gao J-Q Transferrin-modified liposome promotes α-mangostin to penetrate the blood–brain barrier. Nanomedicine. 2016;12:421–430. doi: 10.1016/j.nano.2015.10.021.
69. Abujamai J, Satar R, Ansari SA Designing and formulation of nanocarriers for "Alzheimer's and Parkinson's" early detection and therapy. CNS Neurol Disord Drug Targets. 2024;23:1251–1262. doi: 10.2174/0118715273297024240201055550.

70. Maussang D, Rip J, van Kregten J, van den Heuvel A, van der Pol S, van der Boom B, Reijerkerk A, Chen L, de Boer M, Gaillard P et al. Glutathione conjugation dose-dependently increases brain-specific liposomal drug delivery in vitro and in vivo. Drug Discov Today Technol. 2016;20:59–69. doi: 10.1016/j.ddtec.2016.09.003.
71. Khare P, Edgecomb SX, Hamadani CM, Tanner EEL, Manickam D Lipid nanoparticle-mediated drug delivery to the brain. Adv Drug Deliv Rev. 2023;197:114861. doi: 10.1016/j.addr.2023.114861.
72. Sun D, Lu Z-R Structure and function of cationic and ionizable lipids for nucleic acid delivery. Pharm Res. 2023;40:27–46. doi: 10.1007/s11095-022-03460-2.
73. Ahmed T Lipid nanoparticle mediated small interfering RNA delivery as a potential therapy for Alzheimer's disease. European Journal of Neuroscience. 2024;59:2915–2954. doi: 10.1111/ejn.16336.
74. Kargaard A, Sluijter JPG, Klumperman B Polymeric siRNA gene delivery – Transfection efficiency versus cytotoxicity. Journal of Controlled Release. 2019;316:263–291. doi: 10.1016/j.jconrel.2019.10.046.
75. Ita K Polyplexes for gene and nucleic acid delivery: Progress and bottlenecks. European Journal of Pharmaceutical Sciences. 2020;150:105358. doi: 10.1016/j.ejps.2020.105358.
76. Gorzkiewicz M, Kopeć O, Janaszewska A, Konopka M, Pędziwiatr-Werbicka E, Tarasenko II, Bezrodnyi VV, Neelov IM, Klajnert-Maculewicz B Poly(lysine) dendrimers form complexes with siRNA and provide its efficient uptake by myeloid cells: Model studies for therapeutic nucleic acid delivery. Int J Mol Sci. 2020;21:3138. doi: 10.3390/ijms21093138.
77. Yang X, Yang W, Xia X, Lei T, Yang Z, Jia W, Zhou Y, Cheng G, Gao H Intranasal delivery of BACE1 siRNA and rapamycin by dual targets modified nanoparticles for Alzheimer's disease therapy. Small. 2022;18. doi: 10.1002/smll.202203182.
78. Lu Z-G, Shen J, Yang J, Wang J-W, Zhao R-C, Zhang T-L, Guo J, Zhang X Nucleic acid drug vectors for diagnosis and treatment of brain diseases. Signal Transduct Target Ther. 2023;8:39. doi: 10.1038/s41392-022-01298-z.
79. Yan L, Gao S, Shui S, Liu S, Qu H, Liu C, Zheng L Small interfering RNA-loaded chitosan hydrochloride/carboxymethyl chitosan nanoparticles for ultrasound-triggered release to hamper colorectal cancer growth in vitro. Int J Biol Macromol. 2020;162:1303–1310. doi: 10.1016/j.ijbiomac.2020.06.246.
80. Redhwan MAM, Samaddar S, Bafail DA, Hard SAAA, Guha S Chitosan/siRNA nanoparticles targeting PARP-1 attenuate neuroinflammation and apoptosis in hyperglycemia-induced oxidative stress in Neuro2a cells. Int J Biol Macromol. 2024;282:136964. doi: 10.1016/j.ijbiomac.2024.136964.
81. Sava V, Fihurka O, Khvorova A, Sanchez-Ramos J Enriched chitosan nanoparticles loaded with siRNA are effective in lowering Huntington's disease gene expression following intranasal administration. Nanomedicine. 2020;24:102119. doi: 10.1016/j.nano.2019.102119.
82. Gao Y, Wang Z-Y, Zhang J, Zhang Y, Huo H, Wang T, Jiang T, Wang S RVG-peptide-linked trimethylated chitosan for delivery of siRNA to the brain. Biomacromolecules. 2014;15:1010–1018. doi: 10.1021/bm401906p.
83. Malhotra M, Tomaro-Duchesneau C, Prakash S Synthesis of TAT peptide-tagged PEGylated chitosan nanoparticles for siRNA delivery targeting neurodegenerative diseases. Biomaterials. 2013;34:1270–1280. doi: 10.1016/j.biomaterials.2012.10.013.
84. Sanchez-Ramos J, Song S, Kong X, Foroutan P, Martinez G, Dominguez-Viqueria W, Mohapatra S, Mohapatra S, Haraszti RA, Khvorova A et al. Chitosan-mangafodipir nanoparticles designed for intranasal delivery of siRNA and DNA to brain. J Drug Deliv Sci Technol. 2018;43:453–460. doi: 10.1016/j.jddst.2017.11.013.
85. Pei M, Xu R, Zhang C, Wang X, Li C, Hu Y Mannose-functionalized antigen nanoparticles for targeted dendritic cells, accelerated endosomal escape and enhanced MHC-i antigen presentation. Colloids Surf B Biointerfaces. 2021;197:111378. doi: 10.1016/j.colsurfb.2020.111378.

86. Cao M, Gao Y, Qiu N, Shen Y, Shen P Folic acid directly modified low molecular weight of polyethyleneimine for targeted pDNA delivery. J Drug Deliv Sci Technol. 2020;56:101522. doi: 10.1016/j.jddst.2020.101522.
87. Park T-E, Singh B, Li H, Lee J-Y, Kang S-K, Choi Y-J, Cho C-S Enhanced BBB permeability of osmotically active poly(mannitol-co-PEI) modified with rabies virus glycoprotein via selective stimulation of caveolar endocytosis for RNAi therapeutics in Alzheimer's disease. Biomaterials. 2015;38:61–71. doi: 10.1016/j.biomaterials.2014.10.068.
88. Zhou Y, Zhu F, Liu Y, Zheng M, Wang Y, Zhang D, Anraku Y, Zou Y, Li J, Wu H et al. Blood-brain barrier–penetrating siRNA nanomedicine for Alzheimer's disease therapy. Sci Adv. 2020;6. doi: 10.1126/sciadv.abc7031.
89. Chen Z, Huang W, Zheng N, Bai Y Design and synthesis of a polyguanidium vector with enhanced DNA binding ability for effective gene delivery at a low N/P ratio. Polym Chem. 2020;11:664–668. doi: 10.1039/C9PY01481K.
90. Kubczak M, Michlewska S, Karimov M, Ewe A, Noske S, Aigner A, Bryszewska M, Ionov M Unmodified and tyrosine-modified polyethylenimines as potential carriers for siRNA: Biophysical characterization and toxicity. Int J Pharm. 2022;614:121468. doi: 10.1016/j.ijpharm.2022.121468.
91. Gurung S, Perocheau D, Touramanidou L, Baruteau J The exosome journey: From biogenesis to uptake and intracellular signalling. Cell Communication and Signaling. 2021;19:47. doi: 10.1186/s12964-021-00730-1.
92. Amiri A, Bagherifar R, Ansari Dezfouli E, Kiaie SH, Jafari R, Ramezani R Exosomes as bio-inspired nanocarriers for RNA delivery: Preparation and applications. J Transl Med. 2022;20:125. doi: 10.1186/s12967-022-03325-7.
93. Alvarez-Erviti L, Seow Y, Yin H, Betts C, Lakhal S, Wood MJA Delivery of siRNA to the mouse brain by systemic injection of targeted exosomes. Nat Biotechnol. 2011;29:341–345. doi: 10.1038/nbt.1807.
94. Li J, Peng H, Zhang W, Li M, Wang N, Peng C, Zhang X, Li Y Enhanced nose-to-brain delivery of combined small interfering RNAs using lesion-recognizing nanoparticles for the synergistic therapy of Alzheimer's disease. ACS Appl Mater Interfaces. 2023;15:53177–53188. doi: 10.1021/acsami.3c08756.
95. Chen Y-A, Lu C-H, Ke C-C, Chiu S-J, Jeng F-S, Chang C-W, Yang B-H, Liu R-S Mesenchymal stem cell-derived exosomes ameliorate Alzheimer's disease pathology and improve cognitive deficits. Biomedicines. 2021;9:594. doi: 10.3390/biomedicines 9060594.
96. Fu Z, Zhang X, Zhou X, Ur-Rehman U, Yu M, Liang H, Guo H, Guo X, Kong Y, Su Y et al. In vivo self-assembled small RNAs as a new generation of RNAi therapeutics. Cell Res. 2021;31:631–648. doi: 10.1038/s41422-021-00491-z.
97. Limoni SK, Moghadam MF, Moazzeni SM, Gomari H, Salimi F Engineered exosomes for targeted transfer of siRNA to HER2 positive breast cancer cells. Appl Biochem Biotechnol. 2019;187:352–364. doi: 10.1007/s12010-018-2813-4.
98. Kang SS, Wu Z, Liu X, Edgington-Mitchell L, Ye K Treating Parkinson's disease via activation of BDNF/TrkB signaling pathways and inhibition of delta-secretase. Neurotherapeutics. 2022;19:1283–1297. doi: 10.1007/s13311-022-01248-1.
99. Zhang W, Hong J, Zheng W, Liu A, Yang Y High glucose exacerbates neuroinflammation and apoptosis at the intermediate stage after post-traumatic brain injury. Aging. 2021;13:16088–16104. doi: 10.18632/aging.203136.
100. Amaldoss MJN, Yang J-L, Koshy P, Unnikrishnan A, Sorrell CC Inorganic nanoparticle-based advanced cancer therapies: Promising combination strategies. Drug Discov Today. 2022;27:103386. doi: 10.1016/j.drudis.2022.103386.
101. Yan C, Zhang J, Huang M, Xiao J, Li N, Wang T, Ling R Design, strategies, and therapeutics in nanoparticle-based siRNA delivery systems for breast cancer. J Mater Chem B. 2023;11:8096–8116. doi: 10.1039/D3TB00278K.

102. Dalmina M, Pittella F, Sierra JA, Souza GRR, Silva AH, Pasa AA, Creczynski-Pasa TB Magnetically responsive hybrid nanoparticles for in vitro siRNA delivery to breast cancer cells. Materials Science and Engineering: C. 2019;99:1182–1190. doi: 10.1016/j.msec.2019.02.026.
103. Israel LL, Galstyan A, Holler E, Ljubimova JY Magnetic iron oxide nanoparticles for imaging, targeting and treatment of primary and metastatic tumors of the brain. Journal of Controlled Release. 2020;320:45–62. doi: 10.1016/j.jconrel.2020.01.009.
104. Carrillo-Jimenez A, Puigdellívol M, Vilalta A, Venero JL, Brown GC, StGeorge-Hyslop P, Burguillos MA Effective knockdown of Gene expression in primary microglia with siRNA and magnetic nanoparticles without cell death or inflammation. Front Cell Neurosci. 2018;12. doi: 10.3389/fncel.2018.00313.
105. Laurent N, Sapet C, Le Gourrierec L, Bertosio E, Zelphati O Nucleic acid delivery using magnetic nanoparticles: The Magnetofection™ technology. Ther Deliv. 2011;2:471–482. doi: 10.4155/tde.11.12.
106. Panda SK, Aggarwal I, Kumar H, Prasad L, Kumar A, Sharma A, Vo D-VN, Van Thuan D, Mishra V Magnetite nanoparticles as sorbents for dye removal: A review. Environ Chem Lett. 2021;19:2487–2525. doi: 10.1007/s10311-020-01173-9.
107. Lopez-Barbosa N, Garcia JG, Cifuentes J, Castro LM, Vargas F, Ostos C, Cardona-Gomez GP, Hernandez AM, Cruz JC Multifunctional magnetite nanoparticles to enable delivery of siRNA for the potential treatment of Alzheimer's. Drug Deliv. 2020;27:864–875. doi: 10.1080/10717544.2020.1775724.
108. Amina SJ, Guo B A review on the synthesis and functionalization of gold nanoparticles as a drug delivery vehicle. Int J Nanomedicine. 2020;15:9823–9857. doi: 10.2147/IJN.S279094.
109. Chou JJ, Berger AG, Jalili-Firoozinezhad S, Hammond PT A design approach for layer-by-layer surface-mediated siRNA delivery. Acta Biomater. 2021;135:331–341. doi: 10.1016/j.actbio.2021.08.042.
110. Chaudhary A, Garg S siRNA delivery using polyelectrolyte-gold nanoassemblies in neuronal cells for BACE1 gene silencing. Materials Science and Engineering: C. 2017;80:18–28. doi: 10.1016/j.msec.2017.05.101.
111. Karmakar AK, Hasan MdS, Sreemani A, Das Jayanta A, Hasan MM, Tithe NA, Biswas P A review on the current progress of layered double hydroxide application in biomedical sectors. The European Physical Journal Plus. 2022;137:801. doi: 10.1140/epjp/s13360-022-02993-0.
112. de Araújo MA, dos Santos Júnior ED, dos Santos BP, dos Santos YDR, Paulino PAT, dos Santos EC, Souza TPM, Anhezini L, Bassi ÊJ, Duzzioni M et al. Layered double hydroxides (LDHs) as efficient and safe carriers for miRNA inhibitors: In vitro and in vivo assessment of biocompatibility. Chem Biol Interact. 2024;391:110874. doi: 10.1016/j.cbi.2024.110874.
113. Li X, Han Z, Wang T, Ma C, Li H, Lei H, Yang Y, Wang Y, Pei Z, Liu Z et al. Cerium oxide nanoparticles with antioxidative neurorestoration for ischemic stroke. Biomaterials. 2022;291:121904. doi: 10.1016/j.biomaterials.2022.121904.
114. Naz S, Beach J, Heckert B, Tummala T, Pashchenko O, Banerjee T, Santra S Cerium oxide nanoparticles: A 'radical' approach to neurodegenerative disease treatment. Nanomedicine. 2017;12:545–553. doi: 10.2217/nnm-2016-0399.

13 Engineering Nanoparticles in Drug Delivery for Alzheimer's Disease Treatment

Divya Bisht, Deena Prakash, and Oshin Verma

13.1 INTRODUCTION

Alzheimer's disease (AD) is a chronic neurodegenerative disorder emerging as a medical challenge globally. AD has characteristic symptoms of memory loss, progressive cognitive impairment, and behavioral changes in the patient. It is commonly seen in elderly people, significantly declining the quality of life along with emotional and economic damage to the family and medical system. Its extensive prevalence encouraged researchers to study about this disorder however the precise etiology of AD is yet to be known. The studies however showed the involvement of diverse complicated mechanisms accounting for the onset and progression of AD including amyloid-beta (Aβ) plaque accumulation, neurofibrillary tangles of hyperphosphorylated tau proteins, chronic neuroinflammation, and oxidative stress as the major ones. The management of AD poses serious challenge as the conventional treatment methods focus completely on suppressing the symptoms providing temporary relief to the patient rather than emphasizing on prevention, control and cure of this neurodegenerative disorder. This gives rise to the need to develop more effective treatment alternatives focusing on holistic therapeutic approaches (Kumar et al., 2015; Chopra et al., 2022; Tatulian, 2022).

In this quest of improved treatment method, nanomedicine emerges as a promising candidate working with combination of nanotechnology and medicine, paving path to address the challenges in the treatment of AD. Application of nanomaterial in the treatment offers properties like small size, high surface area-to-volume ratio, and ability to be functionalized for the diagnosis, treatment, and management of AD. Due to their small size (1 to 100 nanometers), nanoparticles easily penetrate the blood–brain barrier (BBB) which act as a major obstacle for other therapeutic methods, preventing them to reach the brain. This characteristic of nanoparticles opens avenues of potentially precise target-specific drug delivery and treatment of various neurodegenerative disorders with enhanced drug bioavailability, reduced instances of side effects, and better therapeutic benefits (Nguyen et al., 2023).

DOI: 10.1201/9781003543381-13

Nanomedicine is the best alternative treatment for AD keeping in consideration the complex pathology of AD as nanoparticles can be customized to deliver various medicinal agents increasing the treatment options and success rate significantly. These medicinal agents can range from traditional drug options to small interfering RNA (siRNA), antisense oligonucleotides, neuroprotective peptides, and various other alternatives which show protective properties for the neural region. Apart from the therapeutic application of nanomedicine, nanoparticles can play a significant role in diagnosis of neurodegenerative diseases as well. Nanotechnology can be used to deliver specific imaging agents and biosensors with high sensitivity facilitating the early diagnosis of AD aiding the timely management of disease.

With recent advancements in nanotechnology, the development of multifunctional nanoparticles facilitates both the diagnosis and treatment of diseases. For example, theranostic nanoparticles are well utilized for their dual functionality as diagnostic and therapeutic agents. This facilitates real-time monitoring as well as treatment of disease. Treatment options like photothermal and photodynamic therapies using photosensitive nanoparticles which get activated in light can be used as cotherapy along with the conventional treatment options. Antioxidant-rich nanoparticles offer another novel treatment method to mitigate oxidative stress-related damage as oxidative damage plays key role in AD-related neuronal damage (Tatulian, 2022; Hu et al., 2023).

All these characteristics of nanomedicine indicate potential applications in the treatment of neurodegenerative diseases. However, this comes with various challenges including the manufacturing hurdles, safety and efficacy issues, regulatory issues, etc. The complex pathology of AD further contributes to these challenges. Nevertheless, the beneficial properties of nanomedicines outweigh all these challenges encouraging the researchers to explore the potential of nanomedicine in the treatment of AD (Khan et al., 2021).

This chapter discusses the promising presence of nanomedicine in the treatment of AD emerging as a potential treatment alternative for AD management. Various aspects of nanomedicine are discussed including types of nanoparticles, various functions, role in diagnosis and treatment, challenges in application of nanomedicines in management of AD, and future prospective of nanomedicine as an effective alternative treatment option.

13.2 ALZHEIMER'S DISEASE & ITS PATHOPHYSIOLOGY

AD is a common disorder in elderly patients progressing as the leading cause of dementia worldwide accounting for 60–70% of cases. It was first reported in 1906 by Dr. Alios Alzheimer and was named after him. AD was defined with combined characteristics of memory loss, behavioral changes, and cognitive dysfunction collectively resulting into difficulty in everyday life, dependency on other people, and death on progression in old age people. With increasing cases of AD every year, this disease demands effective prevention, timely diagnosis, and efficient treatment strategies posing a challenge to the healthcare system (Tatulian, 2022).

The complex mechanism of AD with interplay of various pathological pathways leads to cognitive dysfunction and impairment of memory in elderly people.

Multifactorial causes of AD include genetic factors, environmental factors, and lifestyle factors collectively accounting for the onset and progression of AD. AD progresses by the accumulation of Aβ plaques, tau protein tangles, inflammation in the brain, and neuronal loss (Kumar et al., 2015; Abubakar et al., 2022).

Amyloid cascade hypothesis is one of the popular hypotheses regarding the pathophysiology of AD focusing on the disruption of equilibrium between the production of Aβ peptides and its clearance from the system which leads to accumulation of these peptides starting the cascade to various pathways leading to onset of AD. These peptides originate on the breakdown of amyloid precursor protein by beta-secretase and gamma-secretase enzymes. The aggregation of Aβ peptides forms plaque in the extracellular matrix of brain initiating the loss of normal neuronal function and onset of toxic processes like oxidative stress and inflammation in the brain (Hardy & Higgins, 1992; Kametani & Hasegawa, 2018).

Tau protein is another important component playing key role in the pathology of AD. This microtubule-associated protein regulates the stability of microtubules in the neurons in normal conditions. However, in AD phosphorylation of these tau proteins leads to the detachment from microtubules forming tangles of tau protein in the neurons. These tangles disrupt cellular transportation causing synaptic dysfunction and neuronal death (Kametani & Hasegawa, 2018).

The accumulation of both Aβ peptides and tau protein tangles triggers the inflammatory response in the brain activating the immune cells like microglia and astrocytes. The immune cells on activation release pro-inflammatory cytokines and reactive oxygen species which contribute to neuronal damage and dysfunction. Prolonged inflammation further exacerbates AD creating a vicious cycle of neuronal damage and accumulation of Aβ peptides and tau protein tangles continuously contributing to the AD (Kametani & Hasegawa, 2018).

Reactive oxygen species released due to inflammation further leads to mitochondrial dysfunction and oxidative stress contributing to the progression of AD. Mitochondrial dysfunction leads to decline in ATP generation and increased free radical production causing damage to crucial cellular components like nucleic acids, proteins, and lipids leading to overall cellular disintegration. Oxidative stress also amplifies the toxic impact of Aβ and tau in AD patients (Rojas-Gutierrez et al., 2017).

Another hypothesis of AD pathophysiology is the cholinergic hypothesis which credits the decline in neurotransmitter acetylcholine as a cause of cognitive dysfunction in AD as this neurotransmitter controls the function of learning and memory in the brain. This deficit of acetylcholine is suggested to be due to the neuronal damage in basal forebrain where production of acetylcholine takes place (Hampel et al., 2019).

Overall, the collective effect of Aβ plaque, tau protein tangles, chronic inflammation, oxidative stress, and neuronal loss cause the onset and progression of damage in the brain inhibiting the neuronal regulation of memory and cognitive function operated at the hippocampus and cerebral cortex region of brain. This leads to memory loss, difficulty in coherent speech, and loss of independence in day-to-day life (Kumar et al., 2015; Abubakar et al., 2022).

13.3 DIAGNOSIS AND TREATMENT OF ALZHEIMER'S DISEASE: A CHALLENGE

AD is a challenge in terms of both its diagnosis and management due to its complex pathology, slow progression, and lack of positive response toward the existing treatment options. The onset and initial progression of AD are silent and non-noticeable years before the symptoms appear on surface. Also, the symptoms are often confused with aging and other neurological conditions making the diagnosis a challenge to the medical professionals. Another challenge is the variable expression of AD in patients. Non-uniform symptoms and heterogeneity of expression complicated the diagnosis further. Diagnostic option at biomarker level includes the imaging of cerebrospinal fluid and positron emission tomography (PET) are available, however their high charges make them difficult to be accessed by patients of low-income group. Therefore, all these complications give rise to urgent demand for more accessible, affordable, and efficient diagnostic options (Khan et al., 2021; Tatulian, 2022).

Similarly, treatment of AD is another challenge due to its complicated pathophysiology as one of the main reasons as it's difficult to treat and correct multiple processes at the same time. However, the site of disease also makes the treatment of AD difficult due to the presence of BBB. BBB is a protective shield between the brain and various therapeutic agents making it difficult for these agents to reach the site and start its effect. The current treatment options focus on suppressing the symptoms rather than working on the root cause of AD, only improving the memory and cognitive function of patients. These treatment methods don't check or reverse the progression of AD. Many of the currently used drugs like cholinesterase inhibitors and N-methyl-D-aspartate (NMDA) receptor antagonists trigger various side effects in patients limiting the application of conventional treatment options further. Therefore, the journey of development of new treatment options against AD must focus on BBB and other challenges for better efficiency and higher success rate in patients (Chopra et al., 2022; Hu et al., 2023).

13.4 NEED FOR BETTER TREATMENT OPTIONS

There is a critical need for better treatment alternatives to AD as the current options having therapeutic effects limited to symptom suppression. Delayed diagnosis of AD by conventional diagnostic tools along with failed therapies pose challenges in management of AD. Nanomedicine emerges as a treatment modality with significant potential with early diagnosis through advanced imaging techniques, effective drug-delivery across the BBB, precise multi-target therapies for complex pathology of AD. Nanotechnology loads therapeutic agents with nanocarriers revolutionizing the treatment of AD. Nanomedicine improve patient outcomes with significant neuroprotection leading to effective management of AD (Se Thoe et al., 2021).

13.5 NANOMEDICINE & ITS KEY FEATURES

Nanomedicine as the name suggests is a combination of nanotechnology and medicine combining the principles of nanotechnology and therapeutic properties of various components leading to advanced methods of diagnosis and treatment of various diseases. Nanomedicine with its small size merely ranging from 1 to 100 nanometers provides them with unique physical, chemical, and biological properties to overcome the various challenges researchers face with conventional medicines (Khan et al., 2021; Chopra et al., 2022).

The characteristic features of nanomedicine that make them a promising candidate for the treatment of AD include nanoscale size, targeted drug delivery system, property to pass BBB, multifunctionality, biocompatibility, lesser side-effects and scope of customization for as per the disease and patient requirements (De Matteis et al., 2018; Soares et al., 2018).

- **Size**: The material used in nanomedicine ranges from 1 to 100 nanometers in size, increasing the chances of them interacting better at cellular and molecular level in the body of patient enhancing the therapeutic outcome against diseases.
- **Drug-delivery**: Target-specific and precise drug delivery is another key feature of nanomedicines increasing the chances of effective treatment also reducing the side effects at the nearby regions in the body. Nanomedicines activate against specific stimuli in patients like certain pH level or in presence of specific biomarkers, making the drug delivery more precise and effective.
- **Permeability to BBB**: The biggest challenge in the treatment of AD is BBB as most conventional medicines fail to cross this barrier thus showing no improvement against AD. Nanomedicines can be specifically designed to cross the BBB increasing its effectiveness many folds.
- **Multifunctionality**: Nanotechnology allow the researchers to integrate multiple therapeutic properties in a single nanomedicine at time combining the diagnostic and treatment feature together enabling the same drug to monitor and cure the disease at the same time. Another example can be a nanomedicine that has both antioxidants and anti-inflammatory properties to combat both inflammation and oxidative stress simultaneously.
- **Biocompatibility**: Nanomedicines are specifically designed using biocompatible materials to avoid toxic immune responses in patients. Small size and biocompatibility aid in better distribution and absorption of these medicines in the body simultaneously reducing the occurrence of adverse effects.
- **Controlled drug release**: Nanomedicine allows the gradual release of drug over a period increasing the therapeutic effect in fewer doses of drug enhancing patient compliance and experience.
- **Customization**: As AD has varied symptoms and effect on different patient, nanomedicine allow a more personalized treatment option with drug and its delivery more tailored to the needs of individual.

13.6 TYPES OF NANOPARTICLES USED IN NANOMEDICINE

Nanomedicines are made of a variety of nanoparticles with diverse characteristics selected according to the requirement of different diseases. The most common types of nanoparticles are polymeric nanoparticles, gold nanoparticles, liposomes, dendrimers, carbon-based nanoparticles, quantum dots, etc.

- **Liposomes**: These are spherical vesicles with lipid bilayer used to deliver both hydrophilic and hydrophobic drugs due to their biocompatibility and property of enhance solubility and stability of drug encapsulated.
- **Polymeric nanoparticles**: These are biodegradable polymers known for their feature of controlled drug release. The common polymer used is poly(lactic-co-glycolic acid) PLGA. These nanoparticles are widely used in drug delivery, gene therapy, and vaccine development.
- **Dendrimers**: As the name indicates these are branched, tree-like structures with large surface area for drug attachment. Dendrimers are utilized for their property to carry multiple therapeutic agents simultaneously. Their surface can also be modified with specific ligands facilitation targeted drug delivery.
- **Gold nanoparticles**: These nanoparticles are mainly used for easy synthesis, significant stability, and versatile functionality with different biomarkers. Gold nanoparticles are currently used in diagnosis, imaging and drug delivery with great success in cancer treatment.
- **Quantum dots**: These are semiconductor nanocrystals with special fluorescent properties making them suitable for imaging and diagnostic purposes. Quantum dots are used for various purposes like tracking drug delivery, detection of biomarker, and imaging for diagnosis.
- **Carbon-based nanoparticles**: Most commonly used carbon-based nanoparticles are carbon nanotubes and graphene oxide for their applications in drug delivery system, as biosensors in diagnostics and imagining.
- **Magnetic nanoparticles**: As the name suggests, these are nanoparticles with magnetic properties, so they can be manipulated using magnetic field from outside the patient body. made of materials like iron oxide and used in targeted drug delivery and imaging techniques like MRI and hyperthermia therapy.
- **Silica nanoparticles**: These are porous nanoparticles made of silica providing a large area for loading of desired drug of choice, and the large surface helps in targeting specific tissues and cells.
- **Solid lipid nanoparticles (SLNs)**: These lipid nanoparticles are composed of solid lipids and provide dual advantage combining the features of both liposomes and polymeric nanoparticles. There nanoparticles are used to deliver controlled amount of hydrophilic or hydrophobic drugs to the target cell/tissues.

These are some common nanoparticles widely used in nanomedicine development. Each with their own peculiar features and limitations, thus the selection of compatible nanoparticles is important in alignment with the disease characteristics, site of drug delivery, individual patient body requirements, etc. (Yohan & Chithrani, 2014; Abdel-Mageed et al., 2021; Chopra et al., 2022).

13.7 ROLE OF NANOMEDICINE IN HEALTHCARE

Nanomedicines have significantly revolutionized the medicine world with enhanced diagnostic and imaging techniques facilitating early detection of lethal diseases and specific onsite delivery of drugs and real-time monitoring of the recovery helping healthcare system in better management of diseases like cancer, neurodegenerative diseases, and cardiovascular disorders. Some of the important applications of nanomedicine are mentioned below:

- **Target-specific drug delivery**: One of the most crucial uses of nanomedicine is drug delivery to specific sites (cells/tissue effected by disease), thus enhancing the efficacy of treatment and reducing the side effects of drug to nearby regions. Nanoparticles of choice for drug-delivery include liposomes, dendrimers, and gold nanoparticles due to their adaptability to target various diseases, particular sites, and specific biomarkers. This property of nanomedicine ensures target delivery, improved treatment outcome, and reduced damage to patient's body.
- **Vaccine development**: Another important role of nanomedicine is in vaccine development. Nanoparticles are designed to carry vaccine with the aim to improve the immune system. Antigens are loaded on the nanoparticles and delivered to the immune cells to boost immunity and the body's defense system. Popular nanovaccines used are against malaria, cancer, influenza, etc. to name a few.
- **Implant development**: Drug and hormonal implants are another important tool of nanomedicine. Nanoparticles are embedded in devices and implants to release therapeutic agents for prolonged duration specifically for patients requiring continuous medication. These implants ensure regular controlled release of drugs for real-time management and improved outcomes.
- **Imaging and diagnosis**: Nanomedicine brings incredible advancement in diagnostic imaging techniques. Nanoparticles like quantum dots, magnetic nanoparticles, gold nanoparticles, etc., are employed for imaging at molecular level, helping early diagnosis and real-time monitoring of diseases like cancer, Alzheimer's, and many cardiovascular disorders. Nanoparticles bind precisely to specific biomarkers for the specific, non-invasive detection and monitoring of disease and drug-delivery progression.
- **Medicine customization**: Nanomedicine offers the unique and innovative feature of personalized medicine tailored as per the genetic, molecular, and disease profile of a patient in particular thus enhancing the therapeutic outcomes as well as customized monitoring of disease-specific to an individual's need facilitating the adjustment of treatment as per requirement and minimizing the adverse effect of these modalities on healthy regions surrounding the diseased area.
- **Gene therapy**: Another remarkable application of nanomedicine is in the form of gene therapy. Nanocarriers deliver therapeutic genes and nucleic acid to the target cells to treat genetic disorders, cancer, and viral infections. Lipid nanoparticles and dendrimers are the nanoparticles of choice to avoid degradation of genetic material with facilitated entry to the specific site producing desired therapeutic effects.

Extensive application of nanomedicine is transforming the world of healthcare, improving the methods of diagnosis, monitoring, and drug delivery. Improved diagnostic tools and tailored therapeutic options offer effective treatment modalities ultimately improving the patient outcome and reducing the burden of various diseases on the healthcare system (Pautler & Brenner, 2010; De Matteis et al., 2018; Delbreil et al., 2022).

13.8 NANOMEDICINE AND ALZHEIMER'S DISEASE

Neurodegenerative diseases like Alzheimer's, Parkinson's, and Huntington's disease are a challenge to healthcare due to the unavailability of effective treatment options. Nanomedicine serves as a promising alternative as it can be engineered to pass the BBB. In brain, these nanomedicines can deliver wide range of therapeutic agents like drugs, genes, and anti-inflammatory and antioxidant agents, directly to the affected site. Nanomedicine also plays a crucial role in imaging and diagnosis of neurodegenerative disease (Khan et al., 2021; Hu et al., 2023).

AD is a complex neurodegenerative disorder with multifactorial pathogenesis making it difficult for the existing treatment modalities to treat this disease effectively. This creates a gap between the incidence of AD and its cure increasing the burden of AD population on healthcare system and decrease quality and expectancy of patient's life. AD treatment needs to address the accumulation of Aβ, tangled tau protein, oxidative stress, and inflammation in the brain. Due to these multiple factors, conventional drugs find it difficult to address these factors simultaneously. Nanomedicine offers tailored treatment to this multifactorial disease with an advanced drug delivery system, improved diagnostic tools, and multifunctional therapeutic options. This chapter dives into the application of nanomedicine in management of AD focusing on the diagnosis, monitoring, and drug delivery (Binda et al., 2020; Chopra et al., 2022).

13.8.1 Nanoparticles in Alzheimer's Disease

As discussed earlier in this chapter, there is a wide range of nanoparticles with their unique and versatile characteristic features. Their small size, varied shapes and other features make them suitable for numerous applications by engineering them with in alignment with different diseases and tailoring them as per individual patients need. Different drugs and other medicinal agents are encapsulated in these nanoparticles to be delivered at the desired destinations in the body. Different nanoparticles are used for the diagnosis and treatment of AD, like liposomes, polymeric nanoparticles, dendrimers, gold nanoparticles, and SLNs as shown in Figure 13.1 (Gupta et al., 2019).

- **Liposomes**: The nanoparticles are loaded with neuroprotective agents targeting various pathological factors like anti-Aβ drugs, or modified with ligands that specifically bind to particular biomarkers of AD in the brain. This ensures targeted treatment with onsite drug delivery. These nanoparticles enhance bioavailability of drug increasing its stability and solubility.
- **Polymeric nanoparticles**: These nanoparticles deliver therapeutic agents like proteins, genes, and other drug molecules for the treatment of Alzheimer's. These nanoparticles are engineered to pass through the BBB and deliver the drug inside the brain and attached antibodies/peptides help in the targeted delivery.

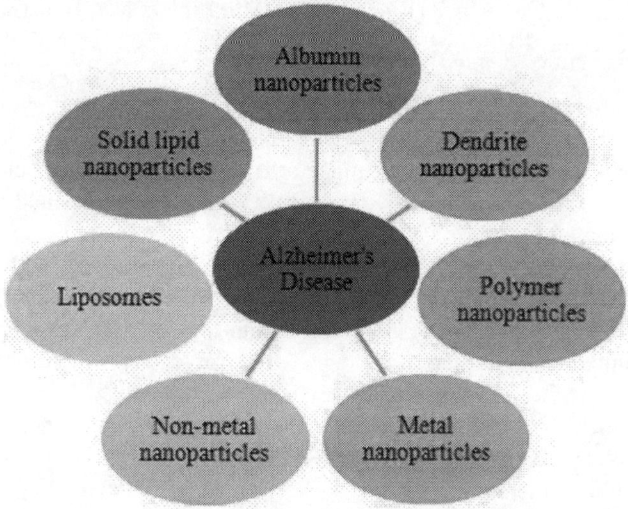

FIGURE 13.1 Commonly used nanoparticles for Alzheimer's disease.

- **Dendrimers**: Dendrimer also have the capacity to cross the BBB making them ideal for the drug delivery in neurodegenerative diseases like Alzheimer's. These nanoparticles encapsulated with drugs and bioactive molecules can be used to target the biomarkers of AD as attachment site delivering precise neuroprotective drug, anti-inflammatory and antioxidant agents combating AD.
- **Gold nanoparticles**: Another potential choice of nanoparticles includes gold nanoparticles due to their characteristic optical and electronic properties as well as their efficacy with wide range of treatment agents for easy encapsulation and delivery. These nanoparticles in AD treatment can be linked with the ligands specific to amyloid plaques or tau tangles, allowing for targeted drug delivery with reduced side effects.
- **SLNs**: These are nanoparticles well known for their high stability and unique properties of controlled drug release making them a great choice for long-term treatments. They can be engineered to cross the BBB and deliver drug to the brain site.

All these nanoparticles are modulated using nanotechnology as per the needs of specific neurodegenerative disorders and also the individual patient molecular, cellular, and genetic requirements (Khan et al., 2021; Hu et al., 2023).

13.9 ADVANTAGES OF NANOMEDICINE IN ALZHEIMER'S TREATMENT

There are various challenges for convention drugs in the treatment of AD, which give rise to the need of alternative treatment options. Nanomedicine considered as a potential candidate as it has numerous properties that are advantageous over the current drugs available for AD (Binda et al., 2020; Ling et al., 2021; Delbreil et al., 2022; Puranik et al., 2023).

- **BBB penetration**: BBB is a major challenge in the treatment of any brain-related disease. It checks the passage of any foreign material to protect the brain from any possible damage or dysfunction. Nanoparticles due to the small size are engineered specifically to pass the BBB and treat AD effectively.
- **Targeted drug delivery**: Nanoparticles can be attached with specific ligands to ensure their attachment to particular biomarkers important in the pathology of AD, like Aβ plaques, tau tangles, oxidative stress, and inflammatory biomarkers. This makes the drug-delivery more precise and effective.
- **Controlled drug release**: One special advantage of using nanoparticles in drug delivery is their ability to release drug gradually over a period of time for sustained therapy with lesser dosage. This makes the treatment process more convenient for the patient.
- **Multifunction drug delivery**: Another special feature of nanomedicine is their capacity to deliver multiple therapeutic agents at the same time focusing on multiple pathological conditions. This multifunctional drug delivery is beneficial in the treatment of AD, which has several factors contributing to its pathology.
- **Enhance solubility and stability**: Therapeutic agents delivered encapsulated in the nanoparticles have better bioavailability as these nanoparticles increase the solubility and stability of these agents thus improving the treatment outcomes.

13.10 TREATMENT METHODS WITH NANOMEDICINE FOR ALZHEIMER'S DISEASE

13.10.1 Nanomedicine in Gene Therapy for Alzheimer's Disease

Gene therapy is the treatment by alteration of genetic material in patient to change/inhibit expression of certain gene and thus curing the disease at the grass-root level. AD as discussed has multifactorial pathology with complex interlinked mechanism of onset and progression of this neurodegenerative disorder. Gene therapy in case of AD targets different genetic or molecular mechanisms to alter its progression. Nanomedicine due to their specific modifications can pass the BBB and deliver the therapeutic gene directly to the effected cells. Gene therapy aims to remove the defective genes, regulate the Aβ production to prevent its accumulation, enhance neurogenesis by delivering different therapeutic gene into the affected region of brain using nanocarriers. Gene therapy with nanomedicine use plasmid DNA/RNA encapsulated with nanocarriers to prevent its degradation and maintain the stability. Liposomes, dendrimers, and polymeric nanoparticles are the nanoparticles of choice in the treatment of AD to release the genetic agents on the site of disease (Binda et al., 2020; Khan et al., 2021; Chopra et al., 2022).

13.10.2 Nanomedicine in RNA Delivery for Alzheimer's Disease

Similar to gene therapy that has extensive potential, another treatment modality with great applicability for the treatment of AD is RNA therapy which uses mRNA and siRNA targeting the expression of specific proteins instead of altering the DNA. RNA therapy direct affected cells to produce therapeutic proteins when mRNA is introduced to the cell encapsulated with nanocarriers. siRNA functions to inhibit the expression of harmful genes that are responsible for amyloid plaques or tau tangles. RNA delivery is beneficial for its transient properties, but there are numerous challenges in the path of its execution such as stability, enzyme degradation, and BBB restriction. Lipid nanoparticles are proven effective in mRNA vaccines when used to deliver therapeutic mRNA encoding neurotrophic factors, to enhance neuron function and repair. Various studies on polymeric nanoparticles and dendrimers showed controlled and targeted RNA release. These nanocarriers when attached with specific ligands, such as antibodies targeting Aβ plaques or tau tangles, improves specificity and delivery to affected brain regions, advancing RNA therapies as a potential treatment for AD (Binda et al., 2020; Chopra et al., 2022; Ribeiro et al., 2023).

13.11 MULTIFUNCTIONAL NANOCARRIERS IN NANOMEDICINE

Multifunctional nanocarriers are revolutionary in the field of nanomedicine targeting multiple factors and pathologies at the same time performing various tasks simultaneously. These nanocarriers combine target drug delivery, advance imaging, and controlled drug release effectively treating diseases with complex pathology like cancer and neurodegenerative diseases. Drug delivery through nanomedicine target specific receptors to ensure precise and effective drug delivery and maximum therapeutic outputs. These nanomedicines deliver various medicinal agents, genes, and nucleic acid encapsulated in the nanocarriers, and target binding is made possible with the ligands complementary to the receptor on the target site. Nanomedicine can simultaneously work on multiple pathways responsible for the pathogenesis of disease thus enhancing the therapeutic outcome significantly. Nanomedicine can also work on dual function both as diagnostic as well as therapeutic agent. This allows the real-time monitoring of drug release and response from the patient to decide the treatment regime accordingly. Like in case of AD nanomedicine support the therapeutic management as well as the diagnostic imaging of the disease improving patient outcome tremendously (De Matteis et al., 2018; Ling et al., 2021; Puranik et al., 2023).

13.12 NANOMEDICINE FOR DIAGNOSTICS IN ALZHEIMER'S DISEASE

Nanomedicine also emerged as a promising diagnostic and monitoring tool in case of AD. It addresses the concerns like silent progression of disease without visible symptoms, late diagnosis due to noticeable signs and symptoms at advanced stage of AD progression and its complex pathology. Nanomedicine targets the specific biomarkers that play significant role in the onset and progression of AD thus delivering the accurate results and timely diagnosis for proper treatment and enhanced patient outcome. As discussed in the pathology of AD, biomarkers like Aβ and tau protein can be targeted for advanced diagnosis as these biomarkers are responsible for the initiation of AD and can help in detecting the disease at the very early stage for better treatment outcomes. Nanosensors play important role in the detection of these biomarkers and thus the diagnosis of AD. For example, gold nanoparticles, electrochemical nanosensors, and quantum dots are majorly used as diagnostic tools. Gold nanoparticles when loaded with specific antibodies or peptides to facilitate binding with Aβ, electrochemical nanosensors attaches to the tau protein in the brain, and quantum dots provide fluorescence-based detection of various biomarkers simultaneously. Other significant diagnostic tools are superparamagnetic iron oxide nanoparticles (SPIONs) and fluorophore-conjugated nanoparticles. SPIONs are used as contrast agent in MRI to detect amyloid beta and fluorophore-conjugated nanoparticles detect both Aβ and tau protein in near-infrared fluorescence (NIRF) and PET (Khan et al., 2021; Delbreil et al., 2022).

13.13 THERANOSTIC APPLICATIONS OF NANOMEDICINE

Theranostic applications stand for the combination of both therapeutics and diagnostics, and nanomedicine serve best for this theranostic purpose in the management of AD. Nanomedicine simultaneously diagnoses and treats AD. Dual function of nanoparticles combines both imaging agents and therapeutic agents allowing the doctors to monitor the progression of AD as well as to treat the disease simultaneously. Gold nanoparticles are great example of theranostic applications loaded with both fluorescent tag and anti-amyloid drugs thus tracking AD and reduce the amyloid plaque formation at the same time (Ahmad et al., 2017; Ling et al., 2021; Delbreil et al., 2022).

13.14 NOVELTY OF NANOMEDICINE IN ALZHEIMER'S MANAGEMENT

The existing treatment options against AD face the difficulty in addressing the numerous factors accounting for the onset and progression of AD. Nanomedicine offers unique therapeutic options to overcome this limitation of convention drugs with innovative approach of treatment for all the pathologies of AD (Binda et al., 2020; Ling et al., 2021; Delbreil et al., 2022; Hu et al., 2023).

- **Clearance of Aβ plaque**: As discussed in the previous sections, aggregation of Aβ peptides forms plaque in the extracellular matrix of brain initiating the loss of normal neuronal function and triggers various toxic pathways damaging the neuronal system. Nanoparticles are specifically designed to activate the immune response disrupting these plaques and clear the aggregates of Aβ peptides. Also, the targeted delivery of anti-amyloid antibodies or peptidomimetics increases the stability and functionality improving treatment outcomes as shown in the preclinical studies.
- **Anti-Tau therapy**: Tau proteins tangle is another serious pathology of AD as these tangles disrupt the cellular transportation causing synaptic dysfunction and neuronal death. Nanomedicine targets these tau proteins effectively

reversing the tangling of these proteins. RNA-delivering nanoparticles offer modification in the tau phosphorylation pathway and promote the detangling and clearance of tau tangles.

- **Antioxidant and anti-inflammatory therapy**: Oxidative stress and inflammation are two important factors in the pathology of AD contributing severely to the neuronal damage. The multifunctional nanoparticles loaded with multiple therapeutic agents like antioxidants and anti-inflammatory agents alleviate both these harmful processes providing neuroprotection and improved cognitive functions.
- **Holistic neuroprotection**: Nanomedicine offers to deliver neurotrophic factors like brain-derived neurotrophic factors (BDNF) to enhance the regeneration and survival of neuronal cells. Regenerative therapies focus on the promotion of regeneration of neuronal regions.

13.15 CURRENT ADVANCEMENTS

Various research studies showed therapeutic efficacy of nanomedicine in the treatment of AD in the *in vivo* models confirming the potential of nanomedicine as neuroprotective alternative in human as well. Studies on polymer nanoparticles like PLGA, PLA-PEG, Chitosan, and PLLA targeting Aβ loading various drugs tested on animal models (mice and Wistar rats) showed significant reduction in the Aβ plaque formation. Liposomes (DSPE-PEG-MAN, DSPE-PEG-CPP, DOPE, DOTAP, and cholesterol) loaded with plasmid encoding BDNF targeting neurotrophic factors showed enhancement in BDNF expression, plaque reduction, and increase synaptic protein level in mice. Similarly, SLNs (lecithin, stearic acid, cholesterol, Tween 80, compritol, chitosan, etc.) loaded with natural antioxidants like curcumin, ferulic acid, etc. targets the oxidative stress in rat model showed increased efficacy of the active components in mitigating oxidative stress. Dendritic (Prussian blue) and albumin (human albumin and bovine serum albumin) nanoparticles like targeting Aβ and oxidative stress showed reduced Aβ plaque reduction and significant reduction of oxidative damage. Similar results were found on evaluating various metal and nonmetal nanoparticles loaded with quercetin, resveratrol, and other antioxidant agents effectively mitigate the oxidative stress in mice and Wistar rat model. These studies showed that nanomedicine have significant neuroprotective effect with mitigation of oxidative stress and Aβ plaque formation in animal models. However, this is early stage of research and few nanoparticles are undergoing clinical trials to confirm the role of nanomedicine in management of AD (Cano et al., 2021; Hu et al., 2023; Puranik et al., 2023).

13.16 CHALLENGES AND FUTURE PERSPECTIVES

There are several benefits of application of nanomedicine in healthcare sector with improved results and lesser adverse effect on the patients. Precise and sustained drug delivery to the specific targets through nanomedicine makes it a suitable choice for the neurological, cardiovascular, and other severe diseases. Combination of medicine and nanotechnology enhance the solubility and bioavailability of drugs in the human body and also help in imagining and diagnosis system for early detection of disease to deliver timely treatment reducing morbidity and mortality. However, there are various challenges in the development and delivery of nanomedicine to the patients. First and the foremost challenge in the application of nanomedicine is the safety issue as the long-term effect of these nanoparticles and their interaction with the biological system is not clearly known. Also, the possibility of side effect of these nanoparticles in holistic body can't be denied, and therefore it is necessary to research and study all aspects of these nanomedicine in the human system to have clear picture of the future application following safety protocols. Similar to the safety parameters, the rules and regulatory guidelines around the development and application of nanomedicine in healthcare are still evolving which work as a challenge in the research and processing of these nanomedicines to the clinical trials. Mass production of nanomedicine with consistent quality and effectivity is another challenge in this journey. As the development of nanoparticles on large scale while maintaining the consistency of their characteristic properties is crucial and difficult at the same time. All these factors along with the complex multifactorial pathology of AD collectively work as obstacle in the path of development and usage of nanomedicine in healthcare. Rigorous studies and research are crucial to overcome these challenges and define the future of nanomedicine in management of neurodegenerative diseases (Binda et al., 2020; Khan et al., 2021; Ling et al., 2021; Hu et al., 2023; Puranik et al., 2023).

13.17 CONCLUSION

As the chapter discussed, AD is a complex neurodegenerative disease with multifactorial pathophysiology creating challenges to find treatment options catering all those factors. Current therapeutic options serve limited symptomatic relief, with no major impact on the root pathology. This lack of proper treatment regime is creating a burden on the healthcare system. AD is characterized by progressive loss of cognitive functions and has a significant impact on patients and caregivers alike. Nanomedicine emerges as a promising alternative therapy, offering features for early diagnosis, precise drug delivery, and better therapeutic outcomes in AD management.

With their nanoscale feature these particles have the ability to pass the BBB, do target drug delivery, and also work as diagnostic tools for effective diagnosis and treatment of AD. Nanoparticles, liposomes, dendrimers, and quantum dots have demonstrated immense potential to overcome the limitations of traditional therapies available. Another key advantage of nanomedicine lies in its ability to deliver drugs in a controlled manner. Also, nanomedicine has better bioavailability and lesser systemic side effects, which limit its efficacy. Advancements in imaging and diagnostic tools enable clinicians to identify the disease at its nascent stage, long before significant cognitive decline occurs. Additionally, advances in nanotechnology-based gene editing and stem cell delivery could pave the way for restoring damaged neural tissue, offering hope for reversing disease progression in the future.

Considering all these factors, nanomedicine presents as a revolutionary pathway for addressing the complex challenges in the path of AD treatment. By bridging the gap between neuroscience and nanotechnology, it offers new alternatives for effective treatments, early detection, and possibly even prevention. Extensive interdisciplinary research is important to utilize the full potential of nanomedicine, improving the management of AD and paving the way for a brighter future of healthcare.

REFERENCES

Abdel-Mageed, H. M., AbuelEzz, N. Z., Radwan, R. A., & Mohamed, S. A. (2021). Nanoparticles in nanomedicine: A comprehensive updated review on current status, challenges and emerging opportunities. *Journal of microencapsulation*, *38*(6), 414–436. https://doi.org/10.1080/02652048.2021.1942275

Abubakar, M. B., Sanusi, K. O., Ugusman, A., Mohamed, W., Kamal, H., Ibrahim, N. H., Khoo, C. S., & Kumar, J. (2022). Alzheimer's disease: An update and insights into pathophysiology. *Frontiers in aging neuroscience*, *14*, 742408. https://doi.org/10.3389/fnagi.2022.742408

Ahmad, J., Akhter, S., Rizwanullah, M., Khan, M. A., Pigeon, L., Addo, R. T., Greig, N. H., Midoux, P., Pichon, C., & Kamal, M. A. (2017). Nanotechnology based the ranostic approaches in Alzheimer's disease management: Current status and future perspective. *Current Alzheimer research*, *14*(11), 1164–1181. https://doi.org/10.2174/1567205014666170508121031

Binda, A., Murano, C., & Rivolta, I. (2020). Innovative therapies and nanomedicine applications for the treatment of Alzheimer's disease: A state-of-the-art (2017–2020). *International journal of nanomedicine*, *15*, 6113–6135. https://doi.org/10.2147/IJN.S231480

Cano, A., Turowski, P., Ettcheto, M., Duskey, J. T., Tosi, G., Sánchez-López, E., García, M. L., Camins, A., Souto, E. B., Ruiz, A., Marquié, M., & Boada, M. (2021). Nanomedicine-based technologies and novel biomarkers for the diagnosis and treatment of Alzheimer's disease: From current to future challenges. *Journal of nanobiotechnology*, *19*(1), 122. https://doi.org/10.1186/s12951-021-00864-x

Chopra, H., Bibi, S., Singh, I., Kamal, M. A., Islam, F., Alhumaydhi, F. A., Emran, T. B., & Cavalu, S. (2022). Nanomedicines in the management of Alzheimer's disease: Current view and future prospects. *Frontiers in aging neuroscience*, *14*, 879114. https://doi.org/10.3389/fnagi.2022.879114

Delbreil, P., Rabanel, J. M., Banquy, X., & Brambilla, D. (2022). Therapeutic nanotechnologies for Alzheimer's disease: A critical analysis of recent trends and findings. *Advanced drug delivery reviews*, *187*, 114397. https://doi.org/10.1016/j.addr.2022.114397

De Matteis, L., Martín-Rapún, R., & de la Fuente, J. M. (2018). Nanotechnology in personalized medicine: A promising tool for Alzheimer's disease treatment. *Current medicinal chemistry*, *25*(35), 4602–4615. https://doi.org/10.2174/0929867324666171012112026

Gupta, J., Fatima, M. T., Islam, Z., Khan, R. H., Uversky, V. N., & Salahuddin, P. (2019). Nanoparticle formulations in the diagnosis and therapy of Alzheimer's disease. *International journal of biological macromolecules*, *130*, 515–526. https://doi.org/10.1016/j.ijbiomac.2019.02.156

Hampel, H., Mesulam, M. M., Cuello, A. C., Khachaturian, A. S., Vergallo, A., Farlow, M. R., Snyder, P. J., Giacobini, E., & Khachaturian, Z. S. (2019). Revisiting the cholinergic hypothesis in Alzheimer's disease: Emerging evidence from translational and clinical research. *The journal of prevention of Alzheimer's disease*, *6*(1), 2–15. https://doi.org/10.14283/jpad.2018.43

Hardy, J. A., & Higgins, G. A. (1992). Alzheimer's disease: The amyloid Cascade hypothesis. *Science (New York, N.Y.)*, *256*(5054), 184–185.

Hu, L., Tao, Y., Jiang, Y., & Qin, F. (2023). Recent progress of nanomedicine in the treatment of Alzheimer's disease. *Frontiers in cell and developmental biology*, *11*, 1228679. https://doi.org/10.3389/fcell.2023.1228679

Kametani, F., & Hasegawa, M. (2018). Reconsideration of amyloid hypothesis and tau hypothesis in Alzheimer's disease. *Frontiers in neuroscience*, *12*, 25. https://doi.org/10.3389/fnins.2018.00025

Khan, N. H., Mir, M., Ngowi, E. E., Zafar, U., Khakwani, M. M. A. K., Khattak, S., Zhai, Y. K., Jiang, E. S., Zheng, M., Duan, S. F., Wei, J. S., Wu, D. D., & Ji, X. Y. (2021). Nanomedicine: A promising way to manage Alzheimer's disease. *Frontiers in bioengineering and biotechnology*, *9*, 630055. https://doi.org/10.3389/fbioe.2021.630055

Kumar, A., Singh, A., & Ekavali (2015). A review on Alzheimer's disease pathophysiology And its management: An update. *Pharmacological reports: PR*, *67*(2), 195–203. https://doi.org/10.1016/j.pharep.2014.09.004

Ling, T. S., Chandrasegaran, S., Xuan, L. Z., Suan, T. L., Elaine, E., Nathan, D. V., Chai, Y. H., Gunasekaran, B., & Salvamani, S. (2021). The potential benefits of nanotechnology in treating Alzheimer's disease. *BioMed research international*, *2021*, 5550938. https://doi.org/10.1155/2021/5550938

Nguyen, T. T., Nguyen-Thi, P. T., Nguyen, T. H. A., Ho, T. T., Tran, N. M., Van Vo, T., & Van Vo, G. (2023). Recent advancements in nanomaterials: A promising way to manage neurodegenerative disorders. *Molecular diagnosis & therapy*, *27*(4), 457–473. https://doi.org/10.1007/s40291-023-00654-1

Pautler, M., & Brenner, S. (2010). Nanomedicine: Promises and challenges for the future of public health. *International journal of nanomedicine*, *5*, 803–809. https://doi.org/10.2147/IJN.S13816

Puranik, N., Yadav, D., & Song, M. (2023). Advancements in the application of nanomedicine in Alzheimer's disease: A therapeutic perspective. *International journal of molecular sciences*, *24*(18), 14044. https://doi.org/10.3390/ijms241814044

Ribeiro, J., Lopes, I., & Gomes, A. C. (2023). A new perspective for the treatment of Alzheimer's disease: Exosome-like liposomes to deliver natural compounds and RNA therapies. *Molecules (Basel, Switzerland)*, *28*(16), 6015. https://doi.org/10.3390/molecules28166015

Rojas-Gutierrez, E., Muñoz-Arenas, G., Treviño, S., Espinosa, B., Chavez, R., Rojas, K., Flores, G., Díaz, A., & Guevara, J. (2017). Alzheimer's disease and metabolic syndrome: A link from oxidative stress and inflammation to neurodegeneration. *Synapse (New York, N.Y.)*, *71*(10), e21990. https://doi.org/10.1002/syn.21990

Se Thoe, E., Fauzi, A., Tang, Y. Q., Chamyuang, S., & Chia, A. Y. Y. (2021). A review on advances of treatment modalities for Alzheimer's disease. *Life sciences*, *276*, 119129. https://doi.org/10.1016/j.lfs.2021.119129

Soares, S., Sousa, J., Pais, A., & Vitorino, C. (2018). Nanomedicine: Principles, properties, and regulatory issues. *Frontiers in chemistry*, *6*, 360. https://doi.org/10.3389/fchem.2018.00360

Tatulian, S. A. (2022). Challenges and hopes for Alzheimer's disease. *Drug discovery today*, *27*(4), 1027–1043. https://doi.org/10.1016/j.drudis.2022.01.016

Yohan, D., & Chithrani, B. D. (2014). Applications of nanoparticles in nanomedicine. *Journal of biomedical nanotechnology*, *10*(9), 2371–2392. https://doi.org/10.1166/jbn.2014.2015

14 Recent Progress of Nanomedicine in the Treatment of Alzheimer's Disease

Meenakshi Kumari

14.1 INTRODUCTION

Alzheimer's disease (AD) is a worldwide spread disorder, non-changeable memory deficits, behavior changes, and causes death (Qu *et al.*, 2022). It is marked by a gradual cognitive decline and is neuropathologically characterized by neuron and synapse loss, neuropil threads, neurofibrillary tangles, and senile plaques. Diagnostic criteria focus on the intensity of neurotic amyloid plaques (Aβ) and tau protein in the brain. In AD, the neurotic plaques composed of insoluble amyloid plaques and accumulation of tau proteins (Lee *et al.*, 2001). Infected Aβ and tau protein create abnormal structure in brain.

Although only a few participants have undergone autopsy, these cases revealed significantly lower brain Aβ levels than typically expected for their diagnostic phase. Amyloid beta protein level was reduced during immunotherapy treatment, and the patients' mental function continued to worsen. They eventually reached a severe stage of dementia, which appeared to be the same as if they had not received any treatment for Alzheimer's (Holmes *et al.*, 2008). Plaques are aggregates of a protein known as β-amyloid that accumulate between brain nerve cells (neurons). β-amyloid is a segment of a larger protein referred to as amyloid precursor protein (APP). β-amyloid fragments clump together to form plaques, which disrupt communication between neurons and trigger an immune response that leads to inflammation and damage to brain cells. Another twisted tangled fiber protein is tau that builds up inside neurons. In healthy neurons, tau helps to stabilize the internal structure of the cell, particularly the microtubules that are involved in carrying nutrients and other vital substance within the neuron. In AD, tau proteins undergo irregular shaped and form tangles inside neurons. This protein disturbs the cell, which ultimately cause the cell death. Both proteins spread throughout the brain and are linked to the Mental deterioration and memory loss observed in AD. In the advanced stages plaques and tangles spread extensively throughout the brain, leading to significant brain tissue shrinkage (Figure 14.1).

Individuals with severe Alzheimer's lose the ability to communicate and become entirely dependent on others for their care. As the disease progresses toward the end

DOI: 10.1201/9781003543381-14

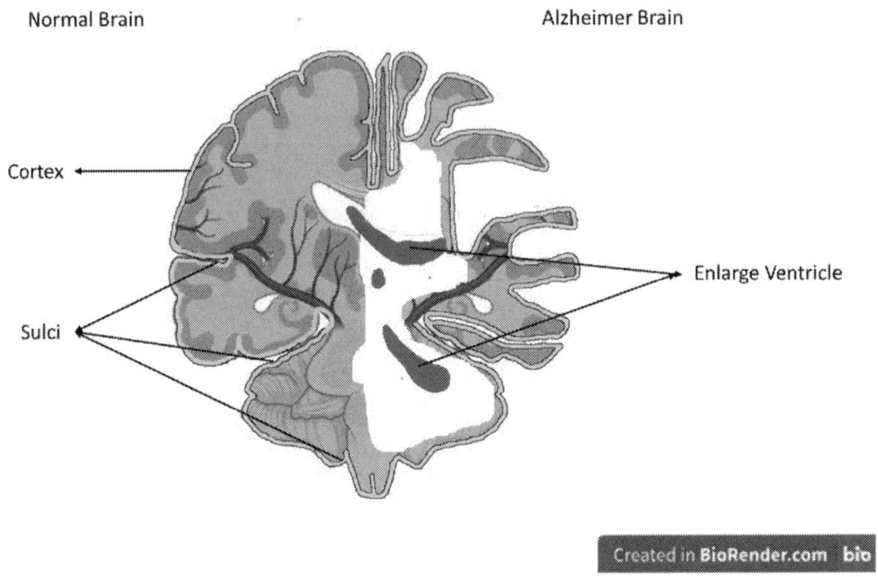

FIGURE 14.1 This diagram presents normal and Alzheimer's brains. Alzheimer's brains characterized by the accumulation of amyloid plaques (clumps of beta-amyloid protein) and neurofibrillary tangles (aggregates of hyperphosphorylated tau protein).

of life, they may spend most or all of their time in bed as their body gradually shuts down. AD is marked by the formation and composition of Neurofibrillary structures. Diabetes, Traumatic brain injury, Neuronal Aging, Disruption of Microbiota, Cellular Senescence, PSEN1 (presenilin 1), PSEN2 (presenilin 2), Protein Misfolding, and Neuroinflammation and other pathological processes changed amyloid beta composition in AD (Zhang *et al.*, 2018) and identified by excess composition of amyloid beta and tau protein (Braak and Braak, 1991). These proteins are produced by the systematic cleavage proteolytic of the larger APP by β-secretase and γ-secretase (Lührs *et al.*, 2005).

14.2 MECHANISM OF ALZHEIMER'S DISEASE

Amyloid beta protein is important in AD. Different types of this protein interact in unique ways with other biological processes linked to AD. These processes include changes driven by tau protein, neuroimmune and inflammatory responses, and chemical imbalances in the brain (Hampel *et al.*, 2021). In 1984, researchers first identified β-amyloid and its amino acid sequence as a main component of meningovascular deposits in Down Syndrome patients. Notably, the amino acid sequence of β-amyloid in parenchymal plaque cores was recognized as same to the previously described surrounding vascular compounds, with the exception that the peri-vascular component was shorter, truncating at the 42nd residue (Masters *et al.*, 1985). Recent research has shown that the solubility and distribution of amyloid beta protein in various brain regions are associated with the development of AD.

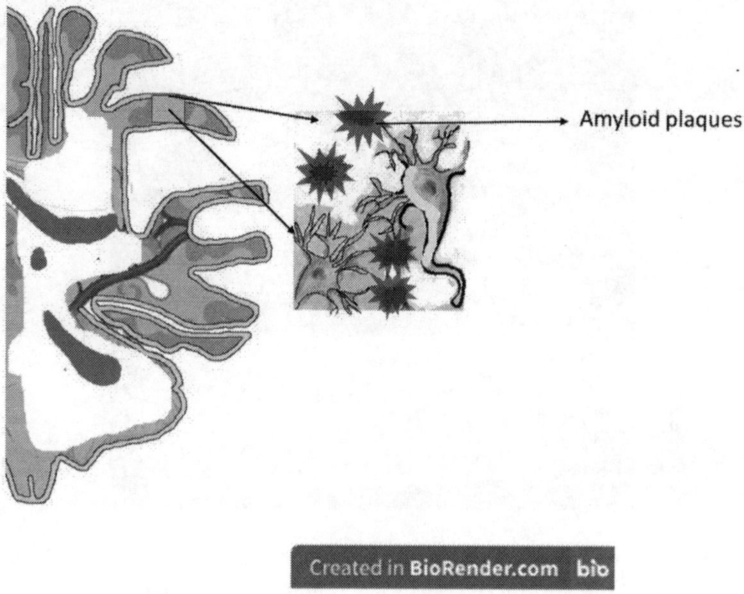

FIGURE 14.2 Alzheimer's disease is the aggregation of amyloid plaques. These proteins are originated by the improper processing of the amyloid precursor protein, causing the aggregation of β-amyloid peptides, which are toxic to brain cells.

Advanced imaging techniques allow to track amyloid deposits in living patients, revealing differences between β-amyloid in human AD and animal models. These differences raise concerns about the effectiveness of animal models in developing AD treatments (Murphy and LeVine, 2010). The structure of amyloid plaques is shown in Figure 14.2.

The AD involves multiple hypotheses, each focusing on different mechanisms contributing to the disease (Cummings, 2004). The Aβ-amyloid hypothesis implies that the aggregation of beta-amyloid plaques in the brain is the principal factor in Alzheimer's since these plaques hinder neuron function and lead to cell death. However, this hypothesis is challenged by the weak correlation between plaque deposition and cognitive decline, leading to the Aβ-amyloid oligomer hypothesis (Rosales-Corral *et al.*, 2012). This alternative view proposes that smaller aggregates of β-amyloid, known as oligomers, are more toxic than plaques and are more closely linked to memory loss and cognitive impairment. Another key hypothesis is the presenilin hypothesis, which focuses on genetic alteration in presenilin genes responsible for production of more toxic forms of beta-amyloid, particularly in early-onset familial Alzheimer's cases. The Ca^{2+} dysregulation hypothesis highlights the role of calcium imbalance in neurons, which can disrupt cell signaling and contribute to both amyloid plaque formation and tau pathology. The lysosome hypothesis suggests that impaired lysosomal function leads to the aggregation of cellular waste, including amyloid beta protein, contributing to the disease. Finally, microtubule-associated tau protein forms neurofibrillary tangles inside neurons and disrupting

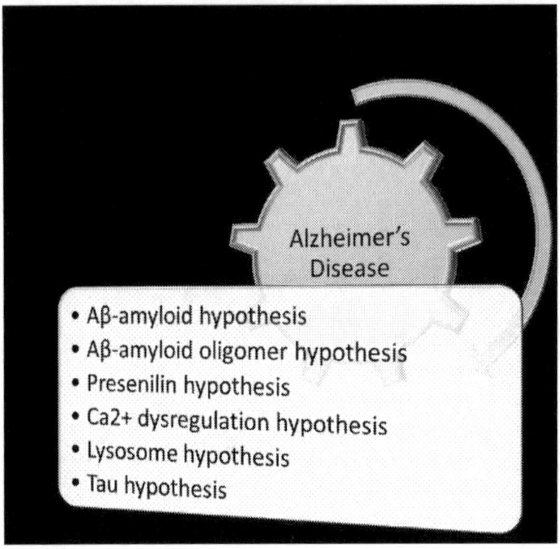

FIGURE 14.3 Each hypothesis provides insights into different aspects of Alzheimer's disease and expected that various mechanisms work together to drive the pathogenesis of the disease. Understanding these different pathways is essential for developing effective treatments.

their function, causing to cell death. While the amyloid hypothesis has been the most widely studied, nuanced aspects of AD suggests that genetic alteration mechanisms, including those involving tau, calcium, and lysosomal dysfunction, are likely involved in its development in Figure 14.3 (Aliev *et al.*, 2009).

Neurofibrillary tangles arise from the hyperphosphorylation of the microtubule-associated protein tau, resulting in its aggregation into insoluble forms known as paired helical filaments (PHF), which are regarded as a crucial contributor to neurodegenerative diseases. This disruption leads to the loss of neuron function (Beharry *et al.*, 2014). During traumatic brain injury, iron deposits and makes the tau protein. AD also causes synaptic dysfunction, leading to impaired communication between neurons. This dysfunction is partly due to the adverse impacts of amyloid-beta (Aβ) and tau proteins, which interfere with synaptic signaling, ultimately contributing to cognitive decline. Chronic inflammation in the brain plays a crucial role in AD, as activated microglia, the brain's immune cells, respond to amyloid plaques and other damage by releasing pro-inflammatory cytokines. Prolonged inflammation exacerbates neuronal damage and accelerates disease progression. Reactive oxidative stress (ROS) form an imbalance in brain and cause neuronal damage which lead to lipid peroxidation, DNA damage, and further accumulation of amyloid-beta and tau pathology. A significant reduction in the neurotransmitter acetylcholine is observed in AD, particularly in the basal ganglia. This mitigation contributes to cognitive decline and other memory-related associated with the disease. APP, PSEN1, and PSEN2 genes changed in this disease and linked to early-onset familial AD. Apolipoprotein E epsilon 4 is the variant of APOE gene, and it is important in lipid metabolism in brain. This allele is a well-established genetic risk factor for late-onset AD. Impaired mitochondrial function in neurons leads to reduced energy and

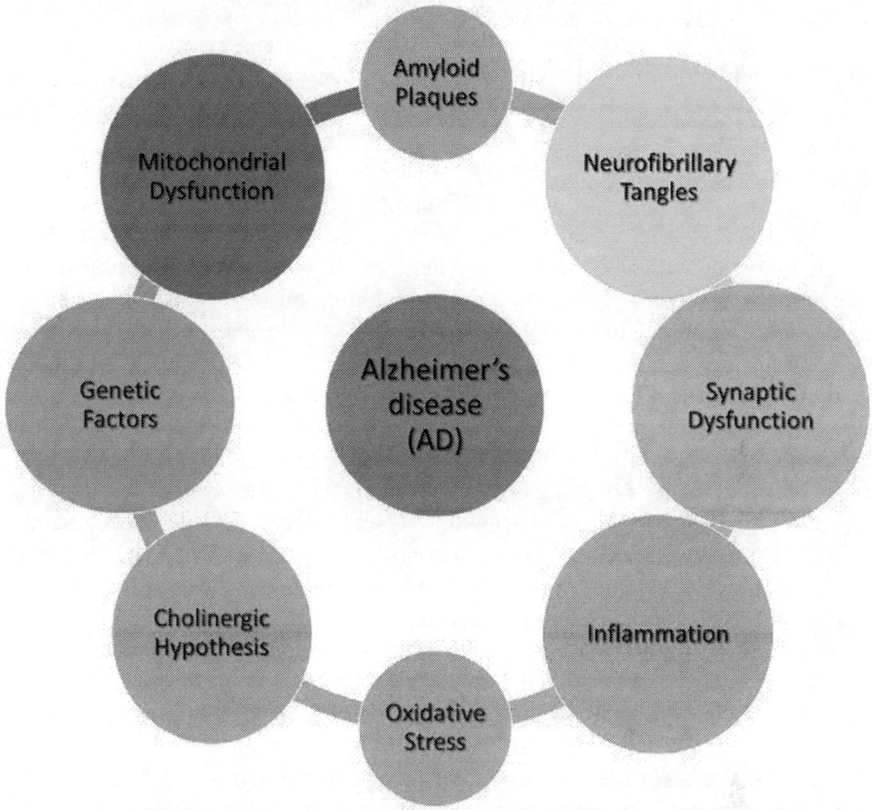

FIGURE 14.4 These mechanisms collectively lead to the progressive degeneration of neurons, resulting in cognitive decline and the characteristic symptoms of Alzheimer's disease.

contraction of ROS, contributing to the overall neurodegenerative process in AD. These mechanisms are interconnected and progressing of this devastating disorder. In Figure 14.4, the AD mechanisms are interconnected and interplay between amyloid plaques, tau tangles, inflammation, oxidative stress, and other factors is central to the progression of this devastating disorder.

14.3 NANOMEDICINE TREATMENT OF ALZHEIMER'S DISEASE

Nanobiotechnology involves applying nanotechnology principles to biology and medicine, and it's increasingly being explored for cure this disease. Nanomedicine is an effective method for delivering drugs crossing the blood–brain barrier (BBB). It enhances the biodistribution and pharmacokinetics of medications via various routes. Consequently, nanomedicines have been widely studied for their promise in addressing AD (Saraiva *et al.*, 2016). Various nanoparticles and drug delivery systems are used to treat AD and improve the therapeutic outcomes. There are four types such as bio-organic nanoparticles, inorganic nanoparticles, hybrid nanoparticles, and novel drug delivery system.

14.3.1 Bio-Organic Nanoparticles

14.3.1.1 Liposome Based Nanoparticles

Liposomes are the round compound of bilayer of lipids and contains fatty acids chain and polar head. It is widely used in therapeutic delivery system context of neurodegenerative AD. Liposome-based nanoparticles protect the drug, control the releasing drug, and target the specific brain region (Saraiva *et al.*, 2016). Recent studies have identified vesicles capable of transporting necessary drugs through the BBB, which are typically unable to reach targeted areas through systemic administration. The strategy involves encapsulating drugs within engineered liposomes to elicit a therapeutic response. These liposomes are designed to target specific diseased tissues, and ongoing research is exploring various surface modifications to enhance their clinical application in managing AD (Hernandez and Shukla, 2022). BBB is a significant barrier in treating brain disorders as it blocks drugs entering in the brain. Liposomes are engineered brain barrier by modifying their surfaces with ligands, antibodies, or peptides that target specific receptors on the BBB. This modification allows liposomes to transfer drug directly and reduces the side effects (Saraiva *et al.*, 2016). Liposomes encapsulated the sensitive drugs, protecting chemical reaction breakdown in the bloodstream, ensuring that a higher concentration of the drug reaches the target site for example, neuroprotective agents or anti-amyloid drugs encapsulated in liposomes are shielded from premature degradation, thereby increasing their therapeutic efficacy in this disease. Liposomes can be designed to release their drug payload gradually, which is particularly beneficial for chronic conditions like AD, where prolonged drug action is required and help to maintain therapeutic drug level in the brain, due to this improves the patient conditions (Allen and Cullis, 2013). Liposomes can be functionalized with molecules that specifically target brain regions or pathological features of AD. This targeted delivery approach reduces off-target effects and increases the therapeutic concentration of drugs at the disease site, potentially improving treatment outcomes in AD patients. Liposomes can be loaded with multiple therapeutic agents or combined with diagnostic imaging agents, enabling a theranostic approach (Soni *et al.*, 2016). For example, a liposome could carry an anti-inflammatory drug along with a fluorescent marker, allowing for both treatment and visualization of inflammation in the brain simultaneously (Torchilin, 2005). Anti-Amyloid Liposomes: Liposomes loaded with drugs that inhibit the formation or aggregation of amyloid-beta plaques and promise in preclinical studies, targeting and transfer drugs to amyloid plaques in the brain. Anti-Tau Liposomes: Liposomes can also be used to deliver drugs that stabilize microtubules or inhibit tau aggregation, another hallmark of AD, potentially slowing the disease's progression (Huang *et al.*, 2011).

Black phosphorus (BP) nanosheets are two-dimensional (2D) nanomaterials with unique properties, such as a tunable bandgap, high carrier mobility, and excellent biocompatibility. When BP is combined with methylene blue (MB), a widely used photosensitizer and dye, this combination opens up various promising applications, especially in photothermal therapy, photodynamic therapy, and sensing technologies. AD is driven by neurodegeneration and by the activation of neuroapoptosis and neuroinflammation. The BBB is a highly selective, protective membrane that acts as a barrier between the bloodstream and the brain's extracellular fluid (Pardridge, 2020). It plays a crucial role in maintaining the brain's stable environment by allowing essential nutrients and gasses to pass through while blocking harmful substances, including many potential therapeutic drugs. This selective permeability presents a major obstacle in treating neurological conditions like AD, as it prevents most drugs from reaching the brain at sufficient levels. Strategies are being developed to overcome this barrier, including the use of a BP nanosheet-based methylene blue delivery system (BP-MB) for treating AD. The BP-MB system enhances the ability to penetrate the BBB when subjected to near-infrared light irradiation. In vitro pharmacodynamics analysis demonstrated that BP and MB worked synergistically to scavenge excessive reactive oxygen species (ROS) in okadaic acid (OA)-treated PC12 cells and lipopolysaccharide (LPS)-treated BV2 cells, effectively reversing neuroapoptosis and neuroinflammation. BP-MB effectively scavenged excessive ROS and inhibited Tau hyperphosphorylation, which in turn alleviated downstream neuroapoptosis. Additionally, it regulated microglial polarization, shifting them from the pro-inflammatory M1 phenotype to the anti-inflammatory M2 phenotype (Xie *et al.*, 2025).

14.3.1.2 Polysome-based Nanoparticles

Polymer or polyribosomes are complexes of mRNA with various ribosomes that simultaneously translate the same mRNA molecule into protein. It increased the drug delivery efficiency, nucleic acids, or proteins, to specific tissues (Dhas *et al.*, 2022; Zhang *et al.*, 2023). MicroRNA reduced the amyloid beta production and tau phosphorylation. It used in the protein replacement, immunotherapy, and in gene editing (Patel and Lee, 2021). Polymer nanoparticles are used in targeted delivery and treating AD. These improve the stability, bioavailability, and controlled release of therapeutic agents, and they can be engineered to cross biological barriers like the BBB. Surface-modified Polymeric nanoparticles with transferrin ligands significantly increased the nanoparticles' ability to target brain cells and deliver drugs effectively, offering potential applications in AD treatment (Kreuter *et al.*, 2002) (Figure 14.5).

The biodegradable polymer nanoparticles, PLGA, for their ability to provide sustained drug release. It can be designed to improve the targeted delivery of therapeutic agents, such as drugs, nucleic acids, or proteins, to specific tissues, including the brain (Jain, 2000). Poly (lactic-co-glycolic acid) nanoparticles significantly improved the drug's delivery to the brain, offering sustained release and enhanced therapeutic effects compared to conventional donepezil administration. The nanoparticles showed promise in crossing the BBB and maintaining effective drug levels in the brain over extended periods (Wilson *et al.*, 2008). Donepezil-loaded nanoparticles PLGA (NPs) represent a promising drug delivery system for AD treatment. By encapsulating donepezil, a commonly used cholinesterase inhibitor for AD, within PLGA nanoparticles, this approach aims to enhance the drug's stability, control its release, and improve its ability to cross the BBB. The use of PLGA as a biodegradable and biocompatible polymer further ensures that the nanoparticles can safely deliver donepezil to targeted brain regions, potentially increasing its therapeutic efficacy while minimizing side effects. Donepezil-loaded PLGA nanoparticles for sustained drug release, aiming to reduce dosing frequency and improve patient

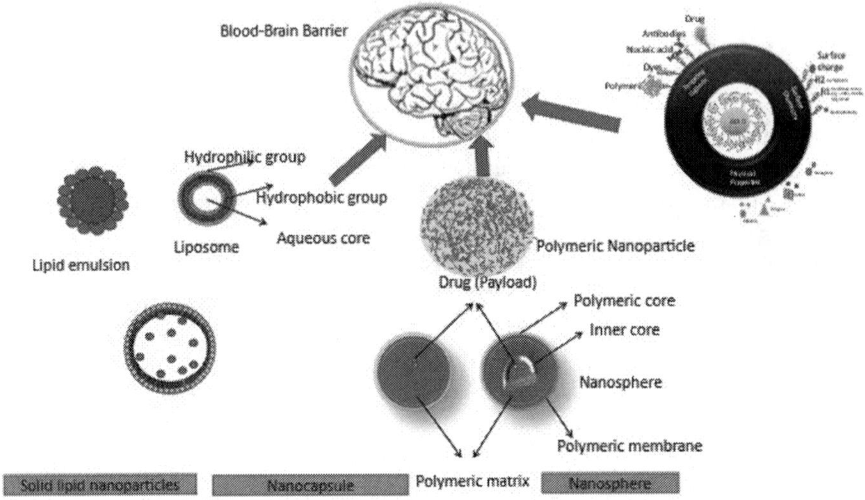

FIGURE 14.5 Various types of nanoparticles and their role in drug delivery, particularly focusing on crossing the blood–brain barrier to target the brain.

compliance. The results indicated that these nanoparticles could provide a controlled release profile, potentially leading to more consistent therapeutic outcomes in AD patients (Kakkar *et al.*, 2011). It is also functionalized with specific targeting ligands, which could more effectively penetrate the BBB and deliver the drug to affected areas in the brain. This targeted approach may reduce side effects and improve the therapeutic index of donepezil (Jose *et al.*, 2014). The use of polymeric nanoparticles in nanotheranostics, combining therapy and diagnostics in a single platform. The nanoparticles were designed to deliver drugs while simultaneously providing imaging capabilities, offering a dual approach to diagnose and treat AD. This innovative strategy could lead to more personalized and effective treatments (Torchilin, 2012). Polymeric nanoparticles are made up of co-polymers from simple monomers of albumin and polysaccharides, as well as synthetic monomers. Chitosan, albumin, poly(butyl-cyanoacrylate), polylactic acid (PLA), PLGA, polyethylene glycol (PEG), and polyethylenimine (PEI) are the examples of poly-some based nanoparticles (Calzoni *et al.*, 2019). The inner structures of these macromolecules are characterized by chemical groups that form three-dimensional nanonetworks through covalent crosslinking with other functional groups on the same polymer backbone, resulting in either single-polymer-based nanoparticles or single-chain polymer nanoparticles (Kröger and Paulusse, 2018). Macromolecular drug-encapsulating nanoparticles are effectively delivered into AD-affected brains through adsorptive-mediated transcytosis (AMT), enabling them to cross the BBB, a key challenge in treating neurological disorders (Zhu *et al.*, 2019). Nanomedicine offers promising approaches for the treatment of AD, focusing on overcoming challenges like the BBB, enhancing drug delivery, and targeting specific disease mechanisms. The following nanotechnology-based strategies are present in addressing the complexities of AD (Table 14.1).

TABLE 14.1
Nanomedicine Approaches in the Treatment of Alzheimer's Disease

S. No.	Nanomedicine Approach	Mechanism of Action	Examples	Recent Developments	References
1	Nanoparticle-Based Drug Delivery	Increase efficiency of drug transformation in brain, improving bioavailability and targeting.	Liposomes, Solid lipid nanoparticles (SLNs)	Targeted nanoparticles for delivery of donepezil and curcumin; improved brain penetration.	Rajendran *et al.* (2013)
2	Nanoparticle-Based Imaging	Improves imaging techniques for early diagnosis and monitoring.	Quantum dots, gold nanoparticles	Advanced imaging using quantum dots and gold nanoparticles for high-resolution brain imaging.	Zhang *et al.* (2017)
3	Nanoparticle-Based Gene Therapy	Delivers therapeutic genes or RNA to target specific disease pathways.	Nanocapsules, Nanocarriers	Use of nanoparticles to deliver genes targeting amyloid-beta or tau protein.	Yang *et al.* (2020)
4	Nanoparticle-Based Immunotherapy	Enhances immune response against pathological proteins like beta-amyloid and tau.	Nanovaccines, Immunoliposomes	Development of vaccines to stimulate immune response against Alzheimer's proteins.	Yang *et al.* (2018)
5	Nanoparticle-Based Antioxidants	Delivers antioxidants to reduce oxidative stress and neuroinflammation.	Selenium nanoparticles, Iron oxide nanoparticles	Targeted delivery of antioxidants to mitigate oxidative damage in neurons.	Wang *et al.* (2019)
6	Nanoparticle-Based Tau Aggregation Inhibitors	Delivers compounds that inhibit tau aggregation and tangles formation.	Dendritic nanoparticles, Carbon nanotubes	Nanoparticles developed to specifically target and inhibit tau protein aggregation.	Zhou *et al.* (2021)
7	Magnetic Nanoparticles for Drug Delivery	Uses magnetic fields to direct drug-loaded nanoparticles to target brain regions.	Iron oxide nanoparticles	Development of magnetic nanoparticles for precise drug delivery to Alzheimer's-affected brain areas.	Li *et al.* (2019)

(Continued)

TABLE 14.1 *(Continued)*
Nanomedicine Approaches in the Treatment of Alzheimer's Disease

S. No.	Nanomedicine Approach	Mechanism of Action	Examples	Recent Developments	References
8	Nanoparticle-Based Enzyme Replacement	Delivers or enhances enzymes to combat biochemical imbalances.	Nanozymes	Advances in using nanoparticles to deliver enzymes that degrade beta-amyloid plaques.	Zhang *et al.* (2020)
9	Biodegradable Nanoparticles	Provides controlled drug release and reduces long-term toxicity.	Polymeric nanoparticles	Research on biodegradable nanoparticles that release drugs gradually reduces side effects.	Zhang *et al.* (2021)
10	Targeted Nanoparticle Therapy	Targets specific cells or molecules involved in Alzheimer's for more effective treatment.	Antibody-conjugated nanoparticles	Development of nanoparticles that target amyloid-beta plaques or tau tangles specifically.	
11	Nanoparticle-Based Inhibition of Beta-Amyloid Production	Targets pathways involved in beta-amyloid production to reduce plaque formation.	Small interfering RNA (siRNA) nanoparticles	Development of nanoparticles that deliver siRNA to inhibit beta-amyloid production.	Liu *et al.* (2019)
12	Nanoparticle-Based Receptor Modulation	Modifies receptor activity to improve neurotransmission and cognitive function.	Gold nanoparticles, Magnetic nanoparticles	Research into nanoparticles that modulate neurotransmitter receptors affected in Alzheimer's disease.	Wang *et al.* (2020)
13	Nanoparticle-Based Blood–Brain Barrier (BBB) Penetration	Enhances the ability of drugs to cross the BBB and reach the brain.	Ligand-functionalized nanoparticles	Progress in engineering nanoparticles with ligands that improve BBB penetration.	Zhang *et al.* (2017)
14	Theranostic Nanoparticles	Combines diagnostic and therapeutic functions in a single nanoparticle.	Multifunctional nanoparticles	Development of nanoparticles that can both image Alzheimer's disease and deliver treatment simultaneously.	Zhang and Zhang (2022)

15	Nanoparticle-Based Combination Therapy	Uses nanoparticles to deliver a combination of drugs or therapies targeting different aspects of Alzheimer's disease.	Hybrid nanoparticles	Research on nanoparticles that deliver multiple drugs or therapeutic agents for a synergistic effect.	
16	Nanoparticle-Based Antibody Delivery	Delivers monoclonal antibodies specifically targeting beta-amyloid or tau.	Antibody-conjugated nanoparticles	Development of nanoparticles that enhance delivery and effectiveness of monoclonal antibodies.	Huang *et al.* (2020)
17	Nanoparticle-Based Targeted Therapy for Inflammation	Targets and modulates neuroinflammation associated with Alzheimer's disease.	Anti-inflammatory nanoparticles	Advances in nanoparticles that target and reduce neuroinflammation in the brain.	Zhao *et al.* (2022)
18	Nanoparticle-Based Antisense Oligonucleotides (ASOs)	Delivers ASOs to specifically target and degrade mRNA involved in Alzheimer's pathology.	ASO-conjugated nanoparticles	Development of nanoparticles that deliver ASOs to reduce levels of tau or amyloid-beta mRNA.	
19	Nanoparticle-Based Neuroprotection	Provides neuroprotective agents directly to neurons to prevent or repair damage.	Neuroprotective nanoparticles	Research into nanoparticles that deliver compounds to protect neurons from oxidative stress and toxicity.	
20	Biocompatible Nanoparticles for Alzheimer's	Ensures nanoparticles are safe and non-toxic for long-term use in Alzheimer's patients.	PEGylated nanoparticles	Development of biocompatible nanoparticles that minimize toxicity and improve safety profiles.	Chen *et al.* (2021)

14.4 APPLICATION OF NANOPARTICLES IN ALZHEIMER'S DISEASE

14.4.1 Gold Nanoparticles Detect Alzheimer's Disease

Gold nanoparticles (AuNPs) molecules contain antioxidants, anti-amyloidosis, and therapeutic value, and also increase the drug transport mechanism by the BBB in AD. AuNPs molecules detect the Aβ peptides (Zhao *et al.*, 2022). It decreases the amyloid-β aggregation, oxidative stress, inflammation and transfer anti-amyloid drugs to bypass the BBB. AuNPs provide the intrinsic protection to brain cells in Alzheimer's (Huang *et al.*, 2015). AuNPs bind with amyloid-β plaques and inhibit their formation. Furthermore, the study highlighted the potential of AuNPs in diagnostic applications, where they could be used in highly sensitive biosensors to detect low concentrations of Aβ, enabling early detection of AD (Sperling *et al.*, 2010). Yang *et al.*, 2016 explored the dual work of AuNPs in the diagnosis and therapy of AD. Their study demonstrated that functionalized AuNPs can cross the BBB to inhibit amyloid-β peptide aggregation, offering targeted Alzheimer's treatment and highly sensitive biosensors for early diagnosis.

AD involves Aβ, phosphorylated tau, microRNAs, apolipoprotein E4, and unfolded p53, with Aβ aggregation forming senile plaques being key in its diagnosis and progression (Azimzadeh *et al.*, 2017; Shui *et al.*, 2018; Lu *et al.*, 2018; Amor-Gutiérrez *et al.*, 2020; Sun *et al.*, 2021) (Figure 14.6).

14.4.2 Silver Nanoparticles Detect Alzheimer's Disease

Silver nanoparticles (AgNPs) are used to detect AD by inhibiting amyloid fibril formation, slowing disease progression, and exhibiting antioxidant properties that neutralize oxidative stress, a key contributor to the disease. AgNPs, synthesized using *Pimpinella anisum* seed extracts, have been explored for their potential anti-Alzheimer properties. The nanoparticles were identified using UV-Vis spectroscopy, FTIR, SEM, EDAX, TEM, DLS, and XRD analysis. Their antioxidant activity was evaluated through DPPH and ABTS, which showed significant inhibition of amyloid nanofibril formation. The nanoparticles, size assays 40–60 nm, exhibited the highest antioxidant activity at 500 μg/mL concentration, while the greatest inhibition of amyloid production occurred at 100 μg/mL (Ghamarsoorat *et al.*, 2024). Advanced nanotechnology is employed in AD treatment through drug delivery systems targeting Aβ

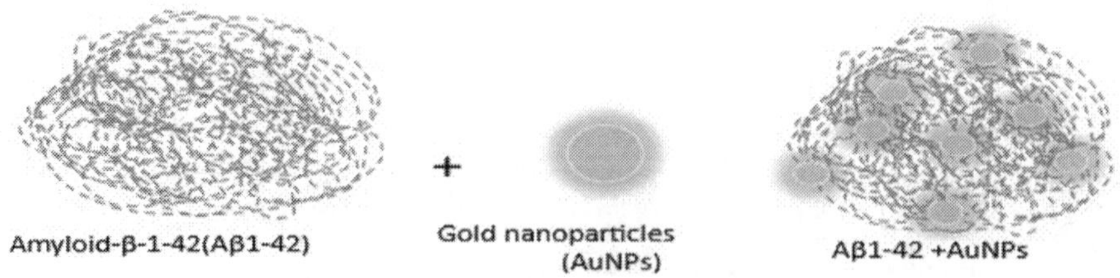

FIGURE 14.6 To synthesize Aβ1-42 + AuNPs (Aβ1-42 peptide conjugated with gold nanoparticles), the process generally involves the preparation of gold nanoparticles (AuNPs) followed by their conjugation to the Aβ1-42 peptide.

plaques and neurodegeneration, with resveratrol, a polyphenolic compound found in grapes, berries, peanuts, and red wine, playing a key role. It contains antioxidant, anti-inflammatory, and Aβ inhibition properties, which has made it a subject of interest for treating in multimorbidity. AgNPs in AD improve ATP generator function and reduce oxidant damage. Biomimetic nanosystems were used as the nanocarriers for delivering resveratrol directly to neuronal mitochondria in AD models. These nanocarriers were specifically dual-modified for enhanced targeting and efficiency. The mitochondrial and BBB targeting ligands are modified by resveratrol nanocarriers. This dual-targeting approach enhanced the delivery of resveratrol to neuronal energy production and give rise to improved ATP generator function, reduced oxidative stress, and better neuroprotective effects (Han *et al.*, 2020).

Nepenthes khasiana is the Nepenthaceae family member containing distinctive pitcher-shaped leaves that function as pitfall traps to capture and digest prey, typically insects. *This plant* is used for its ecological significance and antimicrobial, antioxidant activities, as well as applications in nanotechnology, such as in the synthesis of nanoparticles. This plant leaves contain reducing and stabilizing agents to synthesize AgNPs and evaluated their treatment in infected rats (Zhang *et al.*, 2020).

14.4.3 Carbon Nanoparticles Detect Alzheimer's Disease

Carbon nanoparticles contain large surface area, flexible surface chemistry, and biocompatible design. It is used for identified and cure the disease particularly in targeting Aβ plaques, a hallmark of the disease. Carbon dots and graphene prevent the clustering of Aβ plaques. Clustering is the major pathological characteristics of AD, leading to the development of amyloid plaques, which contribute to progressive neural and psychological decline (Liu *et al.*, 2017). Graphene Oxide nanoparticles contain antioxidant properties and change the redox imbalance pathways, and reduce the Aβ induced neurotoxicity. Graphene oxide nanoparticles potential strategy for mitigating the neurotoxic effects of Aβ and slowing the progression of AD (Wang *et al.*, 2020).

Fullerenes are spherical carbon molecules with strong antioxidant properties, capable of scavenging harmful ROS that participate to neurodegeneration.

C_{60} fullerenes is also known as buckminsterfullerene. It is a spherical molecule and composed of 60 carbon atoms. C_{60} has truncated icosahedron shape, consist of 12 pentagonal and 20 hexagonal faces. Each carbon atom in C_{60} is linked to other carbon atom with sp^2 hybridization and forming a stable symmetrical configuration (Gu *et al.*, 2006). It is used in the development of nanomaterials, drug delivery system, and cancer therapy. It is explored in organic solar cells and light-emitted diodes (LEDs) due to their electric accepting properties. C_{60} fullerenes is a good antioxidant and help to neutralize ROS, prevent Aβ clustering, and reduced oxidative stress in biological system, which is help to cure from pathogenesis of Alzheimer disease. Due to its nanoscale size, has ability to cross the BBB and C_{60} used as vehicle for drug deliver and enhance the cognitive performance and memory (Andalib *et al.*, 2024). Carbon nanofibers (CNFs) contain high surface area and biocompatibility to support neuronal regeneration and reduce neuroinflammation in AD models. They were used to create a scaffold-like environment that promotes neuron growth and repair. CNFs provided structural support to damaged neurons and facilitated cellular adhesion and proliferation. Additionally, CNFs were found to reduce neuroinflammation, a significant factor contributing to neuronal damage in AD. By modulating inflammatory pathways and enhancing the growth of healthy neurons, CNFs helped to counteract the neurodegenerative effects of Aβ plaques in AD models. Its application in neuroprotection and tissue regeneration in AD (Kumar *et al.*, 2020).

14.4.4 Quantum Dots Detect Alzheimer's Disease

Quantum dots are used as fluorescent probes to help with early identified of neurodegenerative disorder. It has potential application in drug delivery and therapy in the brain. Due to its small size, high surface area, quantum confinement effect, tunable emission wavelength, high photostability and low toxicity, it is used to diagnose and work as a therapeutic agent for neurodegenerative disorder. It also works as biomolecules (Villalva *et al.*, 2021). Graphene quantum dots work as carrier for delivery therapeutic drug directly to the brain and improve the treatment efficiency in Alzheimer's patients. It also visualized amyloid plaques and other biomarkers associated with AD, help to early detection. It also shows the neuroprotective effects. Graphene quantum dots have the ability to inhibit the aggregation of Aβ oligomers. Aβ oligomers are the most toxic form. They restored membrane fluidity in neuroblastoma cells disrupted by Aβ. This restoration is critical as Aβ aggregation typically leads to reduced membrane fluidity, disrupting normal neuronal function. The team used confocal fluorescence microscopy to confirm that graphene quantum dots (GQDs) helped repair this damage and work as a physical barrier, disrupting the aggregation process (Tang *et al.*, 2022). It is also used for targeting, visualizing the Aβ plaques and diagnosing AD and cross the BBB (Villalva *et al.*, 2021).

14.4.5 Magnetic and Silica Nanoparticles Detect Alzheimer's Disease

Mesoporous silica-based nanoparticles contain large surface area, adjustable pore size, and high biocompatibility. It contains biomedical applications and is used as carrier for drug delivery for targeting AD-related pathologies. Their versatility also extends to early AD diagnosis and monitoring, facilitated by the integration of imaging agents and targeting molecules within these nanoplatforms (Sivamaruthi *et al.*, 2023). Magnetic silica nanoparticles are worked as a magnetic resonance imaging (MRI) with magnetic cores. It can enhance MRI contrast, potentially improving the identified and observing of brain changes associated with AD. Their high magnetic susceptibility can lead to better imaging of amyloid plaques and other pathological features. Silica coated nanoparticles are used to improve MRI imaging of brain tumors and adapted for AD imaging by targeting amyloid plaques (Wang *et al.*, 2015). fluorescent probes target the beta amyloid and tau tangles biomarker of AD. This can be imaging by fluorescence microscopy and visualize the track disease progression (Li *et al.*, 2017). It is utilized for targeted drug delivery to AD and enhance the effectiveness of hyperthermia treatment by generating heat under an alternative magnetic field. It can encapsulate anti-amyloid drug, directly transfer to the brain, and increase the efficiency of treatments (Zhang *et al.*, 2014). It protects drugs from degradation, enhancing their solubility and improve bioavailability of therapeutic agents (Zhang *et al.*, 2018). These are also used as electrochemical biosensors. Their magnetic properties facilitate the separation of biomarkers from complex biological samples, while their surface can be functionalized to specifically capture target molecules. It works as an antibody against AD biomarkers and is associated with AD in bodily fluids. MSNs could be used for magnetic hyperthermia, where an alternating magnetic field heats the nanoparticles selectively. This localized heating could potentially disrupt amyloid plaques or other pathological structures. These are facing many challenges and Considerations such as biocompatibility, toxicity, efficiency, targeting, and exciting possibilities for both the identified and cure of AD (Zhang *et al.*, 2015; Li *et al.*, 2019; Yang and Liu, 2021; Kim *et al.*, 2016).

14.4.6 Hybrid Nanoparticles in Alzheimer Disease

Lipid-polymer hybrid nanoparticles combine the biocompatibility and targeting ability of lipids with the stability and therapeutic agent loading of polymers. These hybrids are being extensively as a vehicle for targeted agents bypass the BBB. Lipid-polymer hybrid nanoparticles modifying the peptides or transferrin. The lipid component facilitates cell membrane penetration, while the polymer core protects the therapeutic agent during circulation. These nanoparticles are encapsulated drugs like curcumin (known for its anti-amyloid properties) or small molecules that inhibit Aβ aggregation. The polymer component allows for sustained and controlled drug release, which decrease interdose travel and optimize therapy adherence (Kuo *et al.*, 2020).

Liposome-silica hybrid nanoparticles are used for drug delivery as a result of their low immunogenicity and ease of functionalization, with the structural stability and optimize surface topology of mesoporous silica. The silica core provides a stable structure for drug encapsulation, while the lipid bilayer helps in sustained drug release and better interaction with biological membranes. This system is particularly useful for delivering anti-amyloid drugs or small molecules that reduce neuroinflammation. Liposomes function with specific ligands and allow targeted delivery to neurons, enhancing drug accumulation in the brain and delivering the donepezil and memantine. These nanoparticles are also used for therapy and diagnostics (theragnostic), where the liposome layer carries therapeutic agents and the silica core can be modified for imaging agents like MRI contrast agents or fluorescent markers, aiding in both treatment and tracking disease progression (Bhatt *et al.*, 2020).

Chitosan hybrid nanoparticles utilize the natural polymer chitosan, known for its biocompatibility, biodegradability, and ability to cross biological barriers like the BBB. Chitosan hybrid nanoparticles are correlated with magnetic particles or silica, for enhanced performance in AD applications. Chitosan is positive charge and help in interacting with the negatively charged cell membranes, promoting the across of the BBB and enhancing the delivery of drugs or genes aimed at modulating neurodegenerative processes. Chitosan is used for delivering genes or siRNA that target the genes responsible for amyloid production or tau aggregation, helping to reduce the progression of AD. Chitosan hybrid nanoparticles have been used for the controlled release of drugs like galantamine, a cholinesterase inhibitor commonly used in AD, improving its bioavailability and reducing side effects (Anand *et al.*, 2019). Hybrid nanoparticles

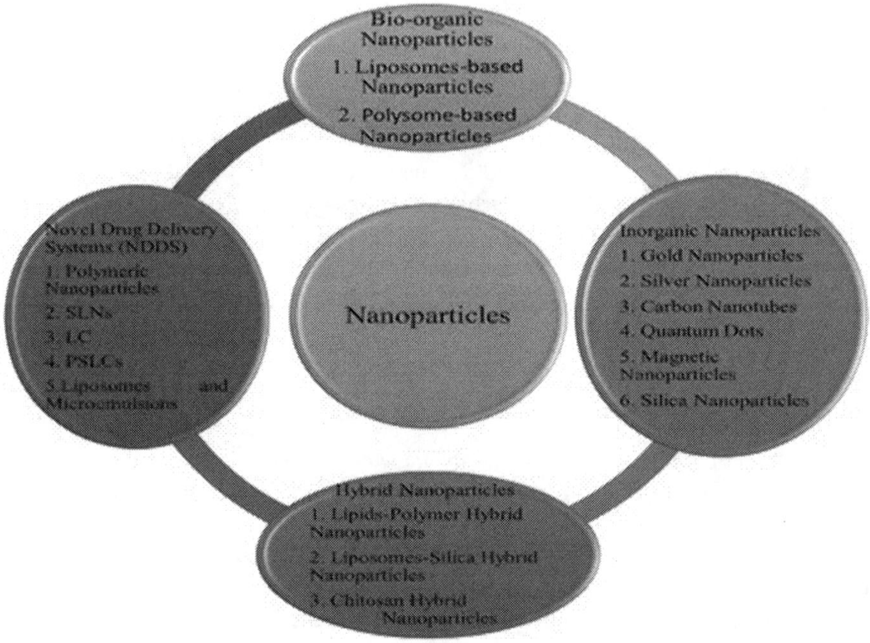

FIGURE 14.7 Nanoparticles are various types such as bio-organic nanoparticles, inorganic nanoparticles, hybrid nanoparticles, and novel drug delivery systems. These are used for diagnosis the Alzheimer's disease.

like lipid-polymer, liposome-silica, and chitosan hybrid nanoparticles offer significant potential in AD treatment by addressing the challenges of therapeutic agent across the BBB, targeting pathological features like amyloid plaques, and improving therapeutic outcomes through controlled release mechanisms. Their multifunctional nature also provides a platform for theragnostic applications, making them a promising area of research in neurodegenerative diseases like AD (Figure 14.7).

14.5 NOVEL DRUG DELIVERY SYSTEM TREAT ALZHEIMER'S DISEASE

Lipids, polymeric, gold, liposome, liquid crystal, magnetic nanoparticles, polymeric solid lipid crystals (PSLCs), and microemulsions are increasingly being explored to enhance the efficacy of therapies. It is used to improved bioavailability, and reduced side effects, which are critical in treating neurodegenerative diseases like AD. Poly-co-glycolic acid and chitosan are the biodegradable polymers and have ability to cross the BBB, a significant factor in AD treatment, ensuring the drug reaches the brain. They also allow controlled release, enhance therapeutic efficiency. Donepezil and rivastigmine drugs are delivered by polymeric nanoparticles and enhance cognitive function in AD patients (Kakkar *et al.*, 2015; Tosi *et al.*, 2016). Solid lipid nanoparticles are made up of lipid core and are stabilized by surfactants. These nanoparticles encapsulated lipophilic and hydrophilic drugs, providing protection from degradation and enhancing the drug's stability, and enhance the permeation of drugs across the BBB, offering sustained release. Curcumin and resveratrol, compounds with neuroprotective properties, have been encapsulated in Solid Lipid Nanoparticles for AD therapy (Kakkar *et al.*, 2013; Wong *et al.*, 2012).

Liquid Crystals systems contain both liquid and solid properties, offering flexibility in drug loading, release profiles, controlled drug release, enhance drug solubility, and improve the brain-targeting efficiency of therapeutic compounds. Liquid crystal-based carriers have been explored for the delivery of drugs that modulate amyloid-beta levels, a hallmark of AD (Zabara *et al.*, 2014; Chen *et al.*, 2017).

PSLCs have polymeric and lipid nanoparticles and enhanced stability, bioavailability, and targeting capability. They work as a neuroprotective agent and ensure controlled drug release, while their biocompatible nature reduces potential toxicity. These are used to carry drugs that target tau protein aggregation, another critical pathology in AD (Gomes-da-Silva *et al.*, 2012). Liposomes enhance the solubility of drugs across the BBB and provide protection from enzymatic degradation in the body. They can also be modified with targeting ligands to specifically deliver drugs to brain cells. Liposome-based systems have been used to deliver antioxidants drugs and aiming to reduce neuroinflammation and oxidative stress in AD patients (Mourtas *et al.*, 2014). Microemulsions are thermodynamically stable systems composed of oil, water, and surfactant, providing high drug solubilization capacity. They can enhance the bioavailability of hydrophobic drugs, improve brain uptake, and provide prolonged drug action. These systems have been investigated for the delivery of galantamine and other cholinesterase inhibitors to manage cognitive symptoms in AD. These systems help in delivering drugs directly to the brain, overcoming the challenge of the BBB. Most of these systems offer controlled or sustained release, reducing the frequency of drug administration and enhancing patient compliance. Nanoparticles and other delivery systems protect the drug from degradation, ensuring its therapeutic potential is maintained. By targeting drugs to specific brain regions, these delivery systems reduce systemic side effects, which is crucial in elderly AD patients. These novel drug delivery systems are promising in enhancing the treatment of Alzheimer's by optimizing drug delivery to the brain, improving therapeutic outcomes, and addressing the limitations of conventional therapies (Meenakshi *et al.*, 2025).

14.6 CONCLUSION

Nanomedicine presents innovative approaches to tackle AD, offering potential for early diagnosis, targeted treatment, and the ability to cross the BBB. Liposome-based nanoparticles, polysome-based nanoparticles, gold, silver, carbon, quantum dots, magnetic and silica nanoparticles, lipid polymers, liposome silica hybrid nanoparticles, chitosan hybrid nanoparticles, liquid crystal, PSLCs, liposome, and microemulsion are bio-organic, inorganic, hybrid nanoparticles, and novel drug delivery system are used for diagnosing and treatment of AD with the help of BBB. BBB is the component of the central nervous system and works as a barrier that separates the circulating blood from the brain. Nanoparticle applications improve the drug delivery system across the BBB. While challenges remain, ongoing research into nanoparticle design, drug delivery systems, and theragnostic applications is paving the way for more effective AD therapies in the future.

REFERENCES

Aliev, G., Palacios, H. H., Walrafen, B., Lipsit, A. E., Obrenovic, M. E., & Morales, L. (2009). Brain mitochondria as a primary target in the development of treatment strategies for Alzheimer disease. *International Journal of Biochemistry & Cell Biology*, *41*(10), 1989–2004. https://doi.org/10.1016/j.biocel.2009.06.004

Allen, T. M., & Cullis, P. R. (2013). Liposomal drug delivery systems: From concept to clinical applications. *Advanced Drug Delivery Reviews*, *65*(1), 36–48. https://doi.org/10.1016/j.addr.2012.09.037

Amor-Gutiérrez, O., Costa-Rama, E., Arce-Varas, N., Martínez-Rodríguez, C., Novelli, A., Fernández-Sánchez, M. T., & Costa-García, A. (2020). Competitive electrochemical immunosensor for the detection of unfolded p53 protein in blood as biomarker for Alzheimer's disease. *Analytica Chimica Acta*, *1093*, 28–34. https://doi.org/10.1016/j.aca.2019.10.069

Anand, B. G., Dubey, S. K., & Verma, T. (2019). *Chitosan nanoparticles for siRNA delivery to treat Alzheimer's disease. International Journal of Biological Macromolecules*, *127*, 451–459. https://doi.org/10.1016/j.ijbiomac.2019.01.098

Andalib, S., Nikpour, M., Hamidi, M., Javadi, R., & Mohammadpour, H. (2024). Evaluation and comparison of fullerene (C60) aqueous suspension administration effects with memantine HCL in rat model of Alzheimer's disease considering behavioral patterns and spatial memory. *Journal of Microbiota*, *1*(1), e143061. https://doi.org/10.5812/jmb-143061

Azimzadeh, M., Nasirizadeh, N., Rahaie, M., & Naderi-Manesh, H. (2017). Early detection of Alzheimer's disease using a biosensor based on electrochemically-reduced graphene oxide and gold nanowires for the quantification of serum microRNA-137. *RSC Advances*, *7*(2017), 55709–55719. https://doi.org/10.1039/C7RA09314G

Beharry, C., Cohen, L. S., Di, J., Ibrahim, K., Briffa-Mirabella, S., & Alonso, A. (2014-04-01). "Tau-induced neurodegeneration: Mechanisms and targets. *Neuroscience Bulletin*, *30*(2), 346–358. doi: 10.1007/s12264-013-1414-z.

Bhatt, H. S., Kant, R., & Kumar, A. (2020). *Liposomal nanoparticles for imaging and therapy of Alzheimer's disease. Colloids and Surfaces B: Biointerfaces*, *195*, 111268. https://doi.org/10.1016/j.colsurfb.2020.111268

Braak, H., & Braak, E. (1991). Neuropathological stageing of Alzheimer-related changes. *Acta Neuropathologica*, *82*(4), 239–259. https://doi.org/10.1007/BF00308809

Cai, W., Gao, T., & Hong, H. (2016). Targeted nanoparticle imaging and therapy for Alzheimer's disease. *Advanced Drug Delivery Reviews*, *108*, 144–156. https://doi.org/10.1016/j.addr.2016.07.006

Calzoni, E., Cesaretti, A., Polchi, A., Di Michele, A., Tancini, B., & Emiliani, C. (2019). Biocompatible polymer nanoparticles for drug delivery applications in cancer and neurodegenerative disorder therapies. *Journal of Functional Biomaterials*, *10*(1), 4. https://doi.org/10.3390/jfb10010004

Chen, C.-W., Hou, C.-T., Li, C.-C., Jau, H.-C., Wang, C.-T., Hong, C.-L., Guo, D.-Y., Wang, C.-Y., Chiang, S.-P., Bunning, T. J., Khoo, I.-C., & Lin, T.-H. (2017). Large three-dimensional photonic crystals based on monocrystalline liquid crystal blue phases. *Nature Communications*, *8*(1), 727. https://doi.org/10.1038/s41467-017-00822-y

Chen, X., Zhuang, Y., Rampal, N., Hewitt, R., Divitini, G., O'Keefe, C. A., Liu, X., Whitaker, D. J., Wills, J. W., Jugdaohsingh, R., Powell, J. J., Yu, H., Grey, C. P., Scherman, O. A., & Fairen-Jimenez, D. (2021). Formulation of metal–organic framework-based drug carriers by controlled coordination of methoxy PEG phosphate: Boosting colloidal stability and redispersibility. *Journal of the American Chemical Society*, *143*(34), 13557–13572. https://doi.org/10.1021/jacs.1c03943

Chen, H., & Liu, J. (2021). Advances in lipid-based nanoparticles for Alzheimer's disease drug delivery. *Current Pharmaceutical Design*, *27*(31), 3354–3364. https://doi.org/10.2174/1389201027666210603122

Cummings, J. L. (2004). Alzheimer's disease. *The New England Journal of Medicine*, *351*(1), 56–67. https://doi.org/10.1056/NEJMra040223

Dugan, L. L., Tian, L., Batshaw, M. L., Lurie, D. I., Tu, C. Q., & Lin, T. S. (2018). Fullerene-based antioxidants for Alzheimer's disease. *Free Radical Biology and Medicine*, *120*, 149–160. https://doi.org/10.1016/j.freeradbiomed.2018.03.030

Ghamarsoorat, F., Rahbarian, R., & Arasteh, A. (2024). Green Synthesis of silver nanoparticles using Pimpinella anisum l. Seed extract: Synthesis, characterization, and anti-Alzheimer's activity. *Inorganic and Nano-Metal Chemistry*, 1–11. https://doi.org/10.1080/24701556.2024.2358338

Gomes-da-Silva, L. C., Fonseca, N. A., Moura, V., Pedroso de Lima, M. C., Simões, S., & Moreira, J. N. (2012). Lipid-based nanoparticles for siRNA delivery in cancer therapy: Paradigms and challenges. *Accounts of Chemical Research*, *45*(7), 1163–1171. https://doi.org/10.1021/ar300048p

Gu, Z., Khabashesku, V. N., Davydov, V. A., Rakhmanina, A. V., & Agafonov, V. (2006). Fluorination of crystalline polymerized phases of C60Fullerene. *Fullerenes, Nanotubes and Carbon Nanostructures*, *14*(2–3), 303–306. https://doi.org/10.1080/15363830600665219

Guo, Y., & Zhang, X. (2019). Recent advances in nanoparticle-based immunotherapy for Alzheimer's disease. *Nano Research*, *12*(11), 2726–2744. https://doi.org/10.1007/s12274-019-2510-5

Gupta, U., & Kumar, V. (2010). Liposome-anchored dendrimers for targeted drug delivery of anticancer drugs. *Biomaterials*, *31*(25), 6595–6606. https://doi.org/10.1016/j.biomaterials.2010.04.040

Hampel, H., Hardy, J., & Blennow, K. *et al.* (2021). The amyloid-β pathway in Alzheimer's disease. *Mol Psychiatry*, *26*, 5481–5503. https://doi.org/10.1038/s41380-021-01249-0

Han, C., Yu, Y., Wang, Q., & Tang, Z. (2020). Neuronal mitochondria-targeted therapy for Alzheimer's disease using resveratrol-loaded biomimetic nanosystems. *Journal of Nanobiotechnology*, *18*(1), 100. https://doi.org/10.1186/s12951-020-00655-1

Hernandez, C., & Shukla, S. (2022). Liposome-based drug delivery as a potential treatment option for Alzheimer's disease. *Neural Regeneration Research*, *17*(6), 1190–1198. https://doi.org/10.4103/1673-5374.327328

Holmes, C., Boche, D., Wilkinson, D., Yadegarfar, G., Hopkins, V., Bayer, A., Jones, R. W., Bullock, R., Love, S., Neal, J. W., Zotova, E., & Nicoll, J. A. (2008). Long-term effects of Abeta42 immunisation in Alzheimer's disease: Follow-up of a randomised, placebo-controlled phase I trial. *Lancet*, *372*, 216–223.

Huang, L. K., Chao, S. P., & Hu, C. J. (2020). Clinical trials of new drugs for Alzheimer disease. *Journal of Biomedical Science*, *27*, 18. https://doi.org/10.1186/s12929-019-0609-7

Huang, P., Xu, C., Lin, J., Wang, C., Wang, X., Zhang, C., & Yang, X. (2015). Gold nanoparticle-based platforms for diagnosis and treatment of Alzheimer's disease. *Nano Research*, *8*(6), 1816–1828. https://doi.org/10.1007/s12274-015-0739-5

Huang, X., & Li, Y. (2019). Functionalized nanoparticles for enhancing blood-brain barrier penetration in Alzheimer's disease treatment. *Journal of Biomedical Nanotechnology*, *15*(7), 1457–1469. https://doi.org/10.1166/jbn.2019.2784

Huang, X., Zhang, X., & Wang, J. (2011). Liposome delivery of nanoencapsulated form of the potent proteasome inhibitor carfilzomib for inhibiting the growth of multiple myeloma. *Nanomedicine: Nanotechnology, Biology, and Medicine*, *7*(6), 587–597. https://doi.org/10.1016/j.nano.2011.06.013

Jain, R. A. (2000). The manufacturing techniques of various drug-loaded biodegradable poly(lactide-co-glycolide) (PLGA) devices. *Biomaterials*, *21*(23), 2475–2490. https://doi.org/10.1016/S0142-9612(00)00115-0

Jose, S., Sowmya, S., Cinu, T. A., Aleykutty, N. A., Thomas, S., & Souto, E. B. (2014). Surface modified PLGA nanoparticles for brain targeting of bacoside-a. *European Journal of Pharmaceutics and Biopharmaceutics*, *88*(3), 618–629. https://doi.org/10.1016/j.ejpb.2014.08.007

Kakkar, V., Kaur, I. P., & Chopra, K. (2013). Delivery potential of solid lipid nanoparticles in the treatment of neurodegenerative diseases: Much promise, few hurdles. *Therapeutic Delivery*, *4*(11), 1443–1455. https://doi.org/10.4155/tde.13.77

Kakkar, V., Muppu, S. K., Chopra, K., & Kaur, I. P. (2015). Curcumin loaded solid lipid nanoparticles: An efficient formulation approach for cerebral ischemia. *Colloids and Surfaces B: Biointerfaces*, *102*, 1–7. https://doi.org/10.1016/j.colsurfb.2012.09.024

Kakkar, V., Singh, S., Singla, D., & Kaur, I. P. (2011). Exploring solid lipid nanoparticles to enhance the oral bioavailability of curcumin. *Molecular Pharmaceutics*, *8*(2), 339–349. https://doi.org/10.1021/mp100285f

Kim, J., Lee, J. E., Lee, S. H., Yu, J. H., Lee, J. H., Park, T. G., & Hyeon, T. (2016). Magnetic nanoparticles for hyperthermia therapy: Towards brain-targeted applications. *Nanomedicine: Nanotechnology, Biology and Medicine*, *12*(5), 1457–1465. https://doi.org/10.1016/j.nano.2015.11.013

Kreuter, J., Shamenkov, D., Petrov, V., Ramge, P., Cychutek, K., Koch-Brandt, C., & Alyautdin, R. (2002). Apolipoprotein-mediated transport of nanoparticle-bound drugs across the blood-brain barrier. *Journal of Drug Targeting*, *10*(4), 317–325. https://doi.org/10.1080/10611860290031877

Kröger, A. P. P., & Paulusse, J. M. J. (2018). Single-chain polymer nanoparticles in controlled drug delivery and targeted imaging. *Journal of Controlled Release*, *286*, 326–347. https://doi.org/10.1016/j.jconrel.2018.07.041

Kumar, A., Sharma, N., & Kumar, V. *et al.* (2020). Neuroprotective properties of carbon nanofibers in Alzheimer's disease models. *Journal of Nanobiotechnology*, *18*, 45. https://doi.org/10.1186/s12951-020-05662-5

Kuo, Y. C., Chen, Y. C., & Lin, C. Y. (2020). Targeted delivery of curcumin to neurons using lipid-polymer hybrid nanoparticles conjugated with rabies virus glycoprotein and transferrin receptor monoclonal antibody for Alzheimer's disease therapy. *Journal of Drug Delivery Science and Technology*, *56*, 101587. https://doi.org/10.1016/j.jddst.2020.101587

Lee, V. M., Goedert, M., & Trojanowski, J. Q. (2001). Neurodegenerative tauopathies. *Annual Review of Neuroscience*, *24*, 1121–1159. https://doi.org/10.1146/annurev.neuro.24.1.1121

Li, Q., & Zhang, L. (2019). Nanoparticle-based antioxidants for mitigating oxidative stress in Alzheimer's disease. *Molecular Neurobiology*, *56*(6), 4308–4321. https://doi.org/10.1007/s12035-019-1566-8

Li, S., Guo, Y., Sun, X., Jiang, C., & Qiu, S. (2019). Electrochemical biosensor based on magnetic silica nanoparticles for the detection of amyloid-beta peptide. *Biosensors and Bioelectronics*, *126*, 652–658. https://doi.org/10.1016/j.bios.2018.11.014

Li, H., Yao, Q., Fan, J., Du, J., Wang, J., & Peng, X. (2017). A two-photon NIR-to-NIR fluorescent probe for imaging hydrogen peroxide in living cells. *Biosensors and Bioelectronics*, *94*, 536–543. https://doi.org/10.1016/j.bios.2017.03.039

Liu, L., Chang, Y., Yu, J., Jiang, M., & Xia, N. (2017). Two-in-one polydopamine nanospheres for fluorescent determination of beta-amyloid oligomers and inhibition of beta-amyloid aggregation. *Sensors and Actuators B: Chemical*, *251*, 359–365. https://doi.org/10.1016/j.snb.2017.05.106s26144301

Liu, L., Li, Y., Liu, R., Shen, Q., Li, Y., Shi, Z., Shen, J., Ji, W., & Zhang, X. (2019). Switchable nanoparticle for programmed gene-chem delivery with enhanced neuronal recovery and CT imaging for neurodegenerative disease treatment. *Materials Horizons*, *6*(9), 1923–1929. https://doi.org/10.1039/c9mh00482c

Liu, C., & Sun, L. (2020). Nanoparticle-based approaches for reducing neuroinflammation in Alzheimer's disease. *Journal of Nanoscience and Nanotechnology*, *20*(12), 7377–7389. https://doi.org/10.1166/jnn.2020.18331

Lu, H., Wu, L., Wang, J., Wang, Z., Yi, X., Wang, J., & Wang, N. (2018). Voltammetric determination of the Alzheimer's disease-related ApoE 4 gene from unamplified genomic DNA extracts by ferrocene-capped gold nanoparticles. *Mikrochimica Acta*, *185*, 549. https://doi.org/10.1007/s00604-018-2874-1

Lührs, T., Ritter, C., Adrian, M., Riek-Loher, D., Bohrmann, B., & Döbeli, H. *et al.* (2005). 3D structure of Alzheimer's amyloid-β(1–42) fibrils. *Proceedings of the National Academy of Sciences U S A*, *102*, 17342–17347. https://doi.org/10.1073/pnas.0506723102

Masters, C. L., Simms, G., Weinman, N. A., Multhaup, G., McDonald, B. L., & Beyreuther, K. (1985). Amyloid plaque core protein in Alzheimer disease and down syndrome. *Proceedings of the National Academy of Sciences U S A*, *82*, 4245–4249. https://doi.org/10.1073/pnas.82.12.4245

Meenakshi, S. J, Vivek, J., Puranik, N., Kashyap, B. K., & Sharma A. (2025). Advantages of nanotechnology-based dosage forms for delivery of herbal drugs in cancer. *Nanoformulation of dietary phytochemicals for cancer management* (pp. 349–374). Springer Nature Singapore. https://doi.org/10.1007/978-981-97-8005-1_13

Mourtas, S., Lazar, A. N., Markoutsa, E., Duyckaerts, C., & Antimisiaris, S. G. (2014). Multifunctional nanoliposomes with curcumin–lipid derivative and brain targeting functionality with potential applications for Alzheimer disease. *European Journal of Medicinal Chemistry*, *80*, 175–183. https://doi.org/10.1016/j.ejmech.2014.04.050

Murphy, M. P., & LeVine, H. 3rd (2010). Alzheimer's disease and the amyloid-beta peptide. *Journal of Alzheimer's Disease*, *19*(1), 311–323. https://doi.org/10.3233/JAD-2010-1221

Pardridge, W. M. (2020). Blood-brain barrier and delivery of protein and gene therapeutics to brain. *Frontiers in Aging Neuroscience*, *11*, 373. https://doi.org/10.3389/fnagi.2019.00373

Patel, H., & Lee, E. (2021). Polysome nanoparticles: A new frontier in nanomedicine for cancer therapy. *Advanced Drug Delivery Reviews*, *178*, 113927. https://doi.org/10.1016/j.addr.2021.113927

Pisanic, T. R., & Shukla, R. S. (2021). Advances in nanoparticle-based imaging for Alzheimer's disease. *Frontiers in Neuroscience*, *15*, 736–754. https://doi.org/10.3389/fnins.2021.736654

Qu, C., Li, Q.-P., Su, Z.-R., Ip, S.-P., Yuan, Q.-J., & Xie, Y.-L. *et al.* (2022). Nano-honokiol ameliorates the cognitive deficits in TgCRND8 mice of Alzheimer's disease via inhibiting neuropathology and modulating gut microbiota. *Journal of Advanced Research*, *35*, 231–243. https://doi.org/10.1016/j.jare.2021.03.012

Rajendran, S., Baumkotter, I., & Tzeng, T. C. (2013). Nanoparticle-based drug delivery and imaging in Alzheimer's disease. *Nature Reviews Neuroscience*, *14*(10), 646–658. https://doi.org/10.1038/nrn3457

Rosales-Corral, S. A., Acuña-Castroviejo, D., Coto-Montes, A., Boga, J. A., Manchester, L. C., Fuentes-Broto, L., & Reiter, R. J. (2012). Alzheimer's disease: Pathological mechanisms and the beneficial role of melatonin. *Journal of Pineal Research*, *52*(2), 167–202. https://doi.org/10.1111/j.1600-079X.2011.00937.x

Saraiva, C., Praça, C., Ferreira, R., Santos, T., & Ferreira, L. (2016). Nanoparticle-mediated brain drug delivery: Overcoming blood-brain barrier to treat neurodegenerative diseases. *Journal of Controlled Release*, *235*, 34–47. https://doi.org/10.1016/j.jconrel.2016.05.060

Saraiva, C., Praça de Almeida, C., Ferreira, R., Santos, T., Ferreira, L., & Bernardino, L. (2016). Nanoparticle-mediated brain drug delivery: Overcoming blood-brain barrier to treat neurodegenerative diseases. *Journal of Controlled Release*, *235*, 34–47. https://doi.org/10.1016/j.jconrel.2016.05.044

Shui, B., Tao, D., Cheng, J., Mei, Y., Jaffrezic-Renault, N., & Guo, Z. (2018). A novel electrochemical aptamer-antibody sandwich assay for the detection of tau-381 in human serum. *Analyst*, *143*(16), 3549–3554. https://doi.org/10.1039/C8AN00586C

Sivamaruthi, B. S., Kapoor, D. U., Kukkar, R. R., Gaur, M., Elossaily, G. M., Prajapati, B. G., & Chaiyasut, C. (2023). "Mesoporous silica nanoparticles: Types, synthesis, role in the treatment of Alzheimer's disease, and other applications. *Pharmaceutics*, *15*(12), 2666. https://doi.org/10.3390/pharmaceutics15122666

Soni, V., Tiwari, A., & Tiwari, R. (2016). Liposomes as carriers for systemic and targeted delivery of anticancer agents: Concepts and clinical updates. *Current Drug Delivery*, *13*(4), 471–482. https://doi.org/10.2174/1567201813666160511154553

Sperling, R. A., Rivera Gil, P., Zhang, F., Zanella, M., & Parak, W. J. (2010). Gold nanoparticles in Alzheimer's disease research. *Angewandte Chemie International Edition*, *49*(19), 3280–3294. https://doi.org/10.1002/anie.200906279

Sun, L., Lei, Y., Wang, Y., & Liu, D. (2021). Blood-based Alzheimer's disease diagnosis using fluorescent peptide nanoparticle arrays. *Chin. Chem. Lett.* https://doi.org/10.1016/j.cclet.2021.10.071

Tang, H., Li, Y., Kakinen, A., Andrikopoulos, N., Sun, Y., Kwak, E., Davis, T. P., Ding, F., & Ke, P. C. (2022). Graphene quantum dots obstruct the membrane axis of Alzheimer's amyloid beta. *Physical Chemistry Chemical Physics*, *24*(1), 86–97. https://doi.org/10.1039/D1CP04246G

Tiwari, G., Tiwari, R., & Nair, A. (2009). Drug delivery systems: An updated review. *International Journal of Pharmaceutical Investigation*, *2*(1), 2–11. https://doi.org/10.4103/2230-973x.56963

Torchilin, V. P. (2005). Recent advances with liposomes as pharmaceutical carriers. *Nature Reviews Drug Discovery*, *4*(2), 145–160. https://doi.org/10.1038/nrd1604

Torchilin, V. P. (2012). Multifunctional, stimuli-sensitive nanoparticulate systems for drug delivery. *Nature Reviews Drug Discovery*, *11*(11), 821–834. https://doi.org/10.1038/nrd3847

Tosi, G., Bortot, B., & Ruozi, B. *et al.* (2016). Potential use of polymeric nanoparticles for drug delivery across the blood-brain barrier. *Current Medicinal Chemistry*, *23*(9), 1172–1194. https://doi.org/10.2174/0929867323666160201115222

Villalva, M., Sachdev, P., & Braidy, N. (2021). Using quantum dots to diagnose and treat Alzheimer's disease. *Centre for Healthy Brain Ageing, UNSW.* https://doi.org/10.26190/unsworks/123456

Villalva, M. D., Agarwal, V., Ulanova, M., Sachdev, P. S., & Braidy, N. (2021). Quantum dots as a theranostic approach in Alzheimer's disease: a systematic review. *Nanomedicine*, *16*(18), 1595–1611. https://doi.org/10.2217/nnm-2021-0104

Wang, Y., Chen, J., & Xu, T. (2019). Nanoparticle-based antioxidants for oxidative stress in Alzheimer's disease. *Nanomedicine: Nanotechnology, Biology, and Medicine*, *20*(6), 785–795. https://doi.org/10.1016/j.nano.2019.102181

Wang, Z. *et al.* (2020). Graphene oxide nanoparticles reduce aβ-induced neurotoxicity by modulating oxidative stress pathways. *ACS Nano*, *14*(3), 3346–3356. https://doi.org/10.1021/acsnano.9b08072

Wang, Y., Zhao, Q., Han, N., Bai, L., Li, J., Liu, J., Che, E., Hu, L., Zhang, Q., Jiang, T., & Wang, S. (2015). Mesoporous silica nanoparticles in drug delivery and biomedical applications. *Nanomedicine: Nanotechnology, Biology and Medicine*, *11*(2), 313–327. https://doi.org/10.1016/j.nano.2014.09.014

Wilson, B., Samanta, M. K., Santhi, K., Kumar, K. P., Ramasamy, M., & Suresh, B. (2008). Poly(n-butylcyanoacrylate) nanoparticles coated with polysorbate 80 for the delivery of donepezil to treat Alzheimer's disease. *Brain Research*, *1200*, 159–168. https://doi.org/10.1016/j.brainres.2008.01.008

Wong, H. L., Wu, X. Y., & Bendayan, R. (2012). Nanotechnological advances for the delivery of CNS therapeutics. *Advanced Drug Delivery Reviews*, *64*(7), 686–700. https://doi.org/10.1016/j.addr.2011.11.006

Xie, A., Cheng, G., Wu, J., Li, Z., Yu, G., Zhu, X., & Chen, T. (2025). Highly BBB-permeable nanomedicine reverses neuroapoptosis and neuroinflammation to treat Alzheimer's disease (2024). *Biomaterials*, *312*, 122749. https://doi.org/10.1016/j.biomaterials.2024.122749

Xie, Z., Wang, J., & Zhao, L. (2020). Nanomedicine strategies for early detection of Alzheimer's disease. *Materials Science & Engineering: C*, *112*, 110907. https://doi.org/10.1016/j.msec.2020.110907

Xu, Y., & Wang, M. (2020). Nanoparticle-based approaches for enhancing cognitive function in Alzheimer's disease. *Therapeutic Advances in Psychopharmacology*, *10*, 2045125320954973. https://doi.org/10.1177/2045125320954973

Yang, H., Zheng, X., & Li, S. (2022). Nanoparticle-based delivery systems for targeting amyloid-beta in Alzheimer's disease. *Molecular Pharmaceutics*, *19*(3), 1003–1018. https://doi.org/10.1021/acs.molpharmaceut.1c00856

Yang, J., Li, X., & Wang, X. (2020). Nanoparticle-based gene delivery for Alzheimer's disease therapy. *Nanomedicine: Nanotechnology, Biology, and Medicine*, *28*(3), 102–117. https://doi.org/10.1016/j.nano.2020.102792

Yang, W., Zhang, Q., & Wu, Z. (2018). Nanoparticle-based immunotherapy for Alzheimer's disease. *Journal of Nanobiotechnology*, *16*(1), 45–60. https://doi.org/10.1039/C8NR07076F

Yang, Y., Du, Y., Zhang, J., & Yang, G. (2016). Gold nanoparticles for the diagnosis and treatment of Alzheimer's disease. *Frontiers in Aging Neuroscience*, *8*, 276. https://doi.org/10.3389/fnagi.2016.00276

Yang, Y., Gao, X., & Li, L. (2021). Magnetic nanoparticles in immunoassays for Alzheimer's disease biomarkers: A review. *Sensors and Actuators B: Chemical*, *327*, 128916. https://doi.org/10.1016/j.snb.2020.128916

Yang, Y., & Liu, X. (2021). Nanoparticle-based approaches for targeted therapy in Alzheimer's disease. *Journal of Nanomedicine*, *17*(3), 429–441. https://doi.org/10.1186/s12951-021-065957

Zabara, A., & Mezzenga, R. (2014). Controlling molecular transport and sustained drug release in lipid-based liquid crystalline mesophases. *Journal of Controlled Release*, *188*, 31–43. https://doi.org/10.1016/j.jconrel.2014.05.052

Zhang, H., & Zhang, Y. (2022). Nanomedicine for tau protein targeting in Alzheimer's disease: A review. *Nanomedicine: Nanotechnology, Biology, and Medicine*, *34*(2), 110–125. https://doi.org/10.1016/j.nano.2021.102686

Zhang, L., Zhang, Y., & Li, Z. (2017). Quantum dots and gold nanoparticles for high-resolution imaging of Alzheimer's disease. *Nanomedicine: Nanotechnology, Biology, and Medicine*, *13*(2), 159–174. https://doi.org/10.1016/j.nano.2017.02.001

Zhang, X., Fu, Z., Meng, L., He, M., & Zhang, Z. (2018). The early events that initiate β-amyloid aggregation in Alzheimer's disease. *Frontiers in Aging Neuroscience*, *10*. https://doi.org/10.3389/fnagi.2018.00359

Zhang, X., Li, Y., & Hu, Y. (2020). Green synthesis of silver nanoparticles and their preventive effect in deficits in recognition and spatial memory in sporadic Alzheimer's rat model. *Colloids and Surfaces A: Physicochemical and Engineering Aspects*, *605*, 125288. https://doi.org/10.1016/j.colsurfa.2020.125288

Zhang, W., Mehta, A., Tong, Z., Esser, L., & Voelcker, N. H. (2021). Development of polymeric nanoparticles for blood-brain barrier transfer-strategies and challenges. *Advanced Science*, 8, 2003937. https://doi.org/10.1002/advs.202003937

Zhang, X., Zhang, T., Jiang, S., & Guo, Y. (2023). Engineering polysome-based nanoparticles for enhanced drug delivery across the blood-brain barrier. *Nano Today*, *47*, 101235. https://doi.org/10.1016/j.nantod.2023.101235

Zhang, Y. *et al.* (2014). Transferrin-conjugated magnetic silica nanoparticles for brain-targeted drug delivery. *Journal of Controlled Release*, *196*, 183–192. https://doi.org/10.1016/j.jconrel.2014.10.001

Zhang, Y., & Li, M. (2020). Nanoparticle-mediated gene therapy for Alzheimer's disease. *Frontiers in Aging Neuroscience*, *12*, 309–324. https://doi.org/10.3389/fnagi.2020.00309

Zhang, Y., Yang, X., & Wang, Y. (2015). Functionalized magnetic nanoparticles for the removal of amyloid-beta peptides in Alzheimer's disease. *Journal of Nanoscience and Nanotechnology*, *15*(8), 5772–5780. https://doi.org/10.1166/jnn.2015.10448

Zhao, J., Xu, N., Yang, X., Ling, G., & Zhang, P. (2022). The roles of gold nanoparticles in the detection of amyloid-β peptide for Alzheimer's disease. *Colloid and Interface Science Communications*, *46*, 100579., ISSN 2215-0382, https://doi.org/10.1016/j.colcom.2021.100579

Zheng, H., & Chen, W. (2021). Nanoparticle-based therapy for tauopathies in Alzheimer's disease. *Neurotherapeutics*, *18*(1), 137–152. https://doi.org/10.1007/s13311-020-00991-6

Zhou, Z., Zhao, Q., & Li, Y. (2021). Nanoparticle-based tau aggregation inhibitors for Alzheimer's disease treatment. *Journal of Controlled Release*, *331*, 82–95. https://doi.org/10.1016/j.nano.2021.102991

Zhu, X., Jin, K., Huang, Y., & Pang, Z. (2019). Brain drug delivery by adsorption-mediated transcytosis. In H. Gao & X. Gao (Eds.), *Brain targeted drug delivery system* (pp. 159–83). Academic Press. https://doi.org/10.1016/B978-0-12-814001-7.00007-X

15 Challenges and Opportunities of Nanomedicines in Clinical Translation

Meenakshi Kumari, Nagaraja Sreeharsha, Prakash Goudanavar, Bharti Sahu, Nidhi Puranik, and Arun Sharma

15.1 INTRODUCTION

The rapidly developing discipline of nanomedicine uses the special qualities of materials at the nanoscale in the diagnosis, treatment, and prevention of various diseases. It is defined as the use of nanotechnology in medicine, which includes the use of nanoparticles (NPs), nanodevices, and nanoscale processes to transport medications, improve imaging, and develop novel treatment approaches [1]. Usually between 1 and 100 nanometers in size, NPs have unique biological, chemical, and physical characteristics that allow for precise molecular and cellular interactions with biological systems [2,3].

Nanomedicine is a broad field that includes drug delivery methods, diagnostic instruments, regenerative medicine, and theranostics, the combination of therapy and diagnostics. Nanomedicine offers the possibility to increase the effectiveness of treatments by customizing NPs to target particular cells or tissues. Furthermore, the potential of nanomedicine to penetrate biological barriers, such as the blood–brain barrier (BBB), creates new therapeutic options for illnesses that have proven difficult to treat with traditional treatments [4].

The field of nanomedicine has evolved from theoretical study to real-world applications, with several diagnostic instruments and medicines based on nanotechnology either in clinical use or undergoing clinical trials [1]. Alzheimer's disease (AD) is a progressive neurodegenerative disorder marked by brain decay, plaque formation, and protein tangles, with treatment limited by the BBB. Nanomedicines offer innovative solutions to enhance drug delivery across the BBB, improving both AD diagnosis and therapy. Recent advances in nanotechnology have transformed AD management, though key challenges remain. Continued research into nanomedicines holds promise for future clinical applications in treating brain diseases like AD [1]. Comparably, the sensitivity and specificity of diagnostic imaging have been

DOI: 10.1201/9781003543381-15

enhanced by NP-based imaging agents, such as iron oxide NPs for magnetic resonance imaging (MRI). MRI is a powerful, non-invasive technique that provides high-resolution images of soft tissues, including the brain. It is highly effective in detecting molecular and structural abnormalities associated with diseases like Alzheimer's. MRI can monitor brain atrophy, plaque deposition, and other pathological changes over time. This makes it a valuable tool for early diagnosis and tracking the progression of neurodegenerative disorders [5,6].

Nanomedicine has emerged as a promising solution, using various nanocarriers—such as polymer NPs, liposomes, and magnetic NPs—to improve drug delivery and therapeutic outcomes. Recent preclinical studies demonstrate the potential of these nanotechnologies in AD management [7]. To guarantee that NPs are used safely in people, it is also necessary to evaluate the long-term safety and biocompatibility of the materials. Nanomedicine has attracted global interest in AD treatment, showing promising results through innovative drug delivery systems (DDSs). Various nanocarriers have been developed to improve treatment effectiveness, including polymer NPs, liposomes, solid lipid NPs, and dendritic and magnetic NPs [8] as shown in Figure 15.1.

The crucial process of transferring cutting-edge research discoveries from the lab into clinical settings so they can be applied to patient care is known as "clinical translation." In terms of nanomedicine, this entails proving the security and effectiveness of nanotechnologies through preclinical research as well as managing the

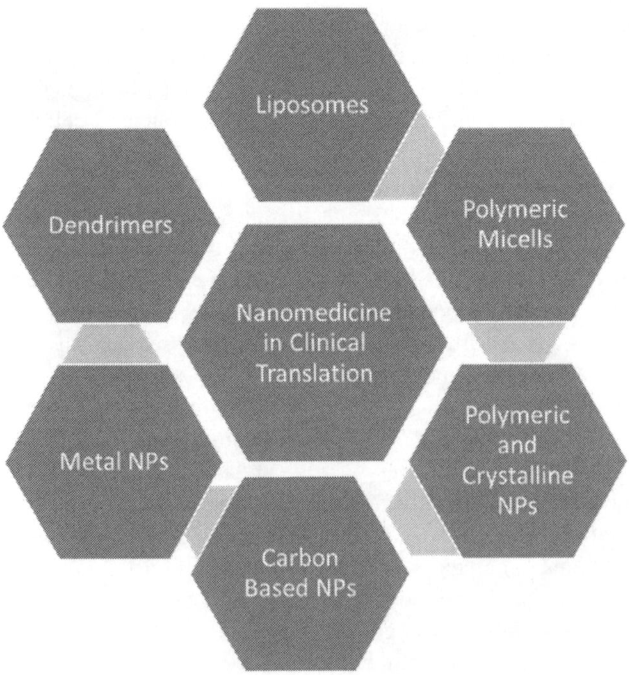

FIGURE 15.1 Nanomaterials in clinical translation of Alzheimer's disease.

intricate regulatory environment, streamlining production processes, and guaranteeing that these technologies can be produced consistently and economically at large scale. Many drugs for AD work well in animal studies but fail in human clinical trials. One reason is that animal models and testing methods are not always reliable or carefully done. To improve translation, the MODEL-AD consortium's Preclinical Testing Core (PTC) established a rigorous screening pipeline with quality control (QC) steps, including drug stability, brain exposure, pharmacokinetics/pharmacodynamics (PK/PD), and imaging (PET/MRI) to assess target engagement and disease modification before behavioral testing. This structured approach ensures reliable results and is available to researchers through the NIA-supported STOP-AD portal, aiming to enhance future AD drug discovery [9].

Many promising innovations fail to advance beyond the experimental stage due to several hurdles, leading to the "valley of death," as it is known, between nanomedicine research and clinical use. These include the challenging nature of synthesizing consistent NPs, the unpredictable nature of NP behavior in intricate biological systems, and the strict guidelines for conducting clinical studies [8]. To close this gap and enable the effective application of nanomedicine in clinical settings, a multidisciplinary team of investigators, physicians, regulators, and business associates must be assembled to tackle these issues. Nanomedicine applies nanotechnology to diagnose, monitor, and treat diseases, offering great potential to transform healthcare. However, its full potential is still unrealized due to unique challenges related to the novel properties of nanomaterials (NMs). These materials present both exciting opportunities and safety concerns that need further study. Closing scientific and regulatory gaps is essential to ensure safe and effective nanomedicine advancements [10].

Nanomedicine offers advanced, targeted treatments through cell-specific therapy, controlled drug release, wearable devices, and personalized medicine, reducing side effects and improving effectiveness. Using technologies like stimuli-responsive NPs and electrochemical sensors, it enables precise drug delivery for diseases like cancer, genetic disorders, and chronic illnesses. While still in the early stages, nanomedicine shows strong potential as a powerful alternative to traditional treatments, with ongoing research supporting its future success [11].

Personalized medicine and nanomedicine are emerging fields aiming to improve treatment outcomes by tailoring therapies to individual patient needs. Personalized medicine customizes treatment based on genetic profiles, while nanomedicine uses nanotechnology for targeted diagnosis and therapy. By combining these approaches, nanomedicines can be adapted to match patient-specific genetic variations, enhancing treatment precision and minimizing side effects [12]. Nanomedicine is anticipated to be a key player in the move towards personalized medicine, in which patient-specific medicines are designed based on their unique traits, as it develops further.

Although there are many obstacles to the clinical translation of nanomedicine, if it is successfully incorporated into healthcare systems, it has the potential to revolutionize the detection and treatment of many different diseases. Global cooperation, innovation, and research are necessary to overcome these obstacles and fully realize the promise of improvement in nanomedicine.

15.2 CHALLENGES IN THE CLINICAL TRANSLATION OF NANOMEDICINE

The use of nanotechnology in medicine, or "nanomedicine," has enormous potential to transform therapies, medication delivery, and diagnostics. Its therapeutic translation, however, is beset by several serious obstacles. These difficulties are seen in many areas, such as pharmacokinetics, safety, regulation, scalability, and ethical issues. We go into further depth about these difficulties below.

15.2.1 Toxicology and Safety

Making sure nanomedicine is safe and reducing toxicity is one of the biggest obstacles to its clinical application. Nanotechnology enhances personalized medicine by improving disease treatment through specially designed NMs. These materials offer advantages like small size, high surface area, and the ability to target specific biological molecules, making them ideal for diagnostics, imaging, and drug delivery. NMs interact with biological systems and highlight examples of nanomedicines in clinical trials. It also addresses key challenges such as toxicity, fabrication difficulties, and regulatory and ethical considerations for developing safe and effective personalized nanomedicines [13]. Because of their special qualities and small size, NPs may behave differently toxicologically than bulk materials. Concerns regarding nanotoxicology are raised by the possibility of oxidative stress, inflammation, and cytotoxicity as a result of NP interaction with biological systems. Predicting and controlling the harmful effects of NPs can be difficult due to their diverse surface chemistry, size, shape, and kind.

The significance of understanding NP behavior within biological systems to ensure the safe application of nanotechnology in medicine. It describes how inorganic NPs interact with cells and organisms, causing altered biodistribution, reactive surface chemistry, and unique solid-state properties combined with mobility. The use of functional nanomagnets allows for controlled drug delivery through mechanical guidance [14].

The use of engineered NMs in medicine is rapidly expanding due to advanced control over their synthesis, enabling diverse biological functions such as drug delivery, imaging, and sensing. These materials offer enhanced performance and new applications, but their interaction with biological systems may cause adverse effects like toxicity, allergies, and genotoxicity, while also facing challenges like corrosion and aggregation in physiological environments. Standard protocols for evaluating nanomaterial safety and effectiveness remain limited, making nanotoxicology a crucial and continuously evolving field [15].

15.2.2 Regulatory Difficulties

NMs are increasingly used in health products, drugs, and medical devices, bringing challenges due to their wide diversity and unique properties. Regulatory inconsistencies hinder the clinical development of nanomedicines despite calls for clearer guidelines. The ANSM's scientific council conducted a multidisciplinary to identify key regulatory concerns and recommended harmonizing international practices to better assess the risk-benefit balance of NMs, ensuring both human and environmental safety while meeting public expectations [16].

The complexity of nanomedicines makes it challenging for them to abide by legal requirements. Characterization of NPs, stability, repeatability, and batch-to-batch variation potential are some of the issues that affect the regulatory approval process. Complementary regulatory issues encompass the absence of standardized testing protocols and the challenge of predicting long-term safety. There is an urgent need for new standards and recommendations that are specifically tailored to nanomedicines. These guidelines ought to address the unique properties of NPs, including their size, shape, surface charge, and interactions with biological systems. Collaboration among academic institutions, industry stakeholders, and regulatory authorities is crucial in developing a comprehensive regulatory framework that ensures the safety and efficacy of nanomedicines.

Since the 1980s, nanomedicine has advanced rapidly, leading to an increasing number of approved nano-based pharmaceutical products used as therapies or targeted DDSs. Currently marketed nanostructures include nanocrystals, liposomes, lipid NPs, PEGylated nanodrugs, protein-based, and metal-based NPs. These innovative systems, along with gene vaccines, hold great potential but face significant regulatory challenges, particularly regarding safety, standardization, and ethical oversight. For nanomedicines, ensuring precise characterization and thorough safety assessments is essential due to their unique interactions with biological systems. Gene vaccines add further complexity, requiring tailored regulations that address vector design, target specificity, and long-term patient monitoring. Ethical considerations such as informed consent, privacy, and intellectual property rights must be carefully balanced with public health priorities. Additionally, high development costs, market risks, and commercial viability concerns limit the success of many nanomedicine products, with only a small number achieving regulatory approval. International cooperation between regulatory bodies, researchers, and industry is crucial to harmonize guidelines and accelerate the development of these therapies. Addressing environmental impacts and societal expectations for safety and efficacy also plays an important role in regulatory discussions. Collaboration with investors is needed to secure funding and confidence in future market profitability. Despite these challenges, the global nanomedicine market is projected to grow, driven by continuous innovation and rising healthcare demands. Successfully navigating regulatory, ethical, and commercial hurdles will be key to realizing the full potential of nanomedicines and gene vaccines in improving global health [17,18].

Nanomedicines and their follow-on versions (nanosimilars) are complex drugs with diverse structures and nanoscale properties, making their regulation and quality evaluation challenging. Traditional generic drug approval methods do not work well for these products due to their complexity. Regulatory agencies like the European Medicines Agency (EMA) and Food and Drug Administration (FDA) have proposed stepwise approaches focusing on critical quality attributes (CQAs), nano-properties, and clinical studies. However, a globally harmonized approval pathway is still lacking, causing differences in regulations. To improve this, collaboration among experts and stakeholders is needed to establish clear standards, ensuring innovation and better patient access [19]. Developers of nanomedicine frequently have difficulties in proving quality, safety, and efficacy in a way that regulatory agencies find acceptable, so new rules and regulations are required. Despite significant research in nanomedicine over the past two decades, fewer than 100 nanomedicines have been approved by the FDA and EMA since 1989, highlighting a major gap between research and market success. Challenges like complex formulation design and manufacturing issues, as seen with the discontinued drug DepoCyt, hinder clinical translation. It also proposes strategies for improving formulation and production through quality-by-design and risk-management approaches to enhance the development and sustainability of nanomedicines [20].

15.2.3 Manufacturing and Scalability

Nanotechnology is increasingly used in drug development, with nanoparticle-based therapeutics offering advantages like overcoming biological barriers, delivering hydrophobic drugs, and targeting disease sites. However, only a few nanomedicines have been clinically approved due to complex design, manufacturing challenges, and strict safety requirements. Minor changes in NPs can affect their safety and efficacy, requiring thorough preclinical and clinical evaluations, especially regarding biodistribution and immune responses. Unlike conventional drugs, nanomedicines face extra regulatory challenges, and clear standards are still evolving [8].

AD is a progressive neurodegenerative disorder with current treatments limited by low bioavailability and poor brain targeting. Intranasal delivery has emerged as a promising, non-invasive alternative, though it faces challenges related to nasal cavity constraints. Nanotechnology-based nanocarriers—such as polymeric NPs, metal NPs, lipid NPs, liposomes, nanoemulsions, quantum dots, and dendrimers—offer improved drug delivery by enhancing bioavailability, crossing the BBB, and targeting the brain effectively. Intranasal nanocarrier systems have the potential to transform Alzheimer's treatment, while emphasizing the need to carefully address regulatory and toxicity issues to ensure safety and effectiveness [21]. Nanomedicine has advanced fields like drug delivery, diagnostics, theranostics, and regenerative medicine, but its future growth faces regulatory challenges due to unclear guidelines. The key factors for the successful clinical translation of nanomedicines, including identifying CQAs, selecting proper analytical methods, defining important process parameters, and using suitable preclinical models. It also emphasizes the need to ensure batch-to-batch consistency and address scale-up challenges for reliable manufacturing. Early collaboration with regulatory agencies is recommended to streamline development and approval processes for future nanomedicines [17].

Nanomedicine holds great potential due to the unique physical and chemical properties of materials at the nanoscale, offering innovative solutions for disease treatment. However, its clinical adoption is limited by the lack of universal standards for nanomaterial characterization and insufficient understanding of how NMs interact with biological molecules like proteins. The nanomaterial characterization and protein interactions, proposes standardized techniques for consistent evaluation, and discusses regulatory challenges in translating nanomedicine to clinical use. Establishing universal standards and deepening biological understanding are key to accelerating nanomedicine's integration into routine medical practice [17]. Figure 15.2 provides an overview of the analytical techniques used for the physicochemical characterization of nanomedicines, highlighting NCL-recommended techniques for the routine evaluation of corresponding parameters.

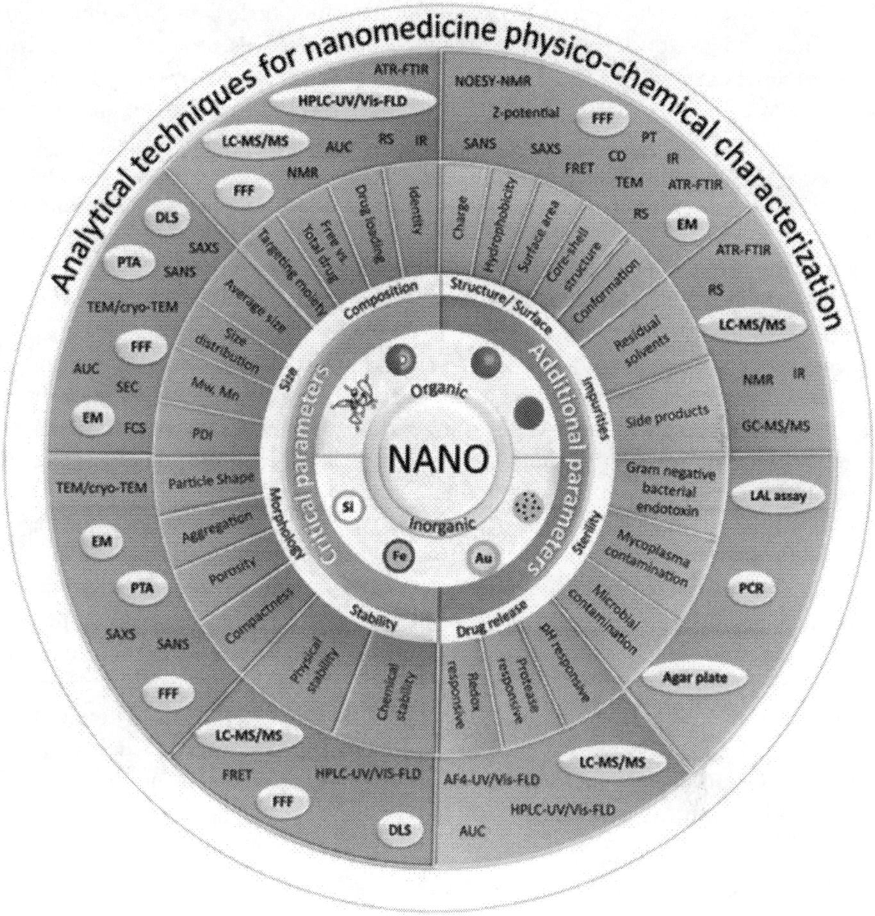

FIGURE 15.2 A schematic representation of critical and additional parameters of nanomedicines and corresponding analytical techniques for their characterization. (Adapted from [18].)

15.2.4 Pharmacokinetics and Biodistribution

NPs have become promising drug carriers due to their high surface-to-volume ratios and unique physicochemical properties, offering fewer side effects than traditional drugs. Nanomedicines are now used for disease detection, tissue repair, and regeneration. Designing effective nanoparticle-based DDSs requires a clear understanding of pharmacokinetics (LADME: liberation, absorption, distribution, metabolism, and elimination). This review explores how the properties of NPs influence their behavior in the body, helping to compare them with conventional medicines. A thorough pharmacokinetic analysis is essential to improve treatment outcomes and advance nanoparticle applications in biomedicine [17]. AD is a neurodegenerative disorder causing cognitive decline, and donepezil is commonly used to treat its symptoms. This study aimed to develop a sustained-release, brain-targeted nanoparticle delivery system for donepezil using poly(lactic-co-glycolic acid) (PLGA). Donepezil-loaded

PLGA NPs were prepared through solvent emulsification diffusion–evaporation and characterized for size, morphology, and drug loading. The NPs, around 90 nm in size with smooth, spherical shapes, showed an initial burst release followed by sustained drug release. In vivo studies demonstrated higher brain uptake of the nanoparticle formulation compared to the regular drug solution. These findings suggest that PLGA NPs could enhance the brain delivery of donepezil for better AD treatment, though further clinical studies are needed [22]. The distribution of NPs within the body is mostly determined by their size, shape, and surface characteristics. AD is the leading cause of dementia in the elderly, marked by β-amyloid plaques, tau tangles, brain shrinkage, and ventricular enlargement. Effective treatment is difficult due to the BBB, which restricts drug delivery to the brain, and challenges like opsonization by plasma proteins. Biodegradable polymeric NPs with surface modifications offer significant potential for crossing the BBB and delivering therapeutic agents to treat neurological disorders such as AD. The effectiveness of brain delivery and treatment can be further improved by optimizing nanoparticle properties, including surfactant concentrations, stabilizers, and amyloid-targeting agents [23].

Nanomedicine and personalized medicine are two emerging fields transforming medical practice. Nanomedicine uses nanotechnology for advanced diagnostics and treatments, while personalized medicine tailors' therapies based on individual patient characteristics, such as genetic profiles, to improve effectiveness and reduce side effects. By combining these approaches, nanomedicines can be customized for patient-specific treatments, enhancing precision in managing various diseases. Nanomedicine and personalized medicine work together to provide tailored treatments based on individual patient profiles, improving effectiveness and reducing side effects. This approach also addresses challenges in advancing nano-personalized therapies into clinical practice [12].

15.2.5 Social and Ethical Concerns

It is necessary to address the ethical and sociological challenges brought up by the clinical translation of nanomedicine. Safety, privacy, and equity are among the ethical issues that are brought up by the application of nanotechnology in medicine. Nanotechnology is increasingly being integrated into clinical medicine, offering new possibilities for treatment, but raising unique ethical challenges that existing bioethics frameworks cannot fully address. A major concern is the lack of clear ethical guidelines and legislation for the safe clinical use of nanotechnology. Public opposition has also grown, driven by uncertainties and fears about the potential risks and implications of these technologies. It compares population concerns with established ethical discussions, seeking to understand whether people are more focused on current or future ethical issues, if their views are shaped by personal values or utility, and whether they assess nanotechnology from an individual or societal perspective [24].

The role of artificial intelligence (AI) in managing AD, a global health challenge characterized by progressive cognitive decline, is becoming increasingly significant. AI offers innovative solutions for early diagnosis, personalized treatment, and caregiver support by analyzing complex data, genetic profiles, and lifestyle factors. Following PRISMA guidelines and utilizing tools such as R programming and the AXIS appraisal tool, research reviews AI's potential to improve outcomes and enhance the quality of life for AD patients. However, important ethical concerns remain, including data privacy, algorithm accuracy, and the risk of depersonalized care. There is a critical need for standardized guidelines and collaborative efforts among policymakers, regulators, and the medical community to ensure the responsible and ethical integration of AI into AD management [25–27]. The way the general public views nanotechnology can have a big impact on how it is applied in medicine. Patients and the general public may become resistant due to worries about the safety and moral ramifications of nanomedicine. Nanotechnology offers promising strategies for improving drug, protein, and anti-amyloid delivery across the BBB in AD treatment. Advances in bioimaging and proteomics also support AD management. However, potential long-term toxicity and large-scale production challenges of NPs need further research. The future of nanomedicine in AD is optimistic, with multifunctional NPs aiming to target inflammation, oxidative stress, tau phosphorylation, and mitochondrial dysfunction. There is also an urgent need for innovative treatments that not only relieve symptoms but also prevent disease progression, improving patients' quality of life [28]. Nanomedicine has emerged as a promising field, using NPs to enhance the diagnosis and treatment of AD by improving drug transport across these barriers. Although significant progress has been made, challenges remain in bringing nanomedicine-based treatments into clinical practice. Continued advancements in this field offer hope for better outcomes in AD management [29]. The rapid growth of nanomedical technology raises significant ethical and legal challenges in disease detection, diagnosis, and treatment [30]. Major characterization and concern in regulation of nanomedicines are represented in Figure 15.3.

Nanomedicine, the application of nanotechnology in medical contexts, holds significant promise for advancing disease detection, diagnosis, and treatment. However, its rapid development introduces various ethical and legal challenges that necessitate careful consideration.

Risk Assessment and Safety Concerns: NPs exhibit unique properties due to their nanoscale size, leading to unpredictable interactions within biological systems. These interactions can result in oxidative stress, inflammation, or immune responses. The long-term effects of NPs remain largely unknown, underscoring the need for comprehensive risk assessments. Existing regulatory frameworks may not be fully equipped to address these unique challenges, necessitating the establishment of specific guidelines for nanomedicine applications [31].

Informed Consent and Patient Autonomy: The complexity of nanomedicine can make it challenging for patients to fully comprehend the potential risks and benefits associated with NP-based treatments. This complexity underscores the importance of obtaining informed consent, ensuring that patients are adequately informed about how their data will be used, stored, and transferred before agreeing to participate in nanomedicine treatments or research [32].

Privacy and Data Security: Nanomedical technologies often rely on the collection and analysis of extensive personal data, including genetic information, to tailor treatments to individual patients. This extensive data collection presents significant risks if not adequately protected, making privacy and data security critical to maintaining trust in the field [31].

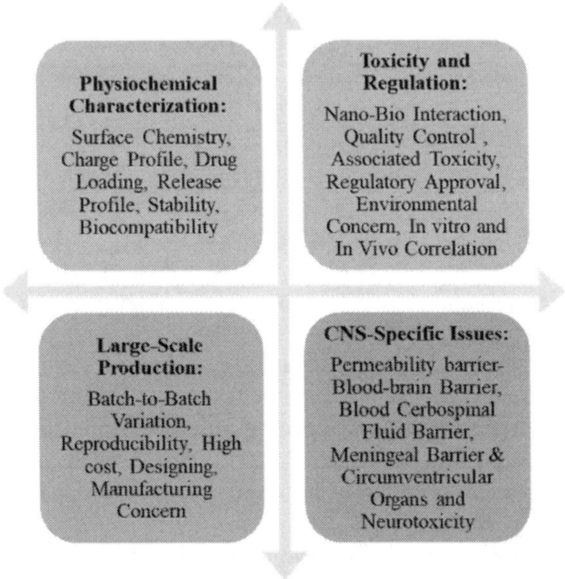

FIGURE 15.3 Biological challenges in the clinical translation of nanomedicine in targeting Central nervous system-associated diseases.

Equitable Access to Nanomedicine: The high costs and sophisticated infrastructure required for nanomedicine could exacerbate existing healthcare disparities. Patients in low-income or marginalized communities may face significant barriers to accessing these advanced treatments. Addressing this issue requires global policies aimed at making treatments more affordable and investments in healthcare infrastructure to ensure equitable access [32].

Application of the Precautionary Principle: Given the uncertainties surrounding the long-term effects of NMs, applying the precautionary principle is crucial. This approach advocates for caution in the development and deployment of nanomedical technologies until their safety is thoroughly validated. Addressing these ethical and legal challenges necessitates a coordinated global effort to establish comprehensive guidelines and regulations [30].

A summary of all major challenges associated with nanomedicine translation is summarized in Figure 15.4.

15.3 OPPORTUNITIES IN CLINICAL TRANSLATION OF NANOMEDICINE

Numerous opportunities in the field of nanomedicine have the potential to completely transform healthcare. The fields of targeted drug delivery, theranostics, breaking down the BBB, and innovative therapeutic modalities are among the most promising ones. These opportunities are thoroughly examined in this section [10].

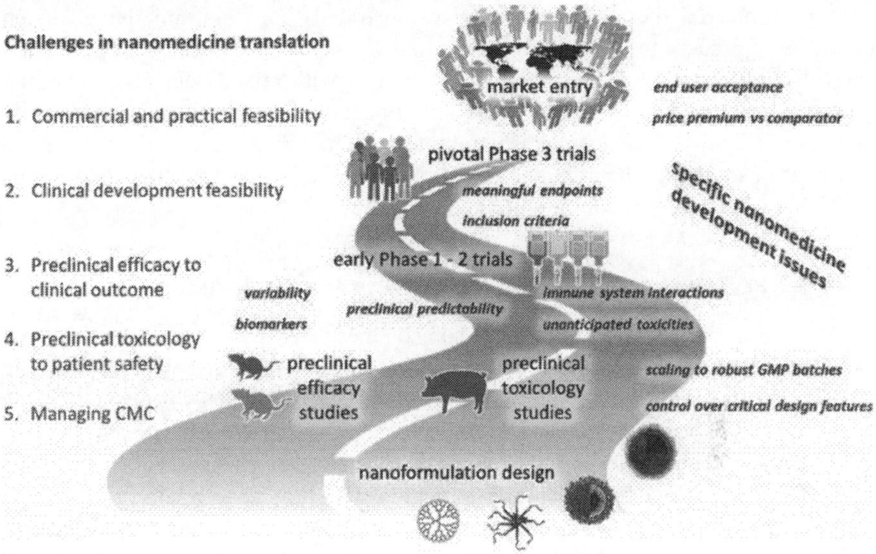

FIGURE 15.4 A summary of challenges in nanomedicine clinical translation. (Adapted from [10].)

15.3.1 Targeted Drug Delivery

Precision medicine is made possible by the notable advances that nanomedicine brings to the field of tailored drug delivery. NPs can deliver drugs to particular cells or tissues in a way that minimizes their negative effects on healthy tissues. One of the main components of precision medicine is this focused approach, which attempts to customize therapies for specific patients according to their genetic, environmental, and lifestyle characteristics. This is made easier by the development of drug delivery methods made possible by nanomedicine, which can be tailored to target certain cell receptors or diseased locations and increase the effectiveness of treatments [11].

15.3.2 Case Studies of Successful Targeted Therapies

Recent advancements in targeted therapies for AD have shown promising results, offering hope for more effective treatments.

Lecanemab (Leqembi) is an FDA-approved monoclonal antibody that targets amyloid-beta plaques in the brain, significantly reducing plaque buildup and slowing cognitive decline in early-stage AD. Lecanemab (Leqembi) is an FDA-approved monoclonal antibody that targets amyloid-beta plaques in the brain, significantly reducing plaque buildup and slowing cognitive decline in early-stage AD. Donanemab (Kisunla): Another monoclonal antibody targeting amyloid plaques, donanemab showed a 35% slowing of cognitive decline in clinical trials. It received approval in Japan for early symptomatic AD, marking a significant milestone in global AD treatment options [33].

A personalized therapy case study demonstrated that a multimodal precision medicine approach, tailored to an individual's specific disease mechanisms, successfully improved cognitive function in a patient with mixed dementia, including AD. A case report detailed the successful treatment of a patient with mixed dementia using a personalized, multimodal therapy approach. This strategy underscores the potential of tailoring interventions based on individual patient profiles, addressing multiple disease mechanisms simultaneously [34].

15.3.3 Potential for Reducing Side Effects and Improving Efficacy

Scientists are increasingly exploring nanomedicine for its vast potential in the diagnosis, treatment, and prevention of various diseases. With promising applications in developing advanced medical tools and techniques, nanotechnology is revolutionizing multiple areas of healthcare, including diagnostics, regenerative medicine, gene therapy, dentistry, oncology, aesthetics, and targeted drug delivery. Extensive data from credible scientific sources have been analyzed to demonstrate how nanotechnology enhances sensitive medical procedures and therapeutic interventions. The future of nanomedicine relies heavily on strong collaboration between clinicians, researchers, and technologists to establish precise, programmable, and innovative healthcare solutions. Despite its growing success, the field still faces challenges due to disease complexity and physiological barriers. Therefore, addressing health, environmental, and ethical concerns related to nanomedicine is essential [35]. Nanotechnology offers a promising solution to overcome the BBB, which limits drug delivery in neurodegenerative diseases like AD, Parkinson's disease (PD), Huntington's disease (HD), and amyotrophic lateral sclerosis (ALS). Lipid-based, polymeric, and inorganic NPs to enhance brain drug transport. Techniques such as surface modifications and targeted ligands improve delivery efficiency. Innovative drug formulations within NPs show positive results in preclinical and clinical studies. Despite progress, challenges remain in safety, scalability, and clinical translation. Continued research may revolutionize NDD treatment [36].

15.3.4 Theranostics

Theranostic compounds are innovative radioactive agents that combine both diagnostic and therapeutic capabilities, allowing for the simultaneous imaging and treatment of diseases. These compounds are administered into the bloodstream, where they target specific cells, enabling imaging techniques like PET scans to detect diseased cells through radiotracers. Beyond diagnosis, these compounds can be enhanced with stronger radioactive elements to actively destroy harmful cells, such as cancer cells. Common examples include I-131 iodine for thyroid cancer, I-131 MIBG for neuroblastomas, and FDA-approved Lutetium-177 DOTATATE for targeted therapies. Theranostic compounds offer multiple benefits, including improved disease detection, precise staging, personalized treatment planning, reduced harm to healthy tissues, and better quality of life for patients. As a rapidly growing field, theranostics plays a vital role in the advancement of personalized medicine, offering new hope for more effective and safer treatments across various diseases [37]. AD remains a major global health challenge, with increasing prevalence and significant economic impact, particularly in aging populations. Despite decades of research, effective diagnostic and therapeutic solutions remain elusive, leaving AD incurable and emphasizing the urgent need for innovative strategies. Recently, theranostic agents have gained attention as a promising approach for AD management. These agents combine both diagnostic and therapeutic functions within a single molecule, enabling real-time monitoring of drug activity, patient response, and pharmacokinetics. This dual functionality makes theranostics highly valuable for advancing personalized medicine and accelerating the development of effective AD treatments. Small-molecule theranostic agents, in particular, show potential to revolutionize the detection and treatment of AD, offering hope for improved clinical outcomes and more efficient research pipelines. With ongoing advancements, theranostics are expected to have a significant and positive impact on future AD clinical practice and can be used to assess the activity of a molecule, the response of the organism, and the pharmacokinetics [38]. Two major obstacles in managing AD are the lack of an easily accessible, reliable early diagnostic method and the absence of effective disease-modifying treatments. The recent success of lecanemab, a monoclonal antibody targeting amyloid-beta, has renewed interest in identifying druggable pathways and reignited small-molecule drug research. Unlike complex and expensive biologics, small molecules offer practical benefits: they are simpler, cost-effective, and can often be taken orally, making early and long-term treatment more feasible. Small-molecule near-infrared (NIR) fluorescent theranostics are gaining significant attention due to their dual ability to diagnose and treat AD simultaneously. These theranostic agents can serve as non-invasive, affordable alternatives to conventional PET imaging, providing real-time diagnostic feedback while delivering therapeutic effects directly to the brain. Recent research has focused on improving their molecular design, synthesis, imaging capabilities, and therapeutic efficacy in both laboratory and animal studies. Overall, fluorescent theranostic agents represent a promising step toward personalized medicine in AD, offering hope for earlier detection, better monitoring, and more effective treatments, with ongoing work aiming to optimize these compounds for future clinical use [39].

15.3.5 Overcoming the Blood–Brain Barrier

Overcoming the BBB is a challenge for treating AD because it limits how drugs can reach the brain. Researchers are developing strategies to improve drug delivery to the brain. The treatment of central nervous system disorders, such as AD and various brain cancers, faces significant challenges due to the protective nature of the BBB, which restricts many therapeutic drugs from effectively reaching the brain. Traditional oral and systemic drug delivery methods often lead to serious side effects or insufficient brain penetration, reducing their therapeutic efficacy. Over the past decade, innovative technologies have been developed to overcome these limitations. The structural and anatomical characteristics of the BBB are examining various experimental models used to study drug transport across the BBB, including *in vitro* (static and dynamic), *in vivo* (microdialysis), and *in situ* (brain perfusion) models. To enhance CNS drug delivery, several advanced formulations have been explored, including NPs (lipid-based, polymeric, magnetic, gold, carbon-based, dendrimers), viral vectors, peptide shuttles, sonoporation with microbubbles, and receptor modulation strategies to bypass efflux transporters. Additionally, intranasal administration offers a non-invasive route to bypass the BBB, while direct brain injections provide localized delivery but are more invasive. By combining these advanced technologies and strategies, researchers aim to develop safer and more effective treatments for severe brain disorders, including neurodegenerative diseases like Alzheimer's, by improving drug delivery to the brain and minimizing systemic side effects [40].

To overcome the challenges posed by the BBB in treating neurological diseases like AD, several advanced strategies have been developed. Nanomedicine uses carriers like liposomes to safely deliver drugs across the BBB. Targeted delivery directs therapeutics to specific brain regions, improving precision and reducing side effects. BBB opening techniques, such as chemical disruption, temporarily increase permeability for drug entry. Nasal drug delivery bypasses the BBB via the olfactory pathway for direct brain access. Intrathecal and intracerebroventricular infusions inject drugs directly into the cerebrospinal fluid. Lastly, targeted ultrasound combined with microbubbles enhances drug transport across the BBB safely. Together, these methods provide promising approaches to improve AD treatment outcomes [41].

Recent case studies and research on AD are focusing on areas like genetic variations linked to the disease, the impact of lifestyle factors on risk, early detection methods, and novel treatment approaches, including investigations into the role of amyloid beta and tau proteins. One case highlighted early-onset Alzheimer's in a young individual, revealing both cognitive decline and physical impairments such as gait disturbances, emphasizing the importance of multidisciplinary care. Research into resilient individuals with genetic risk factors, like apolipoprotein E (APOE) variants, has uncovered potential protective brain mechanisms that delay cognitive symptoms. Another case involving a musician with Alzheimer's demonstrated the disease's impact on complex motor skills essential to their profession. Recent studies have also identified specific genetic variations linked to higher or lower AD risk, particularly APOE alleles, guiding predictions and treatments. Promising clinical trials are targeting amyloid beta plaques and tau tangles, the hallmark proteins of AD pathology. Additionally, lifestyle factors such as regular exercise, a healthy diet, mental stimulation, and social engagement have been shown to reduce AD risk. Advances in early detection now focus on blood-based biomarkers like phosphorylated tau and amyloid beta, while cutting-edge neuroimaging techniques such as PET scans allow precise visualization of brain changes, supporting earlier diagnosis and personalized treatment strategies [42]. AI techniques also applied to neuroimaging are improving early diagnosis and management of AD, though challenges like data standardization and ethical considerations remain [43].

15.3.6 Novel Therapeutic Modalities

Novel therapeutic strategies for AD focus on multiple approaches, including anti-inflammatory therapies to reduce neuroinflammation, anti-amyloid therapies targeting amyloid-beta plaques, and brain stimulation techniques like transcranial magnetic stimulation to enhance cognitive function. Additionally, innovative methods such as stem cell therapies aim to regenerate damaged neurons, genetic modulation seeks to correct or suppress harmful gene expressions, and non-pharmacological interventions like cognitive training, diet, and exercise are being explored to support brain health and slow disease progression. AD is a growing concern with limited effective treatments, prompting research into novel therapies like anti-amyloid, anti-tau, anti-inflammatory agents, neuroprotective drugs, and brain stimulation [44]. Recent research is shifting toward alternative therapeutic strategies, such as tau-targeted therapies, anti-inflammatory approaches, gene therapy, and stem cell treatments, which address other critical aspects of AD pathology. These emerging methods aim to provide more effective, multi-targeted treatments, offering new hope for improving patient outcomes and managing the complexity of AD [45].

15.4 CASE STUDIES OF SUCCESSFUL CLINICAL TRANSLATION

Preclinical studies are crucial for advancing AD treatments, but over-reliance on single-target approaches, particularly the amyloid hypothesis, has slowed progress and led to repeated clinical trial failures. To enhance translation from preclinical studies to effective therapies, the field must broaden its focus beyond amyloid, refine study methods, and consider complex pathogenic pathways to develop more successful anti-dementia treatments [46].

New therapeutic strategies, including cell transplantation and immune modulation, have demonstrated encouraging outcomes in various preclinical models of AD. However, translating these approaches into effective clinical treatments has often fallen short of expectations. Traditional herbal extracts, such as *Bacopa monnieri* and remedies from traditional Chinese medicine, have shown neuroprotective potential in animal studies, yet these findings require further refinement and validation before successful application in human trials. Likewise, phytochemicals like nano-curcumin and S-allyl-cysteine (SAC) have exhibited promising antioxidant and anti-inflammatory effects in experimental models. Despite these advances, there remains a noticeable hesitance to initiate large-scale clinical trials involving herbal extracts, largely due to unresolved concerns regarding their safety profiles, precise mechanisms of action, and long-term efficacy. Addressing these challenges through rigorous research and standardized protocols may unlock the full therapeutic potential of these natural compounds in future AD treatments [46,47].

15.4.1 FDA-Approved Nanomedicines

AD management has progressed with the approval of various pharmacological treatments and the exploration of nanomedicine-based therapies. FDA-approved medications such as Aricept (donepezil), Exelon Patch (rivastigmine), Namenda (memantine), and Namzaric (a combination of memantine and donepezil) aim to alleviate symptoms and slow cognitive decline in AD patients [48]. Recent advancements include the approval of Leqembi (lecanemab) and Kisunla (donanemab), both of which target amyloid-beta plaques to decelerate disease progression in early-stage AD. Concurrently, nanomedicine offers promising avenues for AD treatment by enhancing drug delivery across the BBB, improving therapeutic efficacy, and reducing side effects. NPs such as polymer-based, lipid-based, and metal-based carriers have been investigated for their potential to deliver therapeutic agents directly to the brain, thereby addressing challenges associated with conventional treatments [49]. These advancements reflect a multifaceted approach to AD therapy, integrating traditional pharmacological treatments with innovative nanotechnology to improve patient outcomes.

Current FDA-approved drugs, such as acetylcholinesterase inhibitors and NMDA receptor antagonists, have limited effectiveness due to poor brain penetration, low bioavailability, and undesirable side effects. To overcome these challenges, innovative DDSs have been developed to enhance the targeted delivery, controlled release, and sustained action of AD medications. These DDSs improve therapeutic efficacy while minimizing side effects, offering promising advances in AD management [50].

15.4.2 Lessons Learned from Their Development and Approval Processes

Key lessons from the development and approval processes of AD treatments highlight several critical challenges and considerations. Clinical trials for AD have faced high failure rates, largely due to the disease's complex mechanisms, limitations of animal models, and inadequate trial designs with small sample sizes, which hinder the accurate assessment of treatment efficacy. Accurate, biomarker-based diagnosis using tools like amyloid PET scans is essential to ensure patients truly have AD, improving trial validity. Research also suggests that early intervention, targeting the disease before significant cognitive decline, may improve outcomes. Additionally, due to the complex pathology of AD, multi-target therapies addressing multiple pathways beyond amyloid-beta may be more effective [51]. Clinical trials must also prioritize patient diversity to ensure results are generalizable to real-world populations. Other key considerations include the limitations of subgroup analyses in interpreting failed trials, challenges in translating findings from animal models to human disease, ensuring adequate drug delivery across the BBB, and evaluating the long-term safety of chronic treatments. Recent developments include the controversial approval of aducanumab, which raised questions about balancing potential benefits against uncertain efficacy and high costs, and a growing focus on developing disease-modifying therapies aimed at slowing or halting AD progression rather than merely managing symptoms [52,53].

15.4.3 Analysis of Ongoing and Recently Completed Clinical Trials

Recent analysis of ongoing and recently completed AD clinical trials indicates a shift towards promising results with several Phase 3 trials showing positive outcomes for anti-amyloid therapies like lecanemab and donanemab, signifying a potential breakthrough in disease-modifying treatments, particularly when targeting patients in early stages of the disease; however, challenges remain regarding access, patient selection, and developing combination therapies to address the complex pathology of AD [54]. Current Alzheimer's clinical trials are emphasizing early intervention, particularly in patients with mild cognitive impairment (MCI), using biomarkers for accurate selection. Anti-amyloid therapies like lecanemab and donanemab have shown promising results in slowing cognitive decline, while research is expanding to other targets such as tau protein, neuroinflammation, and neuroprotection. Combination therapies are being explored to address the disease's complexity. Despite advancements, challenges remain, including high treatment costs and improving early diagnosis. Recent progress also highlights the growing use of PET scans, blood biomarkers, and innovative treatments like gene and stem cell therapies [55].

15.4.4 Industry-Academic Collaborations

Industry-academic collaborations are essential for developing new treatments for AD. These collaborations can involve data sharing, establishing standards, and developing biomarkers. Advancing therapeutic strategies for AD requires collaboration between academia, industry, and regulatory bodies to develop reliable biomarkers. These biomarkers are crucial for early detection, patient selection, monitoring drug safety, and measuring treatment effectiveness. Establishing standardized biomarker networks will help accelerate clinical trials, improve regulatory approvals, and ultimately reduce the global impact of AD [56].

A study presents a successful collaboration between academic researchers and industry professionals using the Donepezil Data Repository, which collected data from 18 randomized controlled trials conducted between 1991 and 2005 on AD. Typically, academic circles are cautious of industry-sponsored data mining, fearing commercial interests might outweigh scientific value. However, in this case, Pfizer and Eisai formed an Expert Working Group consisting of seven top Alzheimer's researchers to guide the analysis. The group identified current clinical and scientific gaps that could be addressed using the database and collaborated closely with company statisticians and clinicians. Leadership was shared, with rotating responsibilities for project oversight and publication preparation. This partnership produced six high-quality manuscripts published in respected journals and several conference presentations, contributing valuable insights to Alzheimer's research [57].

15.5 FUTURE DIRECTIONS IN NANOMEDICINE TRANSLATION

Nanomedicine holds significant promise for advancing AD treatment, particularly in overcoming challenges like the BBB that impede effective drug delivery. Recent studies have demonstrated the potential of NPs to facilitate targeted delivery of therapeutic agents to the brain, thereby enhancing treatment efficacy [29]. Future research directions in this field include the development of multifunctional NPs capable of simultaneous diagnosis and therapy, known as theranostics. These advanced systems aim to provide real-time monitoring of disease progression and therapeutic response, enabling personalized treatment strategies [8]. Additionally, exploring alternative administration routes, such as intranasal delivery, offers a promising avenue for bypassing the BBB. This method has shown potential in enhancing drug bioavailability in the brain, presenting a non-invasive approach to AD treatment [17].

15.5.1 Interdisciplinary Collaboration

Interdisciplinary collaboration for AD involves a team of professionals from different fields working together to provide care. This approach is beneficial because no single specialty can address the many challenges of dementia [58]. Collaborative efforts between academia, industry, and regulatory bodies are essential to address the translational challenges of nanomedicine in AD therapy. Establishing standardized protocols for evaluating the safety, efficacy, and long-term effects of nanomedicines is crucial for their successful integration into clinical practice. Interdisciplinary collaboration plays a crucial role in the effective care and management of AD by bringing together a diverse team of professionals to address the complex physical, cognitive, emotional, and social challenges faced by patients. Specialists such as memory care experts, physical and occupational therapists, nutritionists, social workers, speech-language pathologists, and spiritual guides work collectively to provide comprehensive, patient-centered care that improves both quality of life and treatment outcomes. Beyond direct care, interdisciplinary teams also contribute to advancing research by developing integrated models of AD, combining insights from multiple fields to better understand the condition. This collaborative approach is essential not only for delivering high-quality, holistic care but also for supporting families and caregivers, ensuring that all aspects of the disease are managed through coordinated and compassionate strategies [59].

15.5.2 Strategies for Fostering Interdisciplinary Research

To promote interdisciplinary research in AD, it is essential to create collaborative research environments that bring together experts from diverse fields such as neuroscience, genetics, psychology, social work, epidemiology, and clinical trials. Establishing cross-disciplinary funding opportunities, facilitating open communication across specialties, and organizing joint workshops and seminars can further strengthen collaboration. Encouraging team-based science approaches and leveraging shared data platforms are also key to integrating knowledge and resources. By uniting varied expertise, researchers can gain a more comprehensive understanding of AD and work toward the development of more effective, innovative interventions [60].

15.5.3 Regulatory Innovation

Regulatory innovation for AD involves improving the way health authorities evaluate and approve new treatments to better address the challenges of this complex condition. One key area of innovation is updating guidelines to reflect the unique nature of Alzheimer's, such as allowing clinical trials to include patients in earlier stages of the disease and focusing on treatments that slow disease progression rather than just manage symptoms. Another important aspect is the development of new outcome measures to more accurately track how a treatment is working. Traditional memory tests may not fully capture the benefits of new therapies, so regulators are encouraging the use of biomarkers, like brain scans or blood tests, and digital tools that monitor cognitive changes over time. In addition, regulatory agencies are considering a wider range of new treatments, including disease-modifying therapies, gene therapies, and immunotherapies, which may require more flexible approval processes. Together, these innovations help create a clearer, faster path for bringing effective Alzheimer's treatments to patients who urgently need them [61].

Cognitive improvements are expected to eventually lead to better daily functioning. However, improvements in functional abilities may take longer to appear compared to cognitive benefits seen with new treatments. Given the serious impact of Alzheimer's on patients and families and its rising prevalence, there is an urgent need for innovative clinical trial designs and better ways to measure treatment success, especially in the early stages of the disease. While recent scientific discoveries have improved our understanding of Alzheimer's and its complex progression, they have also raised new challenges for drug development. The FDA has expressed its commitment to supporting innovative strategies to assess new drugs, recognizing the urgent need for effective therapies as the global population continues to age [61].

15.5.4 Proposals for Improving the Approval Process for Nanomedicines

AD is the leading cause of memory loss in older adults, with its prevalence increasing due to the aging global population. Currently, there are no highly effective treatments for AD, mainly because of challenges like low drug effectiveness, poor bioavailability, and difficulty delivering drugs across the BBB. In response to these challenges, nanomedicine has emerged as a promising approach for AD treatment. Various types of nanocarriers—including polymer NPs, liposomes, solid lipid NPs, dendritic NPs, biomimetic NPs, and magnetic NPs—have been explored to improve drug delivery and effectiveness [8].

15.5.5 Technological Advancements

Technological advancements are playing an increasingly important role in the fight against AD. Innovations such as AI, wearable sensors, and advanced imaging technologies are helping to improve early diagnosis, personalize patient care, and support better health outcomes. AI can analyze large amounts of data, such as brain scans and medical records, to detect early signs of Alzheimer's that may be difficult for doctors to identify. Wearable sensors monitor patients' daily activities, sleep patterns, and movement, providing real-time information that can help track changes in behavior and cognitive function. Imaging technologies, like PET and MRI scans, offer detailed views of the brain, allowing for the detection of abnormalities associated with Alzheimer's at earlier stages. Together, these technologies not only support earlier and more accurate diagnoses but also help healthcare providers develop tailored treatment plans, ultimately aiming to slow disease progression and improve the quality of life for patients [62].

15.5.6 Role of Artificial Intelligence and Machine Learning in Nanomedicine Research

AD is a neurocognitive disorder and a major cause of dementia, with its global impact growing each year according to the World Health Organization. With the rapid development of technology, AI has become increasingly important in medical diagnostics, including areas such as medical image analysis, drug development, personalized treatment planning, and disease prediction. In particular, deep learning, a key area of AI, is helping to address medical challenges by supporting the early detection, diagnosis, and treatment of AD [25].

15.5.7 Personalized Medicine

Personalized medicine for AD is an individualized approach to treatment and prevention that considers a person's specific genetic makeup, lifestyle factors, and environmental influences. Instead of using a one-size-fits-all strategy, personalized medicine aims to identify the unique characteristics and subtypes of Alzheimer's in each patient. By understanding these differences, researchers and doctors can develop targeted therapies designed to work more effectively for each individual. This approach not only helps in selecting the most appropriate treatments but also supports early intervention and prevention strategies, ultimately aiming to slow disease progression and improve the overall quality of life for people living with Alzheimer's [63].

15.5.8 Challenges and Opportunities in Customized Nanomedicine

AD is a major global public health concern, made difficult to treat due to its complex symptoms, unclear mechanisms, and long asymptomatic preclinical stage. Despite ongoing clinical trials, many Alzheimer's drugs fail to produce consistent patient responses and may cause serious side effects, making the disease a strong candidate for personalized medicine. Nanotechnology plays a key role in advancing personalized treatment for AD. Personalized medicine focuses on creating tailored therapies based on a person's genetics, disease progression, and individual responses to drugs. Improved detection techniques are essential to gather the data needed to predict and monitor treatment outcomes. In this context, bionanosensors are already showing high sensitivity in detecting important AD biomarkers, while functionalized NPs are being developed to improve drug delivery, enhance targeting, and reduce side effects by using lower doses [64].

15.6 CONCLUSION

The journey from laboratory research to clinical application in nanomedicine is involved with several key challenges. One of the most significant challenges in nanomedicine is ensuring safety and minimizing toxicity. The unique properties of NPs, while beneficial, also introduce complexities in predicting their behavior in biological systems, necessitating rigorous safety assessments. The consistent production of safe and effective nanomedicines might be hampered by scalability and manufacturing challenges, which include problems with large-scale production, standardization, and QC. Moreover, the clinical translation process is made more complex by issues with pharmacokinetics, biodistribution, ethics, and society.

Notwithstanding these obstacles, nanomedicine has enormous potential to revolutionize healthcare in the future. By enabling targeted drug delivery, personalized medicine, and theranostics, nanomedicine has the potential to completely transform illness diagnosis, treatment, and prevention. Nanomedicine has the potential to significantly improve patient outcomes and lower healthcare costs. There are a few essential procedures that must be taken to fully utilize nanomedicine. To bridge the gap that exists between clinical practice, industry, and scientific research, multidisciplinary collaboration must first be fostered. At first, working together can hasten the creation of novel solutions and expedite the conversion of research into practical uses. Secondly, regulatory frameworks need to change to better suit the special needs of nanomedicine. This entails creating precise norms and implementing flexible regulatory tactics that can keep up with changes in technology. Ultimately, continuous research and development funding is essential to the field's advancement, the resolution of current issues, and the discovery of new horizons in nanomedicine.

REFERENCES

1. Patra JK, Das G, Fraceto LF, Campos EVR, Rodriguez-Torres MDP, Acosta-Torres LS et al. Nano based drug delivery systems: Recent developments and future prospects. Journal of Nanobiotechnology 2018 16:12018;16():1–33. https://doi.org/10.1186/S12951-018-0392-8.
2. Altammar KA. A review on nanoparticles: Characteristics, synthesis, applications, and challenges. Front Microbiol 2023;14:1155622. https://doi.org/10.3389/FMICB.2023.1155622
3. Khan I, Saeed K, Khan I. Nanoparticles: Properties, applications and toxicities. Arabian Journal of Chemistry 2019;12:908–31. https://doi.org/10.1016/J.ARABJC.2017.05.011.
4. Kurul F, Turkmen H, Cetin AE, Topkaya SN. Nanomedicine: How nanomaterials are transforming drug delivery, bio-imaging, and diagnosis. Next Nanotechnology 2025;7:100129. https://doi.org/10.1016/J.NXNANO.2024.100129.
5. Estelrich J, Sánchez-Martín MJ, Busquets MA. Nanoparticles in magnetic resonance imaging: From simple to dual contrast agents. Int J Nanomedicine 2015;10:1727. https://doi.org/10.2147/IJN.S76501.
6. Fatima H, Kim KS. Iron-based magnetic nanoparticles for magnetic resonance imaging. Advanced Powder Technology 2018;29:2678–85. https://doi.org/10.1016/J.APT.2018.07.017.
7. Etheridge ML, Campbell SA, Erdman AG, Haynes CL, Wolf SM, McCullough J. The big picture on nanomedicine: The state of investigational and approved nanomedicine products. Nanomedicine 2013;9:1–14. https://doi.org/10.1016/J.NANO.2012.05.013.
8. Desai N. Challenges in development of nanoparticle-based therapeutics. AAPS J 2012;14:282. https://doi.org/10.1208/S12248-012-9339-4.
9. Metselaar JM, Lammers T. Challenges in nanomedicine clinical translation. Drug Deliv Transl Res 2020;10:721–5. https://doi.org/10.1007/S13346-020-00740-5/FIGURES/1
10. Chenthamara D, Subramaniam S, Ramakrishnan SG, Krishnaswamy S, Essa MM, Lin FH et al. Therapeutic efficacy of nanoparticles and routes of administration. Biomaterials Research 2019 23:1 2019;23:1–29. https://doi.org/10.1186/S40824-019-0166-X.
11. Mitchell MJ, Billingsley MM, Haley RM, Wechsler ME, Peppas NA, Langer R Engineering precision nanoparticles for drug delivery. Nature Reviews Drug Discovery 2020 20:2 2020;20:101–24. https://doi.org/10.1038/s41573-020-0090-8.
12. Alghamdi MA, Fallica AN, Virzì N, Kesharwani P, Pittalà V, Greish K The promise of nanotechnology in personalized medicine. J Pers Med 2022;12:673. https://doi.org/10.3390/JPM12050673.
13. Zhang XQ, Xu X, Bertrand N, Pridgen E, Swami A, Farokhzad OC Interactions of nanomaterials and biological systems: Implications to personalized nanomedicine. Adv Drug Deliv Rev 2012;64:1363–84. https://doi.org/10.1016/J.ADDR.2012.08.005.
14. Stark WJ, Stark WJ Nanoparticles in biological systems. Angewandte Chemie International Edition 2011;50:1242–58. https://doi.org/10.1002/ANIE.200906684.

15. Pelaz B, Charron G, Pfeiffer C, Zhao Y, De La Fuente JM, Liang XJ et al. Interfacing engineered nanoparticles with biological systems: Anticipating adverse Nano–Bio interactions. Small 2013;9:1573–84. https://doi.org/10.1002/SMLL.201201229.
16. Oualikene-Gonin W, Sautou V, Ezan E, Bastos H, Bellissant E, Belgodère L et al. Regulatory assessment of nano-enabled health products in public health interest. Position of the Scientific Advisory Board of the French National Agency for the Safety of Medicines and Health Products. Front Public Health 2023;11:1125577. https://doi.org/10.3389/FPUBH.2023.1125577/BIBTEX
17. Đorđević S, Gonzalez MM, Conejos-Sánchez I, Carreira B, Pozzi S, Acúrcio RC et al. Current hurdles to the translation of nanomedicines from bench to the clinic. Drug Deliv Transl Res 2021;12:500. https://doi.org/10.1007/S13346-021-01024-2.
18. Farjadian F, Ghasemi A, Gohari O, Roointan A, Karimi M, Hamblin MR Nanopharmaceuticals and nanomedicines currently on the market: Challenges and opportunities. Nanomedicine 2018;14:93. https://doi.org/10.2217/NNM-2018-0120.
19. Mühlebach S Regulatory challenges of nanomedicines and their follow-on versions: A generic or similar approach? Adv Drug Deliv Rev 2018;131:122–31. https://doi.org/10.1016/J.ADDR.2018.06.024.
20. Zhang X, Chan HW, Shao Z, Wang Q, Chow S, Chow SF Navigating translational research in nanomedicine: A strategic guide to formulation and manufacturing. Int J Pharm 2025;671:125202. https://doi.org/10.1016/J.IJPHARM.2025.125202.
21. Dighe S, Jog S, Momin M, Sawarkar S, Omri A Intranasal drug delivery by nanotechnology: Advances in and challenges for Alzheimer's disease management. Pharmaceutics 2024, Vol 16, Page 58 2023;16:58. https://doi.org/10.3390/PHARMACEUTICS16010058.
22. Al Asmari AK, Ullah Z, Tariq M, Fatani A Preparation, characterization, and in vivo evaluation of intranasally administered liposomal formulation of donepezil. Drug Des Devel Ther 2016;10:205–15. https://doi.org/10.2147/DDDT.S93937.
23. Roney C, Kulkarni P, Arora V, Antich P, Bonte F, Wu A et al. Targeted nanoparticles for drug delivery through the blood-brain barrier for Alzheimer's disease. J Control Release 2005;108:193–214. https://doi.org/10.1016/J.JCONREL.2005.07.024.
24. Antoniac L-D, Huţul T-D, Karner-Huţuleac A, Toader E, Turcu C, Iacob A et al. Ethical challenges in nanomedicine and their impact on population acceptance. Journal of Intercultural Management and Ethics 2024;7:55–69. https://doi.org/10.35478/JIME.2024.1.06
25. Zhang W, Li Y, Ren W, Liu B Artificial intelligence technology in Alzheimer's disease research. Intractable Rare Dis Res 2023;12:208–12. https://doi.org/10.5582/IRDR.2023.01091.
26. Abdelfattah A, Sajjad W, Soomro IA, Tariq M, Maqbool L, Rafique AA Harnessing artificial intelligence in early detection and diagnosis of Alzheimer's disease: Current and future applications. Indus Journal of Bioscience Research 2025;3:199–212. https://doi.org/10.70749/IJBR.V3I2.665
27. Cheng F, Wang F, Tang J, Zhou Y, Fu Z, Zhang P et al. Artificial intelligence and open science in discovery of disease-modifying medicines for Alzheimer's disease. Cell Rep Med 2024;5:101379. https://doi.org/10.1016/J.XCRM.2023.101379.
28. Cao Y, Zhang R. The application of nanotechnology in treatment of Alzheimer's disease. Front Bioeng Biotechnol 2022;10. https://doi.org/10.3389/fbioe.2022.1042986.
29. Puranik N, Yadav D, Song M Advancements in the application of nanomedicine in Alzheimer's disease: A therapeutic perspective. International Journal of Molecular Sciences 2023, Vol 24, Page 14044 2023;24:14044. https://doi.org/10.3390/IJMS241814044.
30. Wasti S, Lee IH, Kim S, Lee JH, Kim H Ethical and legal challenges in nanomedical innovations: A scoping review. Front Genet 2023;14:1163392. https://doi.org/10.3389/FGENE.2023.1163392/FULL

31. Resnik DB, Tinkle SS Ethics in nanomedicine. Nanomedicine (Lond) 2007;2:345–50. https://doi.org/10.2217/17435889.2.3.345.
32. Resnik DB, Tinkle SS Ethical issues in clinical trials involving nanomedicine. Contemp Clin Trials 2007;28:433–41. https://doi.org/10.1016/J.CCT.2006.11.001.
33. Altorki N, Wang X, Stinchcombe TE Lecanemab in early Alzheimer's disease. New England Journal of Medicine 2023;388:1630–2. https://doi.org/10.1056/NEJMC2301380
34. Ross MK, Raji C, Lokken KL, Bredesen DE, Roach JC, Funk CC et al. Case study: A precision medicine approach to multifactorial dementia and Alzheimer's disease. J Alzheimers Dis Parkinsonism 2021;11:018.
35. Malik S, Muhammad K, Waheed Y Emerging applications of nanotechnology in healthcare and medicine. Molecules 2023;28:6624. https://doi.org/10.3390/MOLECULES28186624.
36. Roghani AK, Garcia RI, Roghani A, Reddy A, Khemka S, Reddy RP et al. Treating Alzheimer's disease using nanoparticle-mediated drug delivery strategies/systems. Ageing Res Rev 2024;97:102291. https://doi.org/10.1016/J.ARR.2024.102291.
37. Burkett BJ, Bartlett DJ, McGarrah PW, Lewis AR, Johnson DR, Berberoğlu K et al. A review of theranostics: Perspectives on emerging approaches and clinical advancements. Radiol Imaging Cancer 2023;5. https://doi.org/10.1148/RYCAN.220157
38. Sarabia-Vallejo Á, López-Alvarado P, Menéndez JC Small-molecule theranostics in Alzheimer's disease. Eur J Med Chem 2023;255. https://doi.org/10.1016/J.EJMECH.2023.115382.
39. Francisco TN, Malafaia D, Melo L, Silva AMS, Albuquerque HMT Recent advances in fluorescent theranostics for Alzheimer's disease: A comprehensive survey on design, synthesis, and properties. ACS Omega 2024;9:13556–91. https://doi.org/10.1021/ACSOMEGA.3C10417.
40. Bors LA, Erdö F Overcoming the blood–brain barrier. Challenges and tricks for CNS drug delivery. Scientia Pharmaceutica 2019, Vol 87, Page 6 2019;87:6. https://doi.org/10.3390/SCIPHARM87010006.
41. Pardridge WM Blood-brain barrier and delivery of protein and Gene therapeutics to brain. Front Aging Neurosci 2020;11. https://doi.org/10.3389/FNAGI.2019.00373
42. Long JM, Holtzman DM Alzheimer disease: An update on pathobiology and treatment strategies. Cell 2019;179:312–39. https://doi.org/10.1016/J.CELL.2019.09.001.
43. Rudroff T, Rainio O, Klén R AI for the prediction of early stages of Alzheimer's disease from neuroimaging biomarkers – A narrative review of a growing field. Neurol Sci 2024;45. https://doi.org/10.1007/S10072-024-07649-8.
44. Yu TW, Lane HY, Lin CH Novel therapeutic approaches for Alzheimer's disease: An updated review. International Journal of Molecular Sciences 2021, Vol 22, Page 8208 2021;22:8208. https://doi.org/10.3390/IJMS22158208.
45. Tondo G, De Marchi F, Bonardi F, Menegon F, Verrini G, Aprile D et al. Novel therapeutic strategies in Alzheimer's disease: Pitfalls and challenges of anti-amyloid therapies and beyond. J Clin Med 2024;13. https://doi.org/10.3390/JCM13113098.
46. Banik A, Brown RE, Bamburg J, Lahiri DK, Khurana D, Friedland RP et al. Translation of pre-clinical studies into successful clinical trials for Alzheimer's disease: What are the roadblocks and how can they be overcome? Journal of Alzheimer's Disease 2015;47:815–43. https://doi.org/10.3233/JAD-150136/ASSET/IMAGES/10.3233_JAD-150136-IMG1.JPG
47. Anand A, Saraf MK, Prabhakar S Antiamnesic effect of b. Monniera on l-NNA induced amnesia involves calmodulin. Neurochem Res 2010;35:1172–81. https://doi.org/10.1007/S11064-010-0171-X.
48. Puranik N, Song M Therapeutic role of heterocyclic compounds in neurodegenerative diseases: Insights from Alzheimer's and Parkinson's diseases. Neurology International 2025, Vol 17, Page 26 2025;17:26. https://doi.org/10.3390/NEUROLINT17020026.

49. Cano A, Turowski P, Ettcheto M, Duskey JT, Tosi G, Sánchez-López E et al. Nanomedicine-based technologies and novel biomarkers for the diagnosis and treatment of Alzheimer's disease: From current to future challenges. J Nanobiotechnology 2021;19. https://doi.org/10.1186/s12951-021-00864-x.
50. Nunes D, Loureiro JA, Pereira MC Drug delivery systems as a strategy to improve the efficacy of FDA-approved Alzheimer's drugs. Pharmaceutics 2022, Vol 14, Page 2296 2022;14:2296. https://doi.org/10.3390/PHARMACEUTICS14112296.
51. Heidebrink JL, Paulson HL Lessons learned from approval of aducanumab for Alzheimer's disease. Annu Rev Med 2024;75:99–111. https://doi.org/10.1146/ANNUREV-MED-051022-043645.
52. Cummings J Lessons learned from Alzheimer disease: Clinical trials with negative outcomes. Clin Transl Sci 2018;11:147–52. https://doi.org/10.1111/CTS.12491.
53. Cummings J, Ritter A, Zhong K Clinical trials for disease-modifying therapies in Alzheimer's disease: A primer, lessons learned, and a blueprint for the future. J Alzheimers Dis 2018;64:S3–22. https://doi.org/10.3233/JAD-179901.
54. Cummings J, Zhou Y, Lee G, Zhong K, Fonseca J, Cheng F Alzheimer's disease drug development pipeline: 2024. Alzheimer's & Dementia: Translational Research & Clinical Interventions 2024;10:e12465. https://doi.org/10.1002/TRC2.12465
55. Boxer AL, Sperling R Accelerating Alzheimer's therapeutic development: The past and future of clinical trials. Cell 2023;186:4757–72. https://doi.org/10.1016/J.CELL.2023.09.023.
56. Hampel H, Frank R, Broich K, Teipel SJ, Katz RG, Hardy J et al. Biomarkers for Alzheimer's disease: Academic, industry and regulatory perspectives. Nat Rev Drug Discov 2010;9:560–74. https://doi.org/10.1038/NRD3115.
57. Jones R, Wilkinson D, Lopez OL, Cummings J, Waldemar G, Zhang R et al. Collaborative research between academia and industry using a large clinical trial database: A case study in Alzheimer's disease. Trials 2011;12:1–9. https://doi.org/10.1186/1745-6215-12-233/TABLES/2
58. Indiveri A, Paton G, Nogaret JFR Optimal solid state neurons. Nat Commun 2019;10:5309. https://doi.org/10.1038/s41467-019-13177-3.
59. Ablinger I, Dressel K, Rott T, Lauer AA, Tiemann M, Batista JP et al. Interdisciplinary approaches to Deal with Alzheimer's disease-from bench to bedside: What feasible options do already exist today? Biomedicines 2022;10. https://doi.org/10.3390/BIOMEDICINES10112922.
60. Galvin JE, Valois L, Zweig Y Collaborative transdisciplinary team approach for dementia care. Neurodegener Dis Manag 2014;4:455–69. https://doi.org/10.2217/NMT.14.47.
61. Kozauer N, Katz R Regulatory innovation and drug development for early-stage Alzheimer's disease. N Engl J Med 2013;368:1169–71. https://doi.org/10.1056/NEJMP1302513.
62. Zhang F, Li Z, Zhang B, Du H, Wang B, Zhang X Multi-modal deep learning model for auxiliary diagnosis of Alzheimer's disease. Neurocomputing 2019;361:185–95. https://doi.org/10.1016/J.NEUCOM.2019.04.093.
63. Arafah A, Khatoon S, Rasool I, Khan A, Rather MA, Abujabal KA et al. The future of precision medicine in the cure of Alzheimer's disease. Biomedicines 2023;11. https://doi.org/10.3390/BIOMEDICINES11020335.
64. De Matteis L, Martín-Rapún R, de la Fuente JM Nanotechnology in personalized medicine: A promising tool for Alzheimer's disease treatment. Curr Med Chem 2018;25:4602–15. https://doi.org/10.2174/0929867324666171012112026.

Index

Note: Locators in *italics* represent figures and **bold** indicate tables in the text.

C

F

G

H

I

L

Q

R

Made in the USA
Las Vegas, NV
19 May 2026

4403525a-9cc7-4f80-8c42-ebf663b17627R02